Recent Advances in

Paediatrics

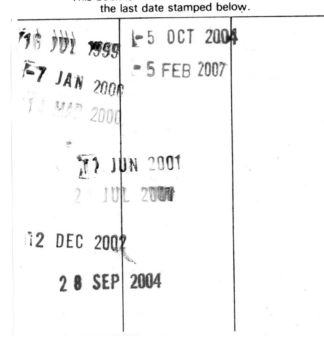

Recent Advances in Paediatrics 16
Edited by T. J. David

Preface

Neonatal necrotizing enterocolitis: progress, problems, and prospects
R. G. Faix, M. Nelson

Biliary atresia
A. Baker, N. Hadzic, A. Dhawan, G. Mieli-Vergani

Screening for congenital dislocation of the hip in the newborn
and young infants
C. Dezateux, S. Godward

Helping the feeding impaired child
E. G. Gisel, R. Birnbaum, S. Schwartz

Lyme disease
P. J. Krause, H. M. Feder, H. Eiffert, H.-J. Christen

Helicobacter pylori and gastroduodenal disorders in children
S. Kugathasan, S. J. Czinn

Insecticide-treated bednets and the prevention of malaria
J. Cattani, C. Lengeler

Genetic basis of asthma and allergic disease
W. O. C. M. Cookson

Immunopathogenesis of allergic diseases
M. F. Hofer, D. Y. M. Leung

Psychosocial factors in epilepsy: the need for psychiatry
D. C. Taylor

Prevention of adolescent substance abuse
M. Sanford, J. A. Morgan

Advances in sodium homeostasis
M. J. Dillon

Paediatric literature review – 1996
T. J. David

Index

ISBN 0-443-05960-8
ISSN 0-309-0140

Look out for *Recent Advances in Paediatrics* 18 in November 1999

NUMBER
17

Recent Advances in
Paediatrics

Edited by

T. J. David MD PhD FRCP FRCPCH DCH

Professor and Head,
Department of Child Health,
University of Manchester;
Honorary Consultant Paediatrician,
Booth Hall Children's Hospital,
Royal Manchester Children's Hospital and St Mary's Hospital,
Manchester, UK

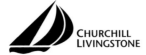

CHURCHILL
LIVINGSTONE

EDINBURGH LONDON NEW YORK PHILADELPHIA SYDNEY TORONTO 1999

CHURCHILL LIVINGSTONE
An imprint of Harcourt Brace & Company Limited

Robert Stevenson House, 1–3 Baxter's Place, Leith Walk, Edinburgh, EH1 3AF

First published 1999

ISBN 0-443-06184-X

ISSN 0-309-0140

British Library Cataloguing in Publication Data
A catalogue record for this book is available from the British Library

Library of Congress Cataloging in Publication Data
A catalog record for this book is available from the Library of Congress

Medical knowledge is constantly changing. As new information becomes available, changes in treatment, procedures, equipment and the use of drugs become necessary. The editors and the publishers have, as far as possible, taken care to ensure that the information given in this text is accurate and up to date. However, readers are strongly advised to confirm that the information, especially with regard to drug usage, complies with current legislation and standards of practice.

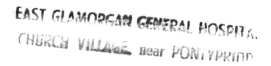
Commissioning Editor – Ellen Green
Project Editor – Jane Shanks
Project Controller – Frances Affleck
Designer – Sarah Cape

The publisher's policy is to use **paper manufactured from sustainable forests**

Printed in China
NPCC/01

Contents

Preface   vi

1. Inhaled corticosteroid toxicity, growth and asthma   1
   G. Russell, T.K. Ninan

2. Bronchopulmonary dysplasia and chronic lung disease of infancy   17
   P.A. Farrell, J.M. Fiascone

3. Skull fracture, subdural haematoma, shaking and impact injury   35
   R. Sunderland

4. Factitious illness by proxy   57
   D.P.H. Jones, C.N. Bools

5. Home safety for children   73
   S. Levene

6. Stabilisation and transport of critically ill children   85
   J. Britto, P. Habibi

7. Hearing screening   115
   J.M. Bamford, A. Davis

8. Advances in the management of the cerebral palsies   129
   M.F. Smith

9. Effects of excessive consumption of soft drinks and declining intake of milk on children's teeth and bones   141
   M.Z. Mughal, F.J. Hill

10. Gastrooesophageal reflux   161
    J.F. del Rosario, S.R. Orenstein

11. Gastrointestinal and hepatobiliary problems in cystic fibrosis   173
    R.J. Rothbaum

12. Low-technology approaches to child care in the third world   193
    D.C. Morley

13. Paediatric care in disaster and refugee settings   211
    N. Banatvala, B. Laurence, T. Healing

14. Paediatric literature review – 1997   229
    T.J. David

Index   257

Preface

The aim of *Recent Advances in Paediatrics* is to provide a review of important topics and help doctors keep abreast of developments. The book is intended for the practising clinician, those in specialty training, and doctors preparing for specialty examinations. The book is sold very widely in Britain, Europe, North America, Asia and Australia, and the contents and authorship are selected with this very broad readership in mind. There are 13 chapters which cover a variety of general paediatric, neonatal and community paediatric areas. As usual, the selection of topics has veered towards those of general rather than special interest.

The final chapter, an annotated literature review, is a personal selection of key articles and useful reviews published in 1997. Comment about a paper is sometimes as important as the original article, so when a paper has been followed by interesting or important correspondence this is also referred to. As with the choice of subjects for the main chapters, the selection of articles has inclined towards those of general rather than special interest. There is, however, special emphasis on community paediatrics and medicine in the tropics, as these two important areas tend to be less well covered in general paediatric journals. Trying to reduce to an acceptable size the short-list of particularly interesting articles is an especially difficult task. Each topic in the literature review section is asterisked in the index, so selected publications on (for example) child abuse can be identified easily, as can any parts of the book that touch on the topic.

Annual publication of this book provides the opportunity to respond to the wishes of readers, and any suggestions for topics to be included in future issues would always be welcome. Please write (or E-mail) to me at the address below.

I am indebted to the authors for their hard work, prompt delivery of manuscripts and patience in dealing with my queries and requests. I would also like to thank my secretaries Angela Smithies and Val Smith, and Gill Haddock of Churchill Livingstone (Harcourt Brace) for all their help, and my wife and sons for all their support.

1998   **Professor T J David**
E-mail: tjd@netcomuk.co.uk
University Department of Child Health, Booth Hall Children's Hospital, Manchester M9 7AA, UK

Contributors

John M. Bamford BA PhD
Professor of Audiology and Education of the Deaf; and Head of the Centre for Human Communication and Deafness, University of Manchester, Manchester, UK

Nicholas Banatvala MBBS MSc MRCP MFPHM
Medical Adviser, MERLIN (Medical Emergency Relief International), London, UK

Christopher N. Bools MB ChB MMedSc MRCPsych
Consultant Child and Family Psychiatrist, Royal United Hospital, Combe Park, Bath, UK

Joseph Britto MBBS MD
Consultant in Paediatric Intensive Care, Imperial College School of Medicine at St Mary's, London, UK

Timothy J. David MD PhD FRCP FRCPCH DCH
Professor, and Head, Department of Child Health, University of Manchester; Honorary Consultant Paediatrician, Booth Hall Children's Hospital, Royal Manchester Children's Hospital and St Mary's Hospital, Manchester, UK

Adrian Davis BSc MSc PhD
Head of Epidemiology, Public Health and Clinical Section, MRC Institute of Hearing Research, Nottingham, UK

J. Fernando del Rosario MD
Assistant Professor of Medicine and Pediatrics, Director, Pediatric Gastroenterology, Allegheny Center for Digestive Health, Allegheny General Hospital, Pittsburgh, PA, USA

Paula A. Farrell MD
Fellow in Neonatal Perinatal Medicine, Division of Newborn Medicine, The Floating Hospital for Children at New England Medical Center, Tufts University School of Medicine, Boston, Massachusetts, USA

John M. Fiascone MD
Medical Director, Neonatal Intensive Care Unit, and Assistant Professor of Pediatrics,

Division of Newborn Medicine, The Floating Hospital for Children at New England Medical Center, Tufts University School of Medicine, Boston, Massachusetts, USA

Parviz Habibi FRCP PhD FRCPCH
Director of Paediatric Intensive Care, Department of Paediatrics, Imperial College School of Medicine at St Mary's, London, UK

Timothy Healing PhD FIBiol
Epidemiologist, MERLIN (Medical Emergency Relief International), London, UK

F.J. Hill MDS FDSRCS (Eng) DOrth RCS (Eng) FDSRCPS (Glasgow)
Consultant in Paediatric Dentistry, The University Dental Hospital of Manchester, Manchester, UK

David P.H. Jones MB ChB FRCPsych DCH D(Obst)RCOG
Consultant Child and Family Psychiatrist and Honorary Senior Lecturer, Park Hospital for Children, Oxford, UK

Bruce Laurence MA MBBS MSc DTM&H
Medical Director, MERLIN (Medical Emergency Relief International), London, UK

Sara Levene MA MRCP FRCPCH
Medical Adviser, Child Accident Prevention Trust, London, UK

David C. Morley CBE MD(Cantab) FRCP
Emeritus Professor of Tropical Child Health, University of London and Centre for International Child Health, University College London, London, UK

M.Z. Mughal MBChB (Liverpool) FRCP (Lond) FRCPCH (UK) DCH (Eng)
Consultant Paediatrician and Honorary Senior Lecturer in Child Health, Department of Paediatrics, Saint Mary's Hospital, Manchester, UK

Titus K Ninan MB MRCP FRCPCH
Department of Medical Paediatrics, Heartlands Hospital, Birmingham, UK

Susan R. Orenstein MD
Professor, Department of Pediatrics, Division of Pediatric Gastroenterology, University of Pittsburgh School of Medicine, Children's Hospital of Pittsburgh, Pennsylvania, USA

Robert J. Rothbaum MD
Associate Professor of Pediatrics, Clinical Director, Division of Pediatric Gastroenterology and Nutrition, Department of Pediatrics, Washington University School of Medicine, St Louis Children's Hospital, St Louis, Missouri, USA

George Russell MB FRCP FRCPE FRCPCH
Reader in Child Health, University of Aberdeen, Consultant in Medical Paediatrics, Royal Aberdeen Children's Hospital, Department of Child Health, University of Aberdeen, Aberdeen, UK

Michael F. Smith MBBS FRCP FRCPCH
Consultant Paediatrician, The Ryegate Children's Centre, The Children's Hospital, Sheffield, UK

Robert Sunderland MD MB ChB FRCP FRCPCH
Consultant Paediatrician, Birmingham Children's Hospital, Birmingham, UK

George Russell Titus K. Ninan

CHAPTER 1

Inhaled corticosteroid toxicity, growth and asthma

Pathologically, the hallmark of bronchial asthma is a chronic inflammatory process involving the airways, a process that to a varying degree is suppressible by corticosteroids. Corticosteroids were originally given systemically both acutely for the relief of attacks of asthma and chronically to prevent relapses. However, it was soon realised that long-term suppression could only be bought at a considerable price in terms of side-effects, and continuous corticosteroid therapy was soon reserved for the most severe and intractable cases.

Paediatricians were particularly concerned that, in children, in addition to all the classical features of Cushingism seen in adults, long-term systemic corticosteroids resulted in stunting of growth. It used to be believed that this effect could be reduced (but not entirely avoided) by the administration of adrenocorticotrophic hormone (ACTH) instead of corticosteroids,[1,2] but the injections were unpopular with patients, side-effects were at least as severe as with ordinary corticosteroids, and dosage was difficult to control because of the adrenal hypertrophy that ensued.

It is, therefore, hardly surprising that, at a time when many cases of childhood asthma could not be controlled without the use of regular oral corticosteroids or ACTH, the introduction of inhaled corticosteroid therapy to clinical practice was welcomed as a major therapeutic development. The substitution of inhaled for oral corticosteroids meant than the great majority of these children were able to discontinue systemic therapy, with immediate and usually very obvious benefits. Beclomethasone dipropionate (Becotide®), budesonide (Pulmicort®) and fluticasone propionate (Flixotide®) are now available for inhaled use in UK; several other molecules are licensed in other countries but will be not considered in this chapter.

George Russell MB FRCP FRCPE FRCPCH
Department of Child Health, University of Aberdeen, Aberdeen AB15 2ZD, UK

Titus K Ninan MB MRCP FRCPCH
Department of Medical Paediatrics, Heartlands Hospital, Birmingham, UK

PHARMACOLOGY OF INHALED CORTICOSTEROIDS

Inhaled corticosteroids have numerous interdependent effects that suppress inflammation, reducing both the number of inflammatory cells and the concentration of inflammatory mediators present in the bronchial secretions. To achieve these effects, the corticosteroid molecule must first penetrate the cell membrane to reach the steroid-binding site on the glucocorticoid receptor, which it then activates.[3] The pharmacokinetics of this process depend primarily on the physicochemical properties of the individual molecules, in particular on their lipid solubility (lipophilicity) which allows easy penetration through cell membranes and is associated more prolonged duration of the anti-inflammatory action.[4] Lipophilicity offers the further advantages of delaying systemic absorption, and enhancing steroid receptor affinity.[3] Beclomethasone has an additional advantage; the dipropionate has relatively weak corticosteroid activity, but is converted within the epithelial cell to the monopropionate which is several times more potent; its properties, therefore, approach those of a pro-drug, i.e. a drug which is inert in itself but which is converted in the body to an active compound.

Bioavailability

Systemic side-effects reflect systemic absorption of the drug from the gut and the lung (Fig. 1.1). Absorption from the gut is influenced by the extent to which the drug is metabolised on passing through the liver, known as first pass metabolism. As indicated in Table 1.1, the three drugs show marked differences in systemic bioavailability when given orally. In contrast, there is no significant difference in the bioavailability of the inhaled portion of the administered dose, 20–25% of the administered dose appearing in the systemic circulation.

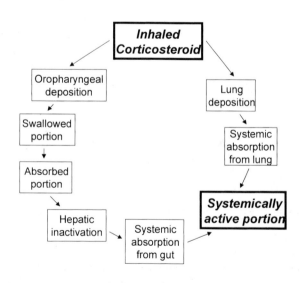

Fig. 1.1 Pharmacokinetics of inhaled corticosteroids.

Table 1.1 Pharmacological differences between the three corticosteroids available for inhaled use in UK

Corticosteroid molecule	Pro-drug	Lipophilicity	Hepatic biotrans-formation	Systemic bioavailability after oral admin.(%)
Hypothetical ideal molecule	+++	+++[a]	+++[a]	0[a]
Beclomethasone dipropionate	++	++	+	< 20
Budesonide	–	+	++	11
Fluticasone propionate	–	+++	+++	< 1

[a]Less important for pro-drug.

Two further factors complicate the above approach to the systemic absorption of inhaled corticosteroids. Firstly, the drugs produce metabolites with varying levels of corticosteroid activity. For instance, very little of an inhaled dose of beclomethasone dipropionate appears in the systemic circulation, but significant quantities of its much more active metabolite, 17-beclomethasone mono-propionate, are found.[5] It is, therefore, simplistic to equate the concentration of the drug itself with the systemic corticosteroid activity resulting from its administration.

A second influence on the systemic bio-availability of inhaled corticosteroid therapy will be the inhaler device used. The traditional metered dose aerosol deposits the major part of its output in the mouth and pharynx, a maximum of 20% being deposited in the lungs. In contrast, when the same metered dose inhaler is used with a large spacer, the proportion deposited in the lung may exceed 30%, and much of the portion deposited in the oropharynx when the inhaler is used alone is now deposited in the spacer, significantly reducing oral bioavailability. Thus, for example, a drug which is readily absorbed from the gut and escapes first pass hepatic metabolism will have much higher systemic activity when given by metered dose aerosol than when given by the same metered dose aerosol together with a spacer. It has also been shown that the pulmonary availability of budesonide is roughly twice as great when it is taken from a Turbohaler® (or Turbuhaler®) than when it is taken from a metered dose aerosol. So, by a simple change in the inhaler device used, the total administered dose can be halved, with obvious benefits in terms of the potential for systemic side-effects. To these predictable effects of various inhalation devices when used by trained well co-ordinated adults must be added the unpredictable results of varying inhaler technique and compliance, variables that are particularly important in children.

The ideal corticosteroid for inhalation

This information allows us to construct blueprints for 'ideal' inhaled corticosteroid molecules. One would be a pro-drug, with little or no potency on its own, being converted to a potent form by enzymes present only in the respiratory epithelial cell. A water soluble pro-drug would readily escape into the systemic circulation, where it would have no effect; provided sufficient were able to cross the cell membrane for local activation, it would be no great disadvantage for a pro-drug to be water soluble. Intestinal absorption would also be unimportant for a completely inert pro-drug, so there would be no clinical reason to worry about the swallowed portion of the administered dose. For corticosteroid molecules that do *not* require further activation, lipophilicity would offer ready penetration across the respiratory epithelial cell, more prolonged duration of action and less ready systemic absorption. The ideal active molecule would either not be absorbed from the gut, or would be totally inactivated on first pass metabolism in the liver. None of the corticosteroids listed in Table 1.1 is either an ideal pro-drug or an ideal active molecule, and there are obvious and apparently major differences between the properties of the three drugs. For instance, Johnson[3] has calculated from published studies that fluticasone propionate has a greater than 10-fold higher lung-to-systemic ratio than budesonide. However, despite these pharmacological differences between the three drugs, in clinical practice the differences are much less clear and remain the subject of claim and counter-claim by their respective manufacturers.

TOXICITY OF INHALED CORTICOSTEROIDS

The initial impression of inhaled corticosteroid therapy was that it was both safe and effective, but it soon became clear that side-effects did occur. The principal purpose of this chapter is to review the potential of inhaled cortico-steroid therapy to produce side-effects, both local and systemic, with particular emphasis on its effects on growth.

Clinical side-effects – local toxicity

Soon after inhaled corticosteroid therapy was introduced, it was recognised that its use was associated with monilial colonisation, although oropharyngeal thrush appears to be less common in children than in adults. Dysphonia, usually attributed to steroid-induced laryngeal myopathy or vocal cord thin-ning, is also less common in children. These effects are easily explained by the high levels of oropharyngeal and upper airway deposition of medication from most inhaler devices, and in the absence of evidence of systemic toxicity are not usually considered to be a cause for concern. Generally, they tend to be less when inhaled corticosteroid therapy is taken through a spacer, and rinsing the mouth after inhalation is also said to be helpful in reducing the incidence of topical side-effects.

Clinical side-effects – systemic toxicity

Occasional patients demonstrate idiosyncratic sensitivity to inhaled cortico-steroid therapy, developing gross features of Cushingism or more subtle signs such as behavioural problems, easy bruising or dermal thinning on normally used doses. These effects disappear on withdrawing the drug, and also often dis-appear when one corticosteroid is substituted for another, suggesting that, in some cases, the problem may lie in the metabolism of, or sensitivity to, individual steroid molecules.

Systemic corticosteroids can cause posterior subcapsular cataracts; these have also been reported in patients on inhaled corticosteroids, but always in patients who have also received oral corticosteroids.[6] A systematic search has now been made for cataracts in more than 300 children who have received corticosteroid therapy only by the inhaled route and they have not been found.[7]

Systemic side-effects – biochemical measurements

Various measurements can be used to look for systemic side-effects following inhaled corticosteroid therapy, including changes in glucose metabolism, suppression of endogenous cortisol production, reduction in adrenal reserve, effects on osteocalcin and other markers of bone metabolism, and effects on growth.

Effects on glucose metabolism

Little attention has been paid to the effects of inhaled corticosteroid therapy on glucose metabolism in children. However, in adults inhaled corticosteroid therapy has been associated with decreased insulin sensitivity and rises in total and high density lipoprotein cholesterol.[8]

Suppression of cortisol production

Early studies of inhaled corticosteroid therapy suggested that its effects on hypothalamic-pituitary-adrenal function were negligible compared to those of the oral corticosteroids it was designed to replace.[9–11] However, studies using more sensitive techniques have shown that inhaled corticosteroid therapy given in normal doses does suppress adrenal function;[12–14] these changes are particularly marked when higher doses are used.[15]

There is, therefore, no doubt that inhaled corticosteroid therapy suppresses adrenal function in children; what is much less clear is whether this suppression is of clinical importance. Decreased cortisol production is a homoeostatic response to the administration of exogenous corticosteroids, representing an attempt to maintain total corticosteroid activity within normal limits, and provided the total corticosteroid activity provided by endogenous cortisol plus the administered corticosteroid is normal, the only danger to the patient lies in an inadequate adrenal reserve.

Effects on adrenal reserve

Adrenal reserve is difficult to assess under normal circumstances, in that it is difficult to find a stressor which would be acceptable ethically, and yet sufficient to stimulate a physiological increase in adrenocortical activity. The short tetracosactrin test is widely used to test adrenal reserve and, although it provides a stimulus vastly greater than that provided by the hypothalamo-pituitary system, it has shown reduced adrenal reserve in some patients on high-dose inhaled corticosteroids.[15] The more physiological low-dose tetracosactrin test reveals an impaired response in about one-third of children taking conventional doses of inhaled corticosteroids.[16]

The clinical significance of this reduction in adrenal reserve remains uncertain and, in adults on inhaled corticosteroid therapy, the stress of hospital admission with severe acute asthma results in an apparently satisfactory adrenocortical response.[17]

Clinical effects of adrenal suppression

Following the introduction of inhaled corticosteroid therapy, numerous workers looked for, but failed to find, any evidence of clinical harm resulting from adrenal suppression. One paper did report adrenal atrophy observed at autopsy in children who had received inhaled corticosteroid therapy,[18] but as these children had also received systemic corticosteroids, it is difficult to attribute their deaths to the inhaled therapy, and there have been no subsequent reports of fatalities. Adrenal suppression is, therefore, common in patients on inhaled corticosteroid therapy, but there is no evidence that it poses any danger to them.

Systemic side-effects – effects on bone metabolism

Bone density

Systemic ticosteroid therapy is associated with reduced bone mineral density, i.e. with osteoporosis, and numerous studies have examined bone metabolism in children, with conflicting results. Asthma itself has no effect on bone mineral density,[19] other than through its effect in delaying bone maturation.[20] In adults, prolonged inhaled corticosteroid therapy has been shown to be associated with reduced bone mass,[21] but most studies on children have shown no effect;[22–24] one study showed an apparent reduction in bone density, but the effect disappeared when bone mineral mass was related to bone age rather than chronological age.[15] Bone mass is at its peak as soon as puberty is complete, but it is not yet known if asthmatic children on inhaled corticosteroids achieve normal peak values.

Biochemical markers of bone metabolism

Studies of bone metabolism using biochemical markers have given inconsistent results. For instance, in one recent study there was evidence of decreases in both bone formation and bone resorption in children on budesonide, but the two were balanced so that there was no net bone loss.[25] In another, serum osteocalcin, a marker of bone formation, was unchanged during treatment with beclomethasone[26], despite the fact that this treatment was associated with a slowing of growth.

Although current knowledge does not permit an unequivocal statement as to the effects of inhaled corticosteroid therapy on the bones of children, we do know that there is a massive accumulation of bone mineral mass during puberty. Although this is commonly regarded as a once-in-a-lifetime opportunity to lay down bone, we also know that there may be some recovery of bone mass in patients recovering from Cushings syndrome, so failure as a result of corticosteroid therapy to achieve the usual pubertal increase in bone mineral mass may not be irreversible. We also know that inhaled corticosteroid therapy, especially at high doses, has an adverse effect on bone density in adults. It is, therefore, reasonable to base our clinical practice on the assumption that inhaled corticosteroid therapy in childhood is likely to have an adverse effect on bone mineral density, thereby predisposing to osteoporosis in adult life. For the clinician, this means that the dose of inhaled corticosteroid therapy should at all times be kept to the minimum required to control the asthma, but not that this therapy should be avoided.

Systemic side-effects – effects on growth

Effects of asthma on growth

There is very little recent literature on the effects of asthma on growth, so it is perhaps fitting to cite Dr Archie Norman's chapter in a previous volume of *Recent Advances in Paediatrics*[27] in which he described the effects of oral prednisolone on growth, presenting data on the heights of the children, all of whom were suffering from severe asthma, before and after corticosteroid therapy. The distribution of their height centiles before starting oral corticosteroid therapy is presented in Figure 1.2 from which it is apparent that asthma had produced considerable stunting of growth before steroids were ever given. A full review of early literature has been provided elsewhere.[28] With modern therapy, including inhaled corticosteroid therapy, asthma of such severity is unusual, but the severity of the asthma has appeared to be an independent variable influencing growth in at least some recent studies of inhaled corticosteroid therapy.[29,30] The adverse effect of severe asthma on growth must, therefore, be considered when interpreting the results of studies, and when deciding on the balance of advantage when prescribing inhaled corticosteroid therapy.

Effects of inhaled corticosteroid therapy on growth

Early studies on inhaled corticosteroid therapy in children suggested that growth was unimpaired.[10,11] Indeed, in many children who had been on long-term oral

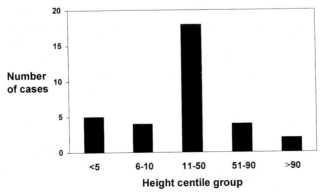

Fig. 1.2 Height distribution of patients with severe chronic asthma before starting oral corticosteroid therapy (based on data of Norman[27]).

corticosteroids, growth was enhanced as they experienced catch-up growth. For some time, therefore, it appeared that the benefits of corticosteroid therapy were now available without the disadvantage of impaired growth. Unfortunately, this comfortable complacency was broken in 1988 by Littlewood and his colleagues who, in a letter to *The Lancet*,[31] reported apparent growth retardation in children treated with inhaled beclomethasone. Their findings did not go unchallenged; it was pointed out that some of the patients were of an age when the pubertal growth spurt would have made the assessment of growth more difficult, and that the study had all the problems associated with any retrospective study. Nevertheless, this letter raised important doubts as to the safety of inhaled corticosteroids, and prompted numerous studies of growth in asthmatic children on these drugs; only a few of these can be touched upon here, and the interested reader is referred to a comprehensive review by Wolthers.[32]

Short-term effects of inhaled corticosteroid therapy on growth

There is now no doubt that inhaled corticosteroids affect growth. Using knemometry, an exquisitely sensitive though rather time-consuming technique for the assessment of tibial growth, clear dose-related growth suppression has been demonstrated immediately after starting treatment with budesonide 800 µg/day[33] (in this study there was no effect from budesonide 200 and 400 µg/day), budesonide 400 and 800 µg/day,[34] beclomethasone 200 and 400 µg/day[35] though not with fluticasone 200 µg/day.[35,36] This effect occurs at all ages, including young children using nebulised corticosteroids,[37] and reflects the systemic potency of the corticosteroid molecule studied. The clinical importance of this initial growth suppression is by no means clear. Its magnitude is so great, amounting in some children to almost complete cessation of growth, that, if it were to persist for any length of time, it would result in severe dwarfism, whereas all the currently available evidence suggests that asthmatic children attain normal adult stature regardless of treatment.[38,39]

Medium-term effects of inhaled corticosteroid therapy on growth

It might be imagined that it would be an easy matter to mount a study to investigate the effects of inhaled corticosteroid therapy on growth. Unfortunately, in practice, this is far from the case. The obstacles to studying this problem include:

1. *The effects of the underlying disease.* As we have seen,[28] asthma itself has effects on growth and bone maturation, as do atopic eczema[40] and allergic rhinitis[41] which are so often associated with asthma. It is difficult, therefore, to determine how much of an observed change is attributable to the disease and how much to its treatment.

2. *The time required to study growth.* Growth is a relatively slow process, and measurement is subject to considerable experimental error. It is, therefore, difficult to assess growth over short periods of time, so prolonged

measurement periods are required. Ideally, height should be measured at relatively frequent intervals over a period of at least 6 months, better still over a year. A best fit line through these serial measurements can then be used to calculate height velocity. Such an arduous regimen is a recipe for non-compliance on the part of patients, and is difficult to incorporate into routine clinical practice. Moreover, inhaled corticosteroid therapy is administered to patients who need it because of uncontrolled asthma; in everyday practice, the dose will have to be adjusted both upwards and downwards to achieve the minimum effective dose, so it difficult to obtain a prolonged study period in which the asthma is stable and the inhaled corticosteroid therapy dosage is constant.

3. *Ethical difficulties.* In an ideal study, the effects of inhaled corticosteroids would be compared with those of an inhaled placebo. However, because active treatment can reasonably be given only to patients who need it, it is impossible to justify giving placebo medication for a prolonged period to patients with equally severe asthma and who are, therefore, clearly in need of active treatment, simply to compare the effects on growth.

These constraints have meant that the great majority of reports on the effects of inhaled corticosteroid therapy on growth have been retrospective studies from hospital asthma clinics, in which the measurements have not been made for research purposes, in which both patients and doctors have been aware of the treatment given, and in which measurements have been compared either with the patients own pre-inhaled corticosteroid therapy measurements, or with standards derived from large population studies, in some cases not even of the same nationality as that of the study patients.

However, growth retardation has now been reported in well designed studies: a comparison of beclomethasone with theophylline,[42] a trial of beclo-methasone given to children to prevent winter-time wheeze,[43] two comparisons of beclomethasone with salmeterol[44,45] and a comparison of fluticasone with cromoglycate.[46] The results of these studies are summarised in Table 1.2. Supporting this evidence are various clinical reports of growth inhibition in children on inhaled corticosteroid therapy, although these are balanced by equally large numbers of studies which have shown no effect, and by a recent meta-analysis[47] of published reports which found no association between the use of inhaled corticosteroid therapy and diminished stature.

On balance, the results of short-term knemometry studies are undeniable, and it is likely that there is also some slight medium-term effect. Any such effect would appear to be small, and of doubtful clinical significance. It is also notable that all the studies listed in Table 1.2, with the exception of the paper on winter wheeze,[43] showed clear evidence of benefit from using inhaled corticosteroids compared to currently available alternatives. In the great majority of children, a small and (as we shall see) almost certainly transient delay in growth will be a reasonable price to pay having well controlled asthma. Moreover, it is difficult to separate with certainty the possible adverse effects of inhaled corticosteroids from the known adverse effects of asthma on growth, and even more difficult to say what the effects of uncontrolled asthma might have been in the absence of inhaled corticosteroids.

Table 2.2 Prospective studies of the effects of inhaled corticosteroid therapy on growth

Ref	Drug used	Dose µg/day	Duration months	Growth effect	General comments
45	BDP	200	12	3.96 cm for BDP versus 5.04 cm for placebo group	Double-blind, randomised parallel group comparison of BDP, salmeterol and placebo. Pubertal and pre-pubertal children recruited. Management contrary to BTS guidelines (salmeterol prescribed as sole preventer). High drop-out rate, especially placebo. BDP group showed significantly slower growth compared to controls ($P = 0.019$) but had less airway responsiveness and fewer interval symptoms
44	BDP	400	12	Height velocity SDS −0.28 in BDP group versus −0.03 in salmeterol group	Double-blind, randomised parallel group comparison of BDP and salmeterol in children with mild to moderate asthma. Management contrary to BTS guidelines (salmeterol prescribed as sole preventer). Clinical effects of BDP vastly better than salmeterol, but growth significantly better on salmeterol ($P = 0.001$)
43	BDP	400	7	2.66 cm in 7 m for BDP versus 3.66 cm for placebo	Double-blind, randomised parallel group trial of BDP in children with virus-induced wheeze during the winter. All prepubertal. Clinical indication for BDP not in accordance with BTS guidelines. Significant growth suppression ($P < 0.0001$), mainly in first 6 weeks
42	BDP	400	12	4.2 cm per year for BDP group versus 5.5 cm for theophylline group (accounted for by effect on boys: 4.5 versus 6.1 cm)	Double-blind, randomised parallel group comparison of BDP and oral theophylline in asthmatic children recruited at age 6–16 years. Significant depression of height velocity in all children ($P = 0.005$), all boys ($P = 0.007$) and prepubescent boys ($P = 0.005$). The differences for pubescent boys and for girls were not significant. Growth rates identical in first and second 6-month periods. Clear evidence of better asthma control on BDP
46	FP	200	144	Height velocity SDS 0.1 in FP group versus 0.5 in cromoglycate group	Prospective randomised open label study comparing fluticasone propionate and cromoglycate. Prepubertal children only. Small numbers. Clinically, fluticasone more effective, and height velocity normal in both groups

Abbreviations: BDP, beclomethasone dipropionate; BUD, budesonide; FP, fluticasone propionate; SDS, standard deviation score (normal average = 0)

Long-term effects of inhaled corticosteroid therapy on growth

The long-term effects of inhaled corticosteroid therapy are even more difficult to assess than the medium-term effects, yet as Wolthers[32] has pointed out, final adult height is the clinically relevant outcome. Sadly, information on final adult height is almost non-existent, although such information as is available is encouraging. Patients studied at the Hammersmith Hospital, UK, in the early days of inhaled corticosteroid therapy were followed to adulthood and showed excellent growth, equalling or exceeding predicted adult height based on parental height measurements.[10] Equally encouraging results have been reported from Australia,[48] USA[38] and Denmark.[39]

One problem in examining growth in asthmatic children is the influence that both asthma and (probably) inhaled corticosteroid therapy have on pubertal development, resulting in a population of children with delayed puberty, in whom the pre-pubertal growth nadir is exaggerated and prolonged, but who eventually achieve satisfactory catch-up growth. In the Australian series,[48] despite significant growth retardation in the mid teens, by the age of 21 years the height of the asthmatic children was indistinguishable from that of the controls.

From this brief overview it can be seen that whilst inhaled corticosteroids have a definite effect on growth when they are first administered, there is no convincing evidence of any adverse effect on eventual adult stature. It therefore seems reasonable to advise that inhaled corticosteroids: (i) should always be used in the minimum effective dose, bearing in mind that the dose-response curve eventually reaches a plateau, and there comes a point (which will vary from child to child) when increasing doses of inhaled corticosteroids will be of no further benefit, although systemic effects will continue to increase; (ii) should not be withheld because of unwarranted fears about effects on growth; but (iii) treated children should have their growth carefully monitored.

DIFFERENCES BETWEEN INDIVIDUAL CORTICOSTEROID MOLECULES

Although there are considerable pharmacological differences between the three drugs used in inhaled corticosteroid therapy (see Table 1.1), these differences have not translated into major differences in clinical efficacy or toxicity. Beclomethasone and budesonide appear to be more or less equipotent, and the choice of drug will as often as not be determined by the choice of inhaler device and the prevailing market price.

Fluticasone has comparable (or possibly slightly greater) therapeutic efficacy at half the dose of the other two drugs, and is, therefore, normally used at half the dose level, which does not in itself offer any particular advantage. Given to children in conventional doses, i.e. up to 200 µg/day, fluticasone has not been associated with adrenal suppression or growth problems, as assessed by either knemometry,[35,36] or stadiometry.[46] It has also been shown to have no effect on growth when used in higher doses for more severe asthma.[49] However, in a paper which attracted heavy criticism in the columns of *The*

Lancet, it was reported that when fluticasone has been used in exceptionally and seemingly inappropriately high doses, growth impairment did occur,[50] confirming that despite the absence of systemic effects from the swallowed portion of the drug, there is significant absorption of active drug from the lung, a feature which it shares with the other inhaled corticosteroids.[51] At present, the balance of the evidence suggests that fluticasone probably does produce fewer systemic effects than the other drugs when used in conventional doses, but there insufficient evidence to be sure that this will translate into greater safety at higher doses.

CONCLUSION

In 1994, when the potential for side effects of inhaled corticosteroid therapy in children was reviewed,[52] the review concluded as follows:

> *Inhaled corticosteroid therapy has improved the lives of countless asthmatic children over the past 20 years and, although we cannot ignore the potential of this form of treatment to produce side effects, we must not allow this to lead to the undertreatment of a common, sometimes disabling, and occasionally fatal, disease. Inhaled corticosteroid therapy may not be the elixir of life, but for most asthmatic children it is more panacea than poison, and is likely to remain a mainstay in their management for many years to come.*

We see no reason to change that verdict.

CONFLICTS OF INTEREST

Both authors have received financial support for research, have been invited to speak at and/or attend international meetings, and have participated in clinical trials organised by Allen & Hanburys (a subsidiary of Glaxo), the manufacturers of Becotide® and Flixotide®, and by Astra, the manufacturers of Pulmicort®.

References

1 Friedman M, Strang LB. Effect of long-term glucocorticoids and corticotrophin on the growth of children. Lancet 1966; ii: 569–572
2 Oberger E, Engström I, Karlberg J. Long-term treatment with glucocorticoids/ACTH in asthmatic children. III. Effects on growth and adult height. Acta Paediatr Scand 1990; 79: 77–83
3 Johnson M. Pharmacodynamics and pharmacokinetics of inhaled glucocorticoids. J Allergy Clin Immunol 1996; 97: 169–176
4 Högger P, Rawert L, Rohdewald P. Dissolution tissue binding and kinetics of receptor binding of inhaled glucocorticoids. Eur Respir J. 1993; 6: 584s
5 Rohdewald P, Rehder S. Plasma levels of beclomethasone dipropionate (BDP) and it 17-monopropionate metabolite (17-BMP) following BDP inhalation. Eur Respir J 1994; 7: 382s
6 Yilmaz A, Akkaya E, Bayramgürler B et al. Frequency of posterior subcapsular cataract (PSC) due to corticosteroid usage in asthma patients. Am J Respir Crit Care Med 1998; 157: A403

Key points for clinical practice

- Inhaled corticosteroid therapy should only be used when it is justified by the severity of the asthma, and in the minimum effective dose.

- Inhaled corticosteroid therapy leads to mild adrenal suppression, with reduced adrenal reserve, but this has no known clinical consequences.

- There is no evidence that inhaled corticosteroid therapy has ever produced a serious or life-threatening side-effect.

- Occasional idiosyncratic reactions can sometimes be abolished by changing the drug used.

- Inhaled corticosteroid therapy has a short-term effect on growth; there is no evidence that this has any effect on adult stature.

- Possible effects on bone mineral density remain to be evaluated in the long term, and represent a threat of unknown magnitude.

- In practice, the differences between the different corticosteroids available for use by the inhaled route are slight, despite substantial differences in their pharmacology and pharmacokinetics; fluticasone may offer slight advantages over beclomethasone and budesonide.

- On current evidence, the very real dangers of not using inhaled corticosteroid therapy far outweigh the largely hypothetical dangers of side effects.

7 AbuEkteish F, Kirkpatrick JNP, Russell G. Posterior subcapsular cataract and inhaled corticosteroid therapy. Thorax 1995; 50: 674–676

8 Kruszynska YT, Greenstone MA, Home PD, Cooke NJ. Effect of high-dose beclomethasone propionate on carbohydrate and lipid metabolism in normal subjects. Thorax 1987; 42: 881–884

9 Harris DM, Martin LE, Harrison C, Jack D. The effect of oral and inhaled beclomethasone dipropionate on adrenal function. Clin Allergy 1973; 3: 243–248

10 Balfour-Lynn L. Growth and childhood asthma. Arch Dis Child 1986; 61: 1049–1055

11 Graff-Lonnevig V, Kraepelien S. Long-term treatment with beclomethasone dipropionate aerosol in asthmatic children with special reference to growth. Allergy 1979; 34: 57–61

12 Law CM, Marchant JL, Honour JW, Preece MA, Warner JO. Nocturnal adrenal suppression in asthmatic children taking inhaled beclomethasone dipropionate. Lancet 1986; i: 942–944

13 Phillip M, Aviram M, Leiberman E et al. Integrated plasma cortisol concentration in children with asthma receiving long-term inhaled corticosteroids. Pediatr Pulmonol 1992; 12: 84–89

14 Goldberg S, Algur N, Levi M et al. Adrenal suppression among asthmatic children receiving chronic therapy with inhaled corticosteroids with and without spacer device. Ann Allergy Asthma Immunol 1996; 76: 234–239

15 Ninan TK, Reid IW, Carter PE, Smail PJ, Russell G. Effects of high doses of inhaled corticosteroids on adrenal function in children with severe persistent asthma. Thorax 1993; 48: 599–602

16 Broide J, Soferman R, Kivity S et al. Low-dose adrenocorticotrophin test reveals impaired adrenal function in patients taking inhaled corticosteroids. J Clin Endocrinol Metab 1995; 80: 1243–1246

17 Brown PH, Blundell G, Greening AP, Crompton GK. High dose inhaled steroid therapy and the cortisol stress response to acute severe asthma. Respir Med 1992; 86: 495–497

18 Mellis CM, Phelan PD. Asthma deaths in children – a continuing problem. Thorax 1977; 32: 29–34

19 Kinberg KA, Hopp RJ, Biven RE, Gallacher JC. Bone mineral density in normal and asthmatic children. J Allergy Clin Immunol 1994; 94: 490–497

20 Boot AM, de Jongste JC, Verberne AAPH, Pols HAP, de Muinck Keizer-Schrama SMPF. Bone mineral density and bone metabolism of prepubertal children with asthma after long-term treatment with inhaled corticosteroids. Pediatr Pulmonol 1997; 24: 379–384

21 Packe GE, Douglas JG, McDonald AF, Robins SP, Reid DM. Bone density in asthmatic patients taking high dose inhaled beclomethasone dipropionate and intermittent systemic steroids. Thorax 1992; 47: 414–417

22 Kerstjens HA, Postma DS, van Doormaal JJ et al. Effects of short-term and long-term treatment with inhaled corticosteroids on bone metabolism in patients with airways obstruction. Thorax 1994; 49: 652–656

23 Hopp RJ, Degan JA, Phelan J, Lappe J, Gallagher GC. Cross-sectional study of bone density in asthmatic children. Pediatr Pulmonol 1995; 20: 189–192

24 Martinati LC, Bertoldo F, Gasperi E, Micelli S, Boner AL. Effect on cortical and trabecular bone mass of different anti-inflammatory treatments in preadolescent children with chronic asthma. Am J Respir Crit Care Med 1996; 153: 232–236

25 Sorva R, Tahtela R, Turpeinen M et al. Changes in bone markers in children with asthma during inhaled budesonide and nedocromil treatments. Acta Paediatr 1996; 85: 1176–1180

26 Doull I, Freezer N, Holgate S. Osteocalcin, growth, and inhaled corticosteroids: a prospective study. Arch Dis Child 1996; 74: 497–501

27 Norman AP. Steroid therapy in asthma. In: Gairdner D. ed. Recent Advances in Paediatrics, vol 3. London: Churchill Livingstone, 1965

28 Russell G. Asthma and growth. Arch Dis Child 1993; 69: 695–698

29 Ninan TK, Russell G. Asthma, inhaled corticosteroid treatment, and growth. Arch Dis Child 1992; 67: 703–705

30 Saha M-T, Laippala P, Lenko HL. Growth of asthmatic children is slower during than before treatment with inhaled glucocorticoids. Acta Paediatr 1997; 86: 138–142

31 Littlewood JM, Johnson AW, Edwards PA, Littlewood AE. Growth retardation in asthmatic children treated with inhaled beclomethasone dipropionate. Lancet 1988; i: 115–116

32 Wolthers OD. Long-, intermediate- and short-term growth studies in asthmatic children treated with inhaled glucocorticosteroids. Eur Respir J 1996; 9: 821–827

33 Wolthers OD, Pedersen S. Controlled study of linear growth in asthmatic children during treatment with inhaled glucocorticosteroids. Pediatrics 1992; 89: 839–842

34 Wolthers OD, Pedersen S. Growth of asthmatic children during treatment with budesonide: a double blind trial. BMJ 1991; 303: 163–165

35 Wolthers OD, Pedersen S. Short term growth during treatment with inhaled fluticasone propionate and beclomethasone dipropionate. Arch Dis Child 1993; 68: 673–676

36 Visser MJ, van Aalderen WMC, Elliott BM, Odink RJ, Brand PLP. Short-term growth in asthmatic children using fluticasone propionate. Chest 1998; 113: 584–586

37 Michaelsen KF, Skov L, Badsberg JH, Jorgensen M. Short-term measurement of linear growth in preterm infants: validation of a hand-held knemometer. Pediatr Res 1991; 30: 464–468

38 Silverstein MD, Yunginger JW, Reed CE et al. Attained adult height after childhood asthma: effect of glucocorticoid therapy. J Allergy Clin Immunol 1997; 99: 466–474

39 Agertoft L, Pedersen S. Final height of asthmatic children treated for 7–11 years with inhaled budesonide. Am J Respir Crit Care Med 1998; 157: A711

40 Massarano AA, Hollis S, Devlin J, David TJ. Growth in atopic eczema. Arch Dis Child 1993; 68: 677–679

41 Ferguson AC, Murray AB, Tze WJ. Short stature and delayed skeletal maturation in children with allergic disease. J Allergy Clin Immunol 1982; 69: 461–466

42 Tinkelman DG, Reed CE, Nelson HS, Offord KP. Aerosol beclomethasone dipropionate compared with theophylline as primary treatment of chronic, mild to moderately severe asthma in children. Pediatrics 1993; 92: 64–77

43 Doull IJ, Freezer NJ, Holgate ST. Growth of prepubertal children with mild asthma treated with inhaled beclomethasone dipropionate. Am J Respir Crit Care Med 1995; 151: 1715–1719

44 Verberne AA, Frost C, Roorda RJ, van der Laag H, Kerrebijn KF. One year treatment with salmeterol compared with beclomethasone in children with asthma. The Dutch Paediatric Asthma Study Group. Am J Respir Crit Care Med 1997; 156: 688–695

45 Simons FE. A comparison of beclomethasone, salmeterol, and placebo in children with asthma. N Engl J Med 1997; 337: 1659–1665

46 Price JF, Russell G, Hindmarsh PC, Weller P, Heaf DP, Williams J. Growth during one year of treatment with fluticasone propionate or sodium cromoglycate in children with asthma. Pediatr Pulmonol 1997; 24: 178–186

47 Allen DB, Mullen M, Mullen B. A meta-analysis of the effect of oral and inhaled corticosteroids on growth. J Allergy Clin Immunol 1994; 93: 967–976

48 Martin A, Landau L, Phelan P. The effects on growth of childhood asthma. Acta Paediatr Scand 1981; 70: 683–688

49 Ubhi BS, Brownlee KG. The clinical effect of long term high dose fluticasone propionate on the growth of severe asthmatic children. Am J Respir Crit Care Med 1998; 157: A711

50 Todd G, Dunlop K, McNaboe J, Ryan MF, Carson D, Shields MD. Growth and adrenal suppression in asthmatic children treated with high-dose fluticasone propionate. Lancet 1996; 348: 27–29

51 Clark DJ, Clark RA, Lipworth BJ. Adrenal suppression with inhaled budesonide and fluticasone propionate given by large volume spacer to asthmatic children. Thorax 1996; 51: 941–943

52 Russell G. Inhaled corticosteroid therapy in children: an assessment of the potential for side effects. Thorax 1994; 49: 1185–1188

Paula A. Farrell John M. Fiascone

CHAPTER 2

Bronchopulmonary dysplasia and chronic lung disease of infancy

The introduction of surfactant therapy and other innovations in the neonatal intensive care unit have resulted in a marked increase in the survival of very low birth weight (VLBW; less than 1500 g) and extremely low birth weight (ELBW; less than 1000 g) infants.[1] Bronchopulmonary dysplasia (BPD) and chronic lung disease of infancy (CLD) are two chronic pulmonary conditions which are the result of incomplete resolution or abnormal repair of lung injury occurring in the neonatal period.[2] Unfortunately, the expectation that surfactant therapy would eliminate any residual lung dysfunction in these infants has not been met, although there is accumulating evidence that such lung dysfunction is less severe than it had been prior to surfactant therapy.[3-5] As a result of increased survival of VLBW and ELBW infants and the failure to completely eliminate BPD and CLD, those caring for children will encounter larger numbers with BPD or CLD. Although BPD and CLD are closely related, they have differing diagnostic criteria[4-6] and convey different information to those who care for these children.[4-6] The spectrum of severity of these conditions is wide. There are some indications that BPD and CLD are second only to asthma among chronic lung diseases in pediatrics.[7] Thus there is ample motivation for those who care for children to be well versed in this condition. This chapter will focus on BPD/CLD as encountered and managed outside the setting of the neonatal intensive care unit.

Paula A. Farrell MD
Division of Newborn Medicine, The Floating Hospital for Children at New England Medical Center, Tufts University School of Medicine, Boston, MA 02111, USA

John M. Fiascone MD
Division of Newborn Medicine, The Floating Hospital for Children at New England Medical Center, Tufts University School of Medicine, Boston, MA 02111, USA

DEFINITIONS, INCIDENCE AND RISK FACTORS

Conceptually BPD and CLD are both the result of incompletely resolved or abnormally repaired lung damage which occurred in the neonatal period. Most children with BPD are born preterm, usually at less than 32 weeks gestational age, and have had surfactant deficiency respiratory distress syndrome (RDS) treated with supplemental oxygen, mechanical ventilation and surfactant replacement therapy.[3,8] Occasionally, children born at more advanced gestational ages and children ventilated for conditions other than RDS will develop BPD. Clinically, uneventful recovery from RDS is shown by resolution of requirement for mechanical ventilation and supplemental oxygen towards the end of the first week of life, while those who develop BPD show improvement as RDS resolves but do not demonstrate complete resolution of their lung disease.[3,8] Chest radiographs mirror this dichotomy in that neonates making an uneventful recovery will show clear lung fields toward the end of the first week of life, while those who will develop BPD generally have hazy lung fields with pulmonary oedema and volume loss.[2,9]

Bronchopulmonary dysplasia can be diagnosed on the 28th day of life in children who continue to require supplemental oxygen, have an abnormal physical examination with tachypnoea, crackles or wheezes and retractions and have an abnormal chest radiograph.[3,5,8] This definition of BPD is useful in making inter-neonatal intensive care unit comparisons of clinical outcomes, in counselling parents and for internal quality control efforts. An infant is said to have chronic lung disease of infancy if, at 36 weeks postconceptional age, there is a continued requirement for supplemental oxygen, an abnormal physical examination as described above and an abnormal chest radiograph.[3,5,6,8] Many infants who meet the criteria for BPD on the 28th day of life will be sufficiently recovered by 36 weeks postconceptional age that they do not meet criteria for the diagnosis of CLD. This is due to the survival of extremely immature babies making BPD a less specific diagnosis. The diagnosis of CLD is a better predictor of clinical respiratory difficulty during the first year of life.[3,6]

Table 2.1 contains data from the authors' institution, the New England Medical Center, obtained between 1992 and 1996. The data show the gestational age-specific incidence of CLD. A similar relationship between birth weight and incidence of CLD is a constant feature in published data. Other important risk factors for CLD and/or BPD in addition to gestational age are presence of RDS and the absence of maternal corticosteroid treatment in preparation for preterm delivery.[4,5]

AETIOLOGY OF LUNG INJURY

The primary aetiological factors in the development of BPD and CLD are: (i) an immature lung; (ii) direct injury to the lung by oxygen and mechanical ventilation (barotrauma or volutrauma); and (iii) injury to the lung which occurs when lung inflammation is initiated by supplemental oxygen and mechanical ventilation.[2,4,5] Ample clinical and experimental data support the following pathogenesis of BPD. When preterm birth is accompanied by RDS

Table 2.1 Gestational age specific incidence of chronic lung disease at the New England Medical Center. (Reproduced with permission from [39])

Gestational age	Neonatal intensive care unit admissions	Percent survival	% chronic lung disease of infancy
23	9	33	67
24	40	58	70
25	56	79	39
26	60	87	21
27	64	92	12
28	99	96	6
29	85	95	6
30	103	98	1
31	169	97	2
32	187	97	0

Data are from patients admitted between 7/92 and 6/96.
Chronic lung disease defined as requirement for supplemental oxygen at 36 week postconceptional age. Note that after 30 weeks gestational age, chronic lung disease becomes very infrequent.

and respiratory failure, the lung is deficient in multiple ways. There is a quantitative deficiency of surfactant; a quantitative deficiency of anti-oxidant defenses and a quantitative deficiency of protease inhibitors.[4,5,9] Mechanical ventilation disrupts epithelial surfaces allowing plasma proteins to enter the airways, stretches and injures the walls of developing small conducting airways and stretches alveolar septa resulting in rupture of these fragile elastin-based structures.[4,5] Supplemental oxygen in the small airways is accompanied by formation of oxygen radicals which damage cell membranes and interior cellular structures.[4,10] The anti-oxidant deficient preterm lung is poorly equipped to handle these oxygen radicals. Mechanical ventilation and supplemental oxygen directly damage the lung and initiate an influx of neutrophils into the lung with consequent lung inflammation. While neonates with RDS routinely have an influx of neutrophils into the lung, those who develop BPD have larger numbers of neutrophils and greater duration of neutrophil influx in comparison to neonates who recover from RDS without complication.[4,5,10] These neutrophils release several degradative enzymes, most prominently neutrophil elastase.[4,5,10] This enzyme digests alveolar septa and other structures within the developing lung.[4,5] The preterm lung is deficient in protease inhibitors and consequently is unable to adequately control neutrophil induced lung damage. Data exist which indicate that children who evolve BPD have more pronounced protease-induced lung damage than infants who recover from RDS without complication.[4,5,10] This protease/antiprotease imbalance is thought to play an important role in the lung injury/abnormal repair that leads to BPD and CLD.[4,5,10]

Once established, the inflammatory cascade has a self-perpetuating aspect as neutrophils recruit more neutrophils into the lung. Thus even as positive airway pressure and supplemental oxygen are withdrawn with the resolution of the child's RDS, continuing inflammation perpetuates the lung damage. A major difference between neonates who recover from RDS without complication and those who develop BPD seems to be the ability to control or down regulate this inflammatory cascade. Several protein and lipid mediators of inflammation are present in lung fluid of patients who develop BPD in greater amounts than found in patients who recover from RDS without complication. Eosinophilic cationic protein, C5a, leukotriene B4, interleukin 8, various other lipid inflammatory mediators, sulphidopeptide leukotrienes and interleukin 6 are but a partial list.[4,5,10]

Although the pathogenesis described above is generally believed to be true, it remains unclear why some neonates resolve RDS in an uncomplicated manner while others develop BPD. It is likely that there is a genetic aspect to the development of BPD as several authors describe a greater risk of BPD in families with a strong history of asthma. There has also been a report of increased risk of BPD in association with the HLA-A2 haplotype.[11–13] Several authors have reported that nutritional status may influence whether RDS resolves in an uncomplicated manner or whether BPD develops. Many important nutrients are transferred from mother to fetus during the third trimester. As such, VLBW and ELBW infants are at a significant nutritional disadvantage, in that their caloric reserves are minimal and they are deficient in several micronutrients, such as selenium, copper, zinc, iron, essential fatty acids and vitamins A and E.[4,5] Also, there is some evidence to indicate that VLBW infants who are colonized with *Ureaplasma urealyticum* are more likely to develop BPD than those not colonized.[4,14]

Conceptually the following equations may be useful in understanding the pathogenesis of BPD:

Immature lung + Mechanical ventilation + Supplemental oxygen
$$= \text{Lung damage and Lung inflammation} \qquad \text{Eq. 1}$$

Lung damage + Lung inflammation + Time
$$= \text{BPD with or without eventual CLD} \qquad \text{Eq. 2}$$

PATHOPHYSIOLOGY AND CLINICAL FINDINGS

Pathological studies have demonstrated abnormalities at all levels of the tracheobronchial tree and pulmonary function studies have reported multiple deficits in lung function.[4,5,15–17] Table 2.2 summarizes these findings. When considering reports of autopsy findings or pulmonary function tests several cautions should be kept in mind: much of the data are from children with particularly severe BPD (e.g. autopsy data), and many of these reports antedate the availability of surfactant therapy, the widespread use of antenatal corticosteroids and other recent innovations in the neonatal intensive care unit. It is not yet clear how generalizable data obtained in previous years will be to patients being cared for with the currently available technology.

Although many abnormalities in pulmonary function tests have been demonstrated in children with BPD, the most consistent finding and the one which seems to be the most clinically important is obstruction of airflow at the level of the small airways.[4,5,16,17] Histological data have demonstrated hypertrophy of smooth muscle in bronchi and bronchioles, large amounts of

Table 2.2 Selected pulmonary abnormalities in bronchopulmonary dysplasia

Location	Pathology	Pathophysiology	Clinical finding
Trachea and proximal bronchi	Tracheomalacia Bronchomalacia Granulation tissue Excessive mucus	Increased airways resistance Expiratory flow limitation	Prolonged expiratory time Wheezing at baseline or often during viral illness Episodes of cyanosis
Smaller airways	Smooth muscle hypertrophy Increased mucus Oedema Narrowing of lumena	Increased expiratory resistance Increased inspiratory resistance Decreased compliance Ventilation/perfusion mismatch	Increased work of breathing Increased oxygen consumption Air trapping Hyperinflation
Acinus	Alveolar simplification Diminished surface area Areas of atelectasis Areas of hyperinflation Oedema	Decreased compliance Ventilation/perfusion mismatch	Increased work of breathing Increased oxygen consumption Supplemental oxygen requirement
Pulmonary vascular bed	Diminished number of vessels Enhanced thickness of medial muscle layer, narrowing of lumena	Pulmonary artery hypertension: fixed and reversible aspects	Possible evolution of cor pulmonale Cyanotic episodes

mucus and the almost universal presence of pulmonary oedema.[4,15] Pulmonary function tests consistently demonstrate elevated resistance to airflow during inspiration and expiration, increased sensitivity to methacholine-induced bronchoconstriction and reversible bronchoconstriction.[4,5,16,17] Many of these findings are similar to those seen in asthma.[4,5,16,17]

The data from pulmonary function tests are consistent with the physical findings in children with BPD or CLD: elevated respiratory rate at rest, retractions, inspiratory crackles, expiratory wheezes and a prolonged expiratory time.[3–5] Airway narrowing leads to ventilation/perfusion mismatch and this accounts for both the hypoxaemia and the relief of hypoxaemia by small amounts of inspired oxygen in children with BPD or CLD.[4,5] As can be anticipated from these findings, children with BPD or CLD have diminished pulmonary reserve. Viral disease which involves the small airways, such as bronchiolitis due to respiratory syncitial virus which leads to further airway narrowing, can rapidly result in frank respiratory failure.[4,5,18] As discussed subsequently, successful pharmacological management of BPD or CLD involves control of pulmonary oedema and relief of bronchoconstriction.

Some children with BPD manifest features of acquired tracheomalacia and/or bronchomalacia.[19] These children have further increased airways resistance and they may have cyanosis on an episodic basis.[4,19] Some children with tracheomalacia have stridor; children with bronchomalacia have wheezing which does not respond to bronchodilators.[4,19]

The most serious pulmonary complication of BPD/CLD is pulmonary vascular disease with the development of cor pulmonale.[4,5,19,20] Severe BPD is accompanied by fibrosis and scarring within the lung. In this setting, there is loss of cross sectional area of the pulmonary capillary bed and the remaining pulmonary vasculature shows increased thickness of the smooth muscle layer and lumenal narrowing. The physiological consequence of this derangement is elevated pulmonary artery pressure.[4,15,19,20] Sustained pulmonary artery hypertension over time can lead to right ventricular hypertrophy and ultimately to cor pulmonale.[4,19,20] Several authors have demonstrated, either by cardiac catheterization or by echocardiography, that some children with severe BPD have elevated pulmonary artery pressure with both fixed and reactive components.[19,20] Administration of supplemental oxygen lowers the pulmonary artery pressure, although not always to normal values. The pulmonary artery pressure is maximally reduced when supplemental oxygen is administered so as to keep pulse oximetry saturation values in the 93–96% range.[4,19,20]

OUTPATIENT MANAGEMENT OF BRONCHOPULMONARY DYSPLASIA AND CHRONIC LUNG DISEASE OF INFANCY

Medical therapies

The medical management of BPD includes the liberal use of low-flow oxygen delivered by nasal cannula, and several categories of medications including diuretics, bronchodilators and methylxanthines. The goal of therapy is to prevent hypoxaemia, minimize respiratory distress and maintain adequate growth. While it is preferable to simplify the treatment plan as much as possible prior to discharge home, some infants with BPD may still require supplemental oxygen and/or medications upon discharge.

Oxygen

Low-flow oxygen delivered by nasal canula is an important modality in the treatment of BPD. It is used to prevent hypoxaemia, pulmonary hypertension and cor pulmonale, and may be necessary to optimize growth.[4,19–22] Oxygen saturation measured via pulse oximetry is a well documented means of monitoring the need for oxygen in infants with BPD. Generally, saturations are kept in the range of 93–96%, although some infants require oxygen saturations greater than 95% in order to prevent complications.[4,5,19–22] Infants with BPD frequently have episodes of desaturation during or after feeding and while sleeping. These periodic episodes of marginal oxygenation or frank hypoxaemia may lead to pulmonary hypertension or cor pulmonale.[4,5,21,22]

Therefore, it is imperative that the infant be monitored in all behavioural states for hypoxaemia or episodic arterial desaturation to determine either that supplemental oxygen is not required or that the appropriate low-flow rate is administered. Infants who are in a home oxygen programme should have frequent visits to the physician to monitor changes in oxygen requirements (again, in various states of behaviour), growth parameters, and assess for complications of inadequate oxygenation. Some home oxygen programmes routinely assess room air oxygen saturation during visits to assess lung function. It is expected that over several months room air oxygen saturation will gradually rise, ultimately allowing discontinuation of home oxygen. Some patients will require supplemental oxygen only during feeding and/or sleep as a prelude to discontinuing oxygen. If the infant is not showing signs of gradual improvement, further assessment is warranted. Lack of progressive improvement in room air oxygen saturations or failure to grow may be secondary to inadequate oxygen support, inadequate doses of medications, poor nutrition, chronic aspiration with gastroesophageal reflux, intercurrent respiratory illness or non-compliance with the home therapy.[4,5,22]

Diuretics

Diuretics are another important adjunct in the treatment of BPD. The rationale for this therapy is based on the almost universal presence of pulmonary oedema in infants with BPD. In addition, multiple studies have shown a short term improvement in pulmonary mechanics after the use of diuretic therapy.[4,5,23,24] Infants with BPD are frequently 'fluid sensitive', leading to respiratory distress with increased feeding volumes to optimize nutrition. Such distress is often minimized by the use of diuretics. The most frequently used diuretics are furosemide, hydrochlorothiazide and spironolactone. Dosing for these medication can be found in Table 2.3.[24] Side effects of this therapy include volume depletion, electrolyte imbalance including hyponatremia, hypokalemia and metabolic alkalosis, hyperglycaemia, hypercalcuria with renal calculi, osteomalacia, and rickets. Infants who are discharged home on diuretics often require supplemental electrolyte therapy to prevent deficiencies and, therefore, need electrolyte levels checked periodically.[4,5,23,24]

There are two general methods for discontinuing diuretic therapy upon discharge. The first would be to allow the infant to 'outgrow' the dose of medication by not adjusting for weight gain. The infant should be closely monitored for evidence of respiratory distress, volume overload, or excessive weight gain, and the dose corrected if needed. The second method would be to continue the diuretics at an appropriate dose until oxygen therapy is no longer necessary and the infant has shown persistent weight gain. At this point, the diuretics may be discontinued and the infant monitored closely. Either of these approaches require parental education and understanding of what would constitute increased respiratory difficulty.[5]

Inhaled bronchodilators

Multiple studies have shown that infants with BPD have short term improvement in pulmonary mechanics after inhaled bronchodilator therapy. Infants with BPD often have a family history of asthma and bronchial hyper-reactivity is a prominent feature of BPD. Inhaled bronchodilator therapy, including β-agonists and anticholinergics, is frequently used in infants with BPD.[23,24] Dosing of these medications can be found in Table 2.3.[23,24] Disadvantages with this mode of therapy include difficulty with administration of the drug and

Table 2.3 Pharmacologic treatment of bronchopulmonary dysplasia and chronic lung disease of infancy

Drug	Dose	Comments
DIURETICS		
Furosemide	1–2 mg/kg/day orally May be divided every 12 h	Most efficacious diuretic, highest frequency of adverse effects. Best diuretic for acute volume overload. Alternate day use may minimize complications but be effective.
Hydrochlor-thiazide	1–2 mg/kg every 12 h	Usually provides adequate diuresis for continuing management. Effect on lung function may require several days. Lower frequency and magnitude of adverse effects compared to furosemide.
Spirono-lactone	1–3 mg/kg/dose orally every 12 h	Generally used with another diuretic to minimize urinary potassium loss and hypokalemia. If used alone, not a very effective diuretic
INHALED BRONCHODILATORS		
Albuterol	Supplied as 0.5% solution, 5 mg/ml. Admin. 0.02–0.04 ml/kg, diluted to 1.5–2.0 ml with normal or 1/2 normal saline every 4–6 h or as needed (0.1–0.2 mg/kg)	Bronchodilator of choice for acute bronchoconstriction. Do not administer if heart rate 180 beats/min, MDI with spacer may be superior to nebulizer
Ipratropium bromide	Supplied as 0.02% solution. Dose is 0.13–0.4 ml/kg, 0.025–0.08 mg/kg up to 0.18 mg in 2–2.5 ml normal saline. Given every 6 h by nebulization	Experience in infants is limited. Do not exceed 0.9 ml of ipratropium solution. May be mixed with albuterol if used within 1 h. Protect from exposure to light
Cromolyn sodium	Given by nebulization. Dose is 20 mg every 6–8 h	Contraindicated during acute respiratory difficulty. Often requires 2–4 weeks to elicit effect
METHYLXANTHINES		
Theophylline	Oral loading dose is 5 mg/kg. Maintenance is 2 mg/kg every 8–12 h	Maintenance requirements vary widely, serum levels should be monitored and kept between 5–12 mg/ml
Caffeine base	10 mg/kg loading dose, 2.5 mg/kg once daily	Convenient dosing schedule for outpatients. Level should be 5–25 μg/ml
Caffeine citrate	20 mg/kg loading dose, 5 mg/kg once daily	Same as for base form of drug.

Note: although dexamethasone has been extensively used within the neonatal intensive care unit for the amelioration of BPD, published experience in outpatients is too limited to permit recommendations.

irregular drug delivery as it is uncertain what percentage of medication is actually delivered to the airways with nebulized or metered dose administration. In addition, infants with tracheomalacia or bronchomalacia may paradoxically worsen with bronchodilator therapy, as the airway bronchoconstriction assists in maintaining a patent airway.[4,5] Side effects of β-agonists include tachycardia, hypertension, tremor and hyperglycaemia. Albuterol, a more selective β_2-agonist, tends to be tolerated better than metaproterenol or isopreterenol.[23,24] As studies have documented only a short-term response to inhaled bronchodilator therapy, an infant should be evaluated for a clear response to this therapy, otherwise the medication should be discontinued.

Inhaled anticholinergic agents, such as ipratropium bromide, antagonize acetylcholine which thereby inhibit parasympathetic-mediated broncho-constriction.[23,24] Ipratropium bromide has fewer side effects because it is an aerosolized solution, and may have a synergistic effect when used in conjunction with a β-agonist.[23,24]

Cromoyln sodium has also been used in infants with BPD. As in patients with asthma, it does not provide direct bronchodilation and, therefore, should not be used acutely. It has been used, however, to prevent airway hyper-reactivity by stabilizing mast cells and preventing histamine release. The effect of cromolyn therapy may take 2–4 weeks to become apparent.[23,24]

Methylxanthines

Methylxanthines such as aminophylline, theophylline, and caffeine are also used for systemic bronchodilator therapy in BPD. These drugs are effective through increasing chemoreceptor sensitivity to carbon dioxide, improved diaphragmatic and skeletal contractility, and improved lung compliance and decreased pulmonary resistance as a direct bronchodilator effect.[23,24] Aminophylline and theophylline have a narrow therapeutic window and, therefore, levels should be monitored carefully. Side effects include gastrointestinal upset, gastroesophageal reflux, agitation, tachycardia, arrhythmias, hyper-reflexia, and seizures. Caffeine has fewer side effects, and a wide therapeutic window. It is unclear if the bronchodilator effect of caffeine is greater than that of theophylline.[23,24] Methylxanthines are also used in the treatment of apnoea of prematurity, a condition which infants usually outgrow prior to discharge home. However, if an infant is discharged home on methylxanthines for BPD, there is a risk that episodes of apnoea may occur upon discontinuing this medication. Frequently, these infants are also on oxygen therapy with a home monitor and, therefore, the infant can be monitored for episodes of apnoea upon discontinuation of the methylxanthine therapy. Should apnoeic episodes occur, the monitor should be continued until 2–3 months have passed without any true apnoeic episodes. There are no data on which to recommend a safe means of discontinuing methylxanthine therapy without the use of a cardiorespiratory monitor. Dosing of these medications are also included in Table 2.3. The outpatient use of methyl-xanthines can be problematical due to the need to monitor levels closely and the risk of apnoea with discontinuation or parental non-compliance. It may be preferable to discontinue this medication prior to discharge home.

Nutritional management

The importance of optimizing nutritional management in infants with bronchopulmonary dysplasia cannot be overemphasized. Adequate nutrition is not only important in maintaining the rapid rate of growth of infants, but also needed for lung repair of the infant with BPD. As a result of increased work of breathing and the need to repair the lung, many of these babies have increased caloric requirements, which can be up to 160–180 kcal/kg/day.[4,5,25,26] However, obtaining these higher caloric requirements may be difficult. These infants are often fluid sensitive, and develop respiratory distress with increased volumes of feedings. The use of increased caloric density of feeding can help to limit the required volume needed to provide the necessary caloric requirements. Powdered formulas can be concentrated with preparation by adding less water. In addition, the formulas can be supplemented with glucose polymers or medium chain fatty acids in order to increase the caloric density. Breast milk can also be supplemented to provide increased caloric density. Weaning from high calorie feeding can begin after the infant has shown adequate and persistent weight gain. The density of the formula can be periodically decreased by 2 cal/oz. The infant must be monitored for continued weight gain with each decrease of calories. If weight gain appears to be excessive, and there is no evidence that this is secondary to inadequate diuretic therapy, then the calories can be weaned more rapidly. Solid foods may be initiated as they would with other infants. Caloric additives frequently used in the management of children with BPD are listed in Table 2.4.[4,5]

MONITORING FOR COMPLICATIONS OF BRONCHOPULMONARY DYSPLASIA AND CHRONIC LUNG DISEASE OF INFANCY

Cardiovascular

Infants with BPD must be monitored for sequelae resulting from their chronic lung disease. Systemic hypertension has been reported in children with BPD. Such hypertension may present after 2–4 months of age, frequently after the infant has been discharged home. Blood pressure should be obtained with each visit to the physician. If hypertension is found, the infant should be evaluated for possible causes. However, these infants may develop hypertension without an identifiable cause. In many of the infants the hypertension is transient, and does not require medications. However, some individuals with prolonged or severe hypertension require antihypertensive therapy.[4] Although the aetiology of this hypertension is unclear, hypoxia and hypercarbia which may have occurred in these infants may lead to increased systemic vascular resistance. Complications of systemic hypertension have been reported, including left ventricular hypertrophy and cerebrovascular accidents, emphasizing the need for monitoring of blood pressure with each visit.[4,27]

Although left ventricular hypertrophy may be secondary to systemic hypertension, in infants with BPD it may occur in the absence of systemic or

Table 2.4 Frequently used nutritional supplements

Supplement	Caloric density and use
Glucose polymers (Polycose Liquid)	4 kcal/ml. Add 0.5 ml/oz formula or breast milk to increase caloric density by 2 kcal/oz
Glucose polymers (Polycose powder)	23 kcal per tablespoon. Add 1/4 teaspoon per ounce of formula to increase caloric density by 2 kcal/oz
Medium-chain triglyceride oil	8 kcal/ml. Add 0.25 ml/oz of formula to increase caloric density by 2 kcal/oz

pulmonary hypertension. This potentially contributes to pulmonary oedema in affected infants.[4] Left ventricular hypertrophy has been shown to be associated with sudden death.[4,27]

Right ventricular hypertrophy, pulmonary artery hypertension, and cor pulmonale can develop in infants with BPD, particularly in those with marginal oxygenation or frequent episodes of desaturations. Cardiac catheterization and echocardiographic studies have shown a decrease in pulmonary vascular resistance with the use of inspired oxygen therapy.[4,19,20] The presence of elevated pulmonary artery pressure and especially the development of cor pulmonale are signs of a very poor prognosis in children with BPD. It is likely that children maintained with borderline oxygenation will more often progress to development of cor pulmonale. In order to prevent this complication, as noted previously, oxygen saturations should be monitored in all behavioural states to identify periods of hypoxaemia, and oxygen should be used liberally in these babies.[19,20]

Growth failure

Growth failure is a significant issue for children with BPD.[4,5,22,25,26] As a group, VLBW infants remain small during at least the first several years of life. They tend to be between the tenth and twenty-fifth percentile for height and weight, but they consistently follow a growth curve.[28] Children with BPD may fail to thrive and exhibit a flattened growth curve, so these infants should be monitored closely for growth failure. Causes of growth failure which relate to BPD or CLD can be placed in two groups: inadequate caloric intake and inadequate oxygenation.[4,5]

Children with BPD or CLD may fail to grow if their oxygenation status is marginal. There are several reports of growth failure associated with parental noncompliance with a home oxygen programme. Growth resumes when supplemental oxygen is restarted in these children.[22] Also, growth failure associated with unsuspected hypoxaemia during sleep has been reversed by the use of supplemental oxygen.[29] Oxygen saturation values in the 93–96% range are generally adequate to support growth.[4,22,29] The infant should be evaluated with a pulse oximeter in all behavioural states for episodes of desaturations. The current medication regimen should be re-assessed to ensure optimal dosing. Also, an assessment should be made for unnecessary medications that may be increasing caloric requirements and could possibly be discontinued. It should be verified that the parents are complying with the current oxygen and medication plan.

Inadequate caloric intake may be relative; children with BPD have increased work of breathing relating to impaired pulmonary mechanics and some require supraphysiological caloric intake (160–180 kcal/kg/day) in order to grow.[4,5,25,26] As such, they may fail to grow with a caloric intake that would easily support growth in a child without BPD. Some children with BPD are poor feeders because of chronic illness and have an inadequate caloric intake because they cannot perform the work associated with feeding. Still other children with BPD will exhibit oral aversive behaviour and struggle to avoid oral intake leading to inadequate caloric intake and great frustration within the home. It is important to distinguish between these situations as hypercaloric feedings will help the first two situations while speech and swallow evaluation and therapy is required to treat oral aversive behaviour.[4,5] An occasional child exhibits such severe oral aversive behaviour that a gastrostomy tube must be placed temporarily to ensure adequate caloric intake. A detailed review of the feeding schedule should be done, including volume of feeds, frequency, and proper preparation of formula should be ensured. The assessment should also include whether the infant is experiencing feeding aversion as noted above. This detailed evaluation of the possible causes of growth failure can assist in identifying a cause, and the management plan can be adjusted accordingly.

Respiratory illness

Viral respiratory illnesses are a frequent problem in infants with BPD. Due to the decreased pulmonary reserve in patients with BPD the ability to tolerate what would otherwise be a minor illness in other infants is drastically reduced. Viral respiratory illnesses in these infants is a significant cause of rehospitalization, and can lead to severe respiratory failure. Many require prolonged hospitalization and up to 25% may require mechanical ventilation.[4,18] The most common pathogen involved is respiratory syncitial virus, but other viruses such as influenza A and B, parainfluenza and adenovirus can also cause severe illness in infants with BPD. Infants at risk are not only those with severe chronic lung disease. Former premature infants without an oxygen requirement and those who had mild respiratory disease also are at risk for severe complications with respiratory illnesses.[30,31] Those at greatest risk for severe respiratory syncitial virus disease are children who currently require, or in the past 6 months required, oxygen therapy.[4,32]

Preventative measurements for infants at risk are effective and include limiting exposure during winter months. This involves limiting day care settings to small situations with no more than 3 children, avoiding passive smoking and deferring hospitalization for elective surgery, such as hernia repair, until after the winter months to prevent nosocomial acquisition.[31,32] Close monitoring for early signs of infection is important as disease can progress rapidly.[18] Parents should be comfortable in assessing for changes in respiratory status, and should be instructed to call immediately with onset of symptoms. Immunizations should be administered according to chronological age, and should include influenza vaccine for infants over 6 months. Family members and caregivers should also be immunized against influenza.

Table 2.5 Criteria for high risk of severe respiratory syncitial virus disease

1.	Children with the diagnosis of BPD, less than 2 years of age , who are still receiving supplemental oxygen or received supplemental oxygen within the 6 months before respiratory syncitial virus season began.
2.	Children born at 28 or less weeks gestation who are younger than one year of age at the start of respiratory syncitial virus season, even if criteria for BPD not met.
3.	Children born at 29–32 weeks gestation who are younger than 6 months old at the start of respiratory syncitial virus season.
4.	Other considerations in determining risk: number of siblings, day care situation, difficulty involved in administration due to travel difficulties or difficulties with intravenous access.

Pertussis vaccine should be withheld only for documented contra-indications, of which there are few.[32]

In 1996, the US Food and Drug Administration approved the use of respiratory syncitial virus IGIV (Respigam®) for the prevention of severe disease in high risk children. This pooled blood product contains a high titer of neutralizing antibodies to respiratory syncitial virus, and is administered intravenously every month during the appropriate season. Table 2.5 lists the criteria for high risk of severe respiratory syncitial virus disease.[32] In several randomized controlled studies, the benefits of Respigam have included a decreased number of lower respiratory tract infections secondary to respiratory syncitial virus, decreased severity of disease, fewer hospitalizations, and decreased number of days in the hospital.[32] An additional benefit has been a decreased occurrence of otitis media in infants receiving monthly infusions. Side effects of Respigam infusions reported to date include transient fluid overload while receiving the infusion which resolves with decreasing the infusion rate or with furosemide, rash and fever.[30,32]

Sudden death

Several publications concerning children with BPD treated before the availability of surfactant therapy indicate a mortality rate of greater than 10% following discharge from the initial hospitalization.[4,5] Some children died from progressive respiratory insufficiency, some from acute deterioration during respiratory syncitial virus disease but some have died suddenly and unexpectedly when they were thought to have been doing well. Thus, infants with BPD are at an increased risk for sudden death, although the magnitude of the risk is not known. Two more recent studies report no post discharge deaths from BPD.[3–5] The actual cause of sudden death in children with BPD, however, may be unclear.[27] Potential mechanisms for the occurrence of sudden death in infants with BPD include intermittent or chronic hypoxaemia, predilection for upper airway obstruction from prolonged intubation, and immaturity of respiratory control centres, where the infant either fails to respond to hypoxia, or has profound apnoea associated with hypoxia despite an initial arousal response.[33] Separate investigations have shown that some children with BPD have unsuspected episodes of hypoxia during sleep and some children with BPD have deficits in arousal from hypoxic challenge.[29,33] These studies further contribute to the basis for the recommendation that oxygenation of children with BPD should be assessed during sleep as well as when awake and the use of supplemental oxygen in the management of BPD should be liberal.[4,5] Pneumograms and sleep studies are not reliable in identifying an infant at risk for sudden death.[4,5] Most infants discharged home with oxygen therapy have home cardiorespiratory monitoring. It should be noted, however, that this has not been proven to decrease the incidence of sudden death in these infants. Parents should be instructed in cardiorespiratory resuscitation prior to the infant being discharged home.

PULMONARY OUTCOME AND RESPIRATORY HEALTH

Information which is available about the pulmonary outcome of children with BPD largely antedates the widespread use of surfactant replacement therapy, antenatal corticosteroid treatment, postnatal dexamethasone for the amelioration of BPD and the increased survival of ELBW infants. As BPD has become a less severe disease within the neonatal intensive care unit,[3] there is reason to believe that the pulmonary outcome of patients being cared for with the current technology will be improved over those cared for even in the relatively recent past.

There are several publications which indicate that premature birth itself, when associated with VLBW, is associated with measurably abnormal lung function in later years without regard to the presence of RDS in the neonatal period.[34] Premature birth per se may alter lung development in a manner which leads to mild airflow obstruction, mild air trapping and increased airway responsiveness as assessed by methacholine challenge.[34] Notably, lung function in the children in these reports was assessed with formal pulmonary function testing, clinically there were no deficits identified.

Several studies have addressed changes in lung function in children with BPD over the first 2–3 years of life and report similar findings.[16,17] Early in infancy, these children have decreased compliance, increased resistance, lowered functional residual capacity, and demonstrable airway hyper-reactivity.[16,17] Respiratory rate is elevated, minute ventilation is elevated and there is increase respiratory effort.[16,17] These deficits improve rapidly, with growth, over the first 6 months and then continue to improve over the duration of the first 2–3 years.[16,17] Values for compliance and functional residual capacity become or closely approximate normal by 2–3 years of age. However, small airways obstruction remains demonstrable and airway hyper-reactivity persists in the majority of children.[16,17]

The majority of school aged children who met criteria for the diagnosis of BPD have clinically normal lung function during their school years. When formally assessed during the school years, children with BPD have shown encouraging results.[35] Total lung capacity and functional residual capacity are normal although residual lung volumes (following forced expiration) are elevated. However, on testing small airways dysfunction persists. Forced expiratory flow rates are often low, although they continue to improve over time.[35] Many, if not most, have bronchial hyper-reactivity demonstrable by methacholine challenge or bronchodilator administration.[35] Overall, it appears that lung growth proceeds in a normal or nearly normal manner but lung dysfunction persists, although this dysfunction requires formal testing to elicit.

Several publications address exercise performance (treadmill or bicycle) in children with BPD who were in the range of 10–15 years of age when studied.[36,37] Studied just before exercise these children showed the same pulmonary abnormalities listed above. They were considered to be doing well and without symptoms. All had normal oxygen saturation at rest. Several of the children with BPD exhibited mild arterial desaturation during exercise, a phenomenon not seen in controls.[37] Some children had lower anaerobic thresholds, and a significant number had exercise-induced wheezing, reduction of forced flow rates and some met criteria for exercise-induced asthma, findings which were not seen in controls.[36,37] In some patients with BPD, ventilatory reserve during peak exercise was limited.[36,37] It is important to note, however, that outside of the laboratory these children were doing well and were not known to be exercise limited. Similar to the situation with school aged children, it appears that older children with BPD do well in the area of exercise, but that formal testing unmasks deficits in lung function.

Finally, there are reports that physician-diagnosed asthma is more common in children with BPD.[11,38] This would be the logical extension of both the understanding of the role lung inflammation in BPD and the common demonstration of hyper-reactive airways when children with BPD undergo pulmonary function testing at advanced ages. The magnitude of the increased frequency of asthma is not easy to determine but has generally been found when studied.[38] On balance, the literature strongly suggests that children with BPD are more likely to be diagnosed as having asthma than children born at full term.[4,5,11,38]

Key points for clinical practice

- Although less severe, bronchopulmonary dysplasia continues to develop in infants with respiratory distress syndrome. It is second only to asthma among chronic lung diseases in pediatrics.

- Aetiological factors include an immature lung; direct injury to the lung by oxygen and mechanical ventilation; and the effects of lung inflammation initiated by oxygen and mechanical ventilation.

- Clinical characteristics are primarily the result of lower airway obstruction due to smooth muscle hypertrophy and bronchoconstriction as well as pulmonary oedema leading to symptoms of respiratory distress. Use of bronchodilator therapy and diuretics can improve these symptoms.

- Inadequate oxygenation and periodic arterial desaturation can lead to severe complications, such as pulmonary vascular disease and cor pulmonale.

Key points for clinical practice (continued)

- Pulse oximetry is ideal for assessing the adequacy of oxygenation; oxygen saturation should be monitored in all behavioural states as desaturation may occur during sleep or associated with feedings. Oxygen saturation values should remain between 93–96%.

- Providing optimal nutritional management is important in resolving chronic lung disease. Infants should be closely monitored for growth failure and a thorough evaluation should be pursued if growth failure occurs.

- Respiratory viral illnesses, especially when due to respiratory syncitial virus, can lead to severe respiratory failure in infants with chronic lung disease. Preventative measures should be emphasized to the family and the infant should be closely monitored for early signs of infection.

References

1 Wegman ME. Annual summary of vital statistics – 1990. Pediatrics 1991; 88: 1081–1092
2 O'Brodovich HM, Mellins RB. Bronchopulmonary dysplasia. Unresolved neonatal acute lung injury. Am Rev Respir Dis 1985; 132: 694–709
3 Rojas MA, Gonzalez A, Bancalari E, Claure N, Poole C, Silva-Neto G. Changing trends in the epidemiology and pathogenesis of neonatal chronic lung disease. J Pediatr 1995; 126: 605–610
4 Abman SH, Groothius JR. Pathophysiology and treatment of bronchopulmonary dysplasia. Pediatr Clin North Am 1944; 41: 277–315
5 Farrell PA, Fiascone JM. Bronchopulmonary dysplasia in the 1990s: a review for the pediatrician. Curr Probl Pediatr 1997; 27: 129–172
6 Shennan AT, Dunn MS, Ohlson A, Lennox K, Hoskins EM. Abnormal pulmonary outcomes in premature infants: predictions from oxygen requirements in the neonatal period. Pediatrics 1988; 82: 527–532
7 Singer I, Yamashita T, Lilien L, Collin M, Baley J. A longitudinal study of developmental outcome of infants with bronchopulmonary dysplasia and very low birth weight. Pediatrics 1997; 100: 987–993
8 Bancalari E, Abdenour GE, Feller R Gannon J. Bronchopulmonary dysplasia: clinical presentation. J Pediatr 1979; 95: 819–823
9 Frank L, Sosenko IRS. Development of lung antioxidant enzyme system in late gestation: possible implications for the prematurely born infant. J Pediatr 1987; 110: 9–14
10 Zimmerman JJ. Bronchoalveolar inflammatory pathophysiology of bronchopulmonary dysplasia. Clin Perinatol 1995; 22: 429–456
11 Smyth JA, Tabachnik E, Duncan WJ, Reilly BJ, Levison H. Pulmonary function and bronchial hyperreactivity in long-term survivors of bronchopulmonary dysplasia. Pediatrics 1981; 68: 336–340
12 Nickerson BG, Taussig LM. Family history of asthma in infants with bronchopulmonary dysplasia. Pediatrics 1980; 65: 1140–1146
13 Clark DA, Pincua LG, Oliphant M, Hubbell C, Oates RP, Davey FR. HLA-A2 and chronic lung disease in neonates. JAMA 1982; 248: 1868–1869

14 Wang EEL, Cassell GH, Sanchez PJ, Regan JA, Payne NR, Liu PP. Ureaplasma urealyticum and chronic lung disease of prematurity: critical appraisal of the literature on causation. Clin Infect Dis 1993; 17 (Suppl): S112–S116

15 Margraf LR, Tomashefski JF, Bruce MC, Dahms BB. Morphometric analysis of the lung in bronchopulmonary dysplasia. Am Rev Respir Dis 1991; 143: 391–400

16 Baldari E, Filippone M, Trevisanuto D, Zanardo V, Zacchello F. Pulmonary function until two years of life in infants with bronchopulmonary dysplasia. Am J Respir Crit Care Med 1997; 155: 149–155

17 Mallory GB, Chaney H, Mutich RL, Motoyama EK. Longitudinal changes in lung function during the first three years of premature infants with moderate to severe bronchopulmonary dysplasia. Pediatr Pulmonol 1991; 11: 8–14

18 Groothius JR, Gutierrez KM, Lauer BM, Respiratory syncitial virus infection in children with BPD. Pediatrics 1988; 82: 199–203

19 Miller RW, Woo P, Kellman RK, Slagle TS. Tracheobronchial abnormalities in infants with bronchopulmonary dysplasia. J Pediatr 1987; 111: 779–782

20 Berman W, Katz R, Yabek SM, Dillon T, Fripp RR, Papile LA. Long-term follow-up of bronchopulmonary dysplasia. J Pediatr 1986; 109: 45–50

21 Moyer-Mileur LJ, Nielsen DW, Pfeffer KD, Witte MK, Chapman DC. Eliminating sleep-associated hypoxemia improves growth in infants with bronchopulmonary dysplasia. Pediatrics 1996; 98: 779–783

22 Groothuis JR, Rosenberg AA. Home oxygen therapy promotes weight gain in infants with bronchopulmonary dysplasia. Am J Dis Child 1987; 141: 992–995

23 Davis JM, Sinkin RA, Aranda JV. Drug therapy for bronchopulmonary dysplasia. Pediatr Pulmonol 1990; 8: 117–125

24 Bernbaum JC. Medical care after discharge. In: Avery GB, Fletcher MA, MacDonald MG. (Eds) Neonatology. Pathophysiology and Management of the Newborn. Philadelphia: JB Lippincott, 1994; 1355–1366

25 Kurzner SI, Garg M, Bautista DB, Sargent CW, Bowman CM, Keens TG. Growth failure in bronchopulmonary dysplasia: elevated metabolic rates and pulmonary mechanics. J Pediatr 1988; 112: 73–80

26 Kurzner SI, Garg M, Bautista DB et al. Growth failure in infants with bronchopulmonary dysplasia: nutrition and elevated resting metabolic expenditure. Pediatrics 1988; 81: 379–384

27 Abman SH, Burchell MF, Schaffer MS, Rosenberg AA. Late sudden unexpected deaths in hospitalized infants with BPD. Am J Dis Child 1989; 143: 815–819

28 Casey PH, Kraemer HC, Bernbaum J, Yogman MW, Sells JC. Growth status and growth rates of a varied sample of low birth weight, preterm infants: a longitudinal cohort study from birth to three years of age. J Pediatr 1991; 119: 599–605

29 Garg M, Kurzner SI, Bautista DB, Keens TG. Clinically unsuspected hypoxia during sleep and feeding in infants with bronchopulmonary dysplasia. Pediatrics 1988; 81: 635–642

30 Meissner HC, Welliver RC, Chartrand, Fulton DR, Rodriguez W, Groothuis JR. Prevention of respiratory syncitial virus infection in high risk infants: consensus opinion on the role of immunoprophylaxis with respiratory syncitial virus hyperimmune globulin. Pediatr Infect Dis J 1996; 15: 1059–1068

31 The PREVENT Study Group. Reduction of respiratory syncitial virus hospitalization among premature infants and infants with bronchopulmonary dysplasia using respiratory syncitial virus immune globulin prophylaxis. Pediatrics 1997; 99: 93–99

32 Committee on Infectious Disease, Committee on Fetus and Newborn, American Academy of Pediatrics. Respiratory syncitial virus immune globulin intravenous: indications for use. Pediatrics 1997; 99: 645–650

33 Garg M, Kurzner SI, Bautista D, Keens TG. Hypoxic arousal responses in infants with bronchopulmonary dysplasia. Pediatrics 1988; 82: 59–63

34 Galdes-Sebaldt M, Sheller JR, Grogaard J, Stahlman M. Prematurity is associated with abnormal airway function in childhood. Pediatr Pulmonol 1989; 7: 259–264

35 Blayney M, Kerem E, Whyte H, O'Brodovich H. Bronchopulmonary dysplasia: improvement in lung function between 7 and 10 years of age. J Pediatr 1991; 118: 201–206

36 Bader D, Ramos AD, Lew CD, Platzker AC, Stabile MW, Keens TG. Childhood sequelae of infant lung disease: exercise and pulmonary function abnormalities after bronchopulmonary dysplasia. J Pediatr 1987; 110: 693–699.

37 Santuz P, Baraldi E, Zaramella P, Filippone M, Zacchello F. Factors limiting exercise performance in long-term survivors of bronchopulmonary dysplasia. Am J Respir Crit Care Med 1995; 152: 1284–1289

38 Palta M, Sadek M, Barnet JH et al. Evaluation of criteria for chronic lung disease in surviving very low birth weight infants. J Pediatr 1998; 132: 57–63

39 Fiascone JM. Advance for Managers of Respiratory Care 1998; 7: 43–47

Robert Sunderland

Skull fracture, subdural haematoma, shaking and impact injury

Scholastikos was approached by a man who had been told on the highest authority that his friend was dead yet the friend protested his vitality. Scholastikos pondered deeply and then replied, æOpinion can always be challenged by Evidence'.

Pelagius of Alexandria, *5th Century BC*

In recent years, child protection has assumed an increasing role in paediatricians' work. This arena is both emotive and emotional. Increasing awareness, improvements in imaging and changes in patterns of disease have allowed attention to be directed at the imperfect ascertainment of child abuse cases within the community. Increased public awareness following a series of high profile cases has led to increased pressure to find and protect all vulnerable children. There is, then, a risk that clinicians become overloaded with uncertain cases and unable to re-evaluate the available evidence. This could lead to a clinical presentation or symptom complex being assumed to be due to abuse unless proved otherwise – inverting the usual principle of studying evidence to establish cause. Exercising opinion or exhibiting prejudice is often mistaken for presentation of evidence. Unquestioningly repeating untested opinion produces dogma, not evidence.

The use of evidence to test historical opinion applies no less to child protection than other clinical areas. By developing and rigorously testing objective criteria, professional standards will be maintained and children protected more effectively. This chapter will, by revisiting previous research, endeavour to advance this process by answering the following questions:

1.   What is known of the epidemiology, presenting features, differential diagnosis, investigation and outcome of skull fracture, subdural haematoma and diffuse axonal injury (DAI)?

Robert Sunderland MD MB ChB FRCP FRCPCH, Consultant Paediatrician, Birmingham Children's Hospital, Steelhouse Lane, Birmingham B4 6NH, UK

2.   What do we know of the minimum forces necessary to cause fractures, subdural haematoma and DAI?

3.   Can such forces be generated by normal nursing, by shaking alone or is impact necessary?

4.   Is it possible to estimate the time of injury from clinical signs at presentation?

Injury to the brain can be irreversible. Increasing lay, press and professional awareness of non-accidental brain injury has highlighted the need to prevent brain injury wherever possible. Much of the scientific research into brain injury is based upon retrospective analysis of human accidents and experimental injuries induced in primates. Extrapolations from such experimental models have assisted advancing knowledge. However, speculative over-interpretation of such models has sometimes led to inappropriate presumption of causation. There is a limited literature on witnessed infant falls, which allows estimation of the forces needed to cause certain injuries. Finally, there is a large body of observational studies which merge into everyday clinical practice. We appreciate that although toddlers fall during development of locomotion, the vast majority suffer no brain injury.

SKULL FRACTURES

Fractures occur when bone is loaded beyond its elastic limit. The load, speed and area of impact determine the severity of injury. Striking the head on a nail or the edge of a metal sink will produce a more serious injury (usually a depressed rather than linear fracture) than the same impact on a flat surface (Fig. 3.1). High velocity impacts create more significant injuries, usually a depressed, stellate or multiple fracture which may cross suture lines. Lesser impact may produce a haematoma, greater impact will not only fracture the skull but also deform and damage the underlying brain. The speed of impact similarly influences the nature of injury sustained. Striking one's head with a metal bar is less pleasant than a sponge bat because of the different rates of deceleration and load. Impact on a stone floor produces more rapid deceleration and more serious injury than landing on soft furnishings.

Force needed to fracture the skull

The force needed to fracture skull bones requires impact; shaking alone will not cause this. Multiple fractures require multiple impacts or crush injury unless tramline fractures (either side of an impacted object) are found. Accidental falls usually result in linear fractures, most commonly in the parietal area. Depressed, growing (leptomeningeal), multiple, stellate, and cross-suture fractures are indicative of higher energy transfers/impact and, in the absence of appropriate history, are considered suspicious of non-accidental injury.[1] The research on which these statements have been based has been criticised[2] as it can contain a circular argument where the likely cause for the fracture (e.g. accidental or non-accidental) is decided by the authors, who then

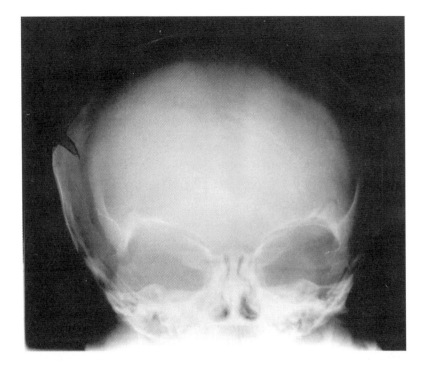

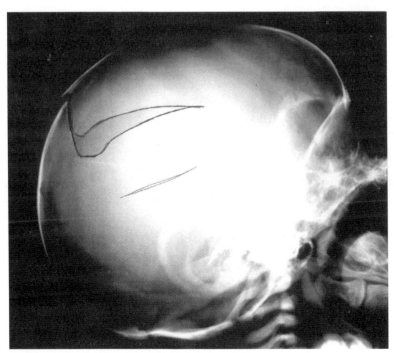

Fig. 3.1 A depressed and linear skull fracture (margins have been highlighted). The history offered was that the carer slipped, banging the infant's head against a protruding nail which caused the depressed fracture. The baby then fell onto a stone floor sustaining the linear fracture. There was no underlying brain damage. Double fractures are often non-accidental and are usually associated with severe brain damage.

proceed to analyse their data and conclude that certain types of fracture are typical of their attributed aetiology. Such work is of necessity dependent upon a limited number of cases which will have been selected by referral and is always dependent upon a diagnosis which involves assumptions about the underlying history which may not have been tested evidentially or established as fact. We have no suspicion when a patient sustains an occipital fracture by a simple backward fall in a public area with many witnesses. Should one react differently when this happens with a single parent alone with a child?

It is self-evident that truly objective research cannot be conducted to identify the forces necessary to cause infant skull fracture. We are dependent upon limited data from mortuary experiments and interpretations of observed accidents. The former may not be directly referrable to the living but from them we know that 80% of stillbirths dropped 18 inches onto a paved floor sustain skull fracture.[3] Infant cadavers dropped 82 cm onto concrete, foam backed linoleum or thin carpet all sustain fracture,[4] interposing 8 cm of camel blanket reduced the skull fracture rate to 16% and 2 cm of rubber as shock absorber reduced the rate to 10%.[5]

The incidence of skull fracture is uncertain. There may be some variation between rural and urban communities, but there is clear consistent gender difference with boys sustaining many more fractures than girls. Children under 2 years have a higher risk of fracture which is attributed variously to higher risk of abuse at this age or increased vulnerability during development. At Birmingham, where the casualty department sees 38,000 children per annum from a local population of 100 000, we treated 51 patients with skull fracture in 1997. There were 21 right parietal, 21 left parietal, 8 occipital and 5 frontal (some children had multiple fractures). Seven of these fractures were depressed, 5 parietal (2 left, 2 right) and 2 were frontal – all except one (which was abusive) involved impact with small heavy objects, such as golf club, stone or edge of radiator. Of these children, 28 were < 1 year old and 5 were aged 1–2 years. Of the total, 13 were female. There was no ethnic predisposition with 43% fractures arising in the 40% of our community who are recent immigrants.

Protective reflexes

The role of protective reflex, landing surface and true free-fall have frequently been misunderstood in studies of head injury. The true impact is calculated from the free fall. Thus, where a child lands on a shoulder, the head is slowed and only travels a few inches further to impact, and the fall is 'broken' by the shoulder acting as a shock absorber. Protective reflexes such as putting an arm up or curling the head forward to take a blow across the upper back are examples of these instinctive shock absorbers which are obviously not reflected in cadaver studies.

Landing surfaces

Landing surfaces which have some flexibility will cause deceleration resulting in less deforming forces upon the skull and, hence, the brain. This may explain why many observed infant falls do not result in injury. One study of over 200 child falls in hospital found only two fractures – a skull fracture with an estimated impact of 39 Newton (N) and a clavicle fracture with an impact of 103 N; many other falls had impacts greater than 100 N yet did not result in serious injury.[6] From this and other observational work has arisen the confident extrapolation that head injury does not occur in falls from less than 5 (or 10) feet. Anyone claiming this should realise that, if suspended inverted blindfolded and with their arms tied, they will sustain a skull fracture if dropped four feet onto a hospital floor.[7,8] Incorporating these figures into common clinical scenarios indicates that an infant weighing 2 kg falling from knee/chair height (45 cm) onto concrete will sustain an impact of 96 N; a toddler falling from waist/worksurface (82 cm) would have an impact of 320 N. Interposing soft timber, carpet then foam for the 82 cm fall would give calculated impacts of 160 N, 107 N, and 64 N respectively. From the calculations of Lyons and Oates[6] giving the minimum identified impact of 39 N as sufficient to cause a linear parietal fracture, one can deduce that the likelihood of producing a skull fracture is high unless protective reflexes intervene. Infants do not have rearward protective reflexes.[9]

Speed and energy of impact

The speed and area of impact affect the distortional forces acting on the skull. A 4 kg weight delivers 40 N. Applying this as a static force onto a child's head may not cause a fracture, but dropping it from a height of 2 feet would. Applying this force across a large area will cause lesser damage than applying it through a point. Thus an infant dropped against a sharp unyielding surface is much more likely to sustain a stellate or depressed fracture than a similar fall onto a floor.

Brain injury

The energy transfers which fracture the skull can also deform and damage the underlying brain. Thus pedestrian accidents, falls from great height or other significant accidental head injuries can result in serious brain injury. Abusive injuries usually have brain damage which give an idea of the likely level of violence. Plain skull x-ray has poor discriminatory power to identify underlying brain injury (sensitivity 65%, negative predictive value 83%), which is better identified by the clinical criteria of persistent vomiting, headache or impaired consciousness (sensitivity 91%, negative predictive value 99%).[10] Severe intracranial injury can occur in the absence of skull fracture.

SUBDURAL HAEMATOMA

Infantile subdural haematoma and diffuse axonal injury are caused by shearing forces. The subdural bleeding occurs when bridging veins which run from the surface of the cerebral hemispheres to the sagittal sinus are torn (Fig. 3.2). Venous blood returns from the cerebral cortex into the nearest available sinus of the dura mater. These cortical veins travel superficially adherent to the deep surface of the arachnoid, crossing the subdural space as bridging veins near the midline and entering the sinus obliquely against the direction of blood

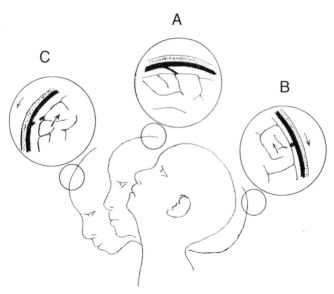

Fig. 3.2 Shaking an infant's head produces inertial rotational movements of the brain. The only connection between the brain and the vault of the skull are the bridging veins which run obliquely forward to the sagittal sinus (**A**). These veins are compressed if the brain moves forward relative to the skull (**B**). If the skull reverses direction, the brain continues to move under inertial forces. When the brain moves backwards, especially if there is repetitive inertial movement, the veins become increasingly strained and eventually shear (**C**) (*Courtesy of J. Sunderland*).

flow.[11] These bridging veins are distensible but not significantly extensible. In the sagittal sinus this means that the bridging veins run forwards, providing a potential tension-release mechanism against forward movement but tethering the brain against backward rotation. Some British and Japanese neurosurgeons have queried the diagnostic argument that subdural haematoma cannot occur in simple rearward falls.[12–14] These anatomical considerations and the epidemiological facts of high incidence in adventurous male toddlers both add doubts to the confident assertion that such a history is not ever credible.

Historically, subdural haematoma was attributed to springing of the skull bones at birth leading to tearing of the vessels or dural tears. Caffey[15] in 1946 first made the association between subdural haematomas and fractures of long bones (often multiple and of different ages). Emerging awareness of the spectrum, scope and scale of child abuse initially met considerable resistance. At that time, many child experts presumed that parents would not injure their own children. Kempe[16] suggested that professional acceptance of the problem dated from his changing the description to the intentionally emotive 'battered baby syndrome'. For some time, attention tended to focus on the fractures. Subdural haematomas were often considered a late manifestation of birth injury. Increasing availability of imaging is changing this emphasis.

Epidemiology

There does not appear to have been a population based study of the incidence of subdural haematoma. Paediatric neurology and neurosurgical textbooks state that subdural haematoma is 'common' in infancy without quoting rates or the denominator population. The distribution of such patients seen will depend upon the nature of the reporting hospital. Specialist hospitals with neurosurgical, neuroimaging and intensive care facilities will have a greater number of referred cases than a District hospital. Our hospital fulfils these criteria draining a local population of 100 000 and a regional population of 1 million children. We have seen 108 children with subdural haematoma in the past four years: 23 due to cerebral tumours, 17 followed witnessed trauma, 15 with vascular malformations, 3 meningitis, 3 metabolic disease, 1 haemophilia, 22 were due to non-accidental injuries, 7 were of uncertain cause and 20 were chronic. These figures may be an under-ascertainment since there is no screening test for subdural haematoma, cases are investigated when they present with evidence of neurological dysfunction. To place these figures in context, we see approximately 1 case of physical abuse per day, 1 case of sexual abuse per week, 50 cases of skull fracture per year (mostly accidents, witnessed falls); our casualty department treats 38 000 children per annum of which 2100 are head injuries.

Liverpool Children's Hospital[10] reported 9269 children attending their casualty department or admitted for head injury between February 1993 and January 1994. They excluded children from outside the city referred for intensive care. There were 6011 skull x-rays revealing 162 fractures and 156 CT scans with 23 intracranial injuries. Of these 23, 15 had a skull fracture and, in the majority, the abnormality was related to this (local oedema or bleeding) but two required evacuation of intracranial haematoma. Among the remainder, there were two with haematomas who died, one from non-accidental injuries. The age distribution of these patients is not given, the authors go on to state that infants (under 2 years) were significantly more likely than older children to have skull fracture but less likely to have intracranial injury. There were 4 deaths, only one was associated with skull fracture and all died as a result of severe intracranial injuries. While forces sufficient to fracture a skull may also cause intracranial injury, other forces can cause similar or worse brain injury without fracture. Of the 23 children with evidence of intracerebral injury, 21 had abnormal neurological signs and the authors conclude that clinical abnormalities are reliable predictors of intracranial injury, whereas skull x-ray is not.

The Geneva Neurosurgical Clinic reported 1812 cases of head trauma in an 8.5 year period among 57 000 resident children aged under 15 years (plus an unspecified number of severe injuries referred in from an unspecified population). There were only 8 cases of subdural haematoma, 4 in infants less than a year. Falling was the most frequent cause of injury, with road accidents the most serious. Babies and toddlers suffered more skull fractures and subdural haematoma from lower estimated energy-transfer injuries than older children. They lost consciousness less but had more frequent seizures and lateralising signs.[17]

A review of 30 child deaths caused by physical abuse in Kuala Lumpur found the commonest cause was intracranial haemorrhage. Of these 17 deaths, only 4 had skull fracture which suggested to the authors the possibility of whiplash shaking injuries being the commonest mechanism. The mean age at death was 2.5 years. Unlike most studies which show an unexplained and strikingly high prevalence of males over females, the Malay study found slightly more girl (17) than boy (13) fatalities. There has been some disquiet that unselected studies might inadvertently contain a number of accidental injuries. This study, by commencing with cases selected for abuse, suggests that there may be no gender difference in abusive fatalities. Among the identified abusers there were features of deprivation, drug or alcohol abuse and aggressive personalities. There was little gender difference among the identified abusers with fathers the commonest followed by mothers then childminders.[18]

Iowa paediatricians and forensic examiners identified 24 infants (under 4 years) with abusive brain injuries in a 4.5 year period.[19] Nine died from their injuries. There was again no gender difference in this study on patients selected for abuse.

Differential diagnoses

The main potential causes for infantile subdural haematoma are trauma, bacterial meningitis, hypernatraemic dehydration, leukaemia, bleeding diathesis and birth injuries. Any condition which results in cerebral atrophy, including inborn errors of metabolism, increases the vulnerability of the bridging veins and thus increases the risk of a subdural haematoma. Where there is unclear, confusing or absent history, these conditions need to be excluded before considering possible traumatic causes.

Trauma

Trauma of some form is considered to be the most common cause. There is, however, confusion in the literature regarding the relative importance of birth injury, accidental fall and non-accidental violence. At present this is leading to controversy which seems unrelated to the available evidence. Large series of subdural haematoma and other brain injury from the pre-CT period have been published where more than half of the injuries were presumed to have arisen from unwitnessed falls. Reviewing this today causes concern, as among these accidental injuries were many of the children with subdural haematoma and retinal haemorrhage.[20.]

Birth trauma

Regardless of the birth route, shearing forces are applied to the head. There are anecdotal reports of subdural haematoma being discovered at routine cranial ultrasound after apparently normal non-traumatic deliveries. There is an apparent assumption that subdural haematoma discovered in the first month of life is attributable to birth injury.[21] In the absence of a prospective cohort of infants screened at birth, such speculation is presumptive. The corollaries, that non-accidental injury is uncommon below this age and that after this age some other explanation is needed, are equally unproved.

Re-bleeding

Subdural haematomas which develop a capsule and mature into chronic haematomas may steadily swell due to the osmotic activity of the degrading

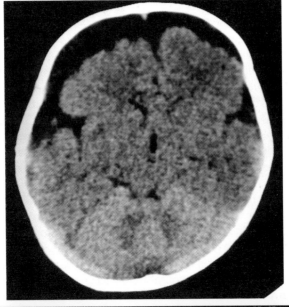

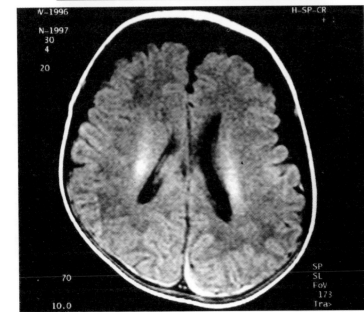

Fig. 3.3 Subdural collections from different causes may appear similar. (**A**) shows a chronic subdural effusion secondary to pneumococcal meningitis. (**B**) is a subdural haemorrhage (black area at top of picture, frontal pole) with rebleed (white streaks at occiput).

contained product. Veins which are crossing the margins of such capsulated haematomas are placed under increased strain and may bleed under minimal stimulation. Children who present with such a symptom complex create a clinical dilemma as the acute presentation gives no clue as to the cause of the initial bleeding.[22]

Retinal haemorrhages

Retinal haemorrhages occur when there is extravasation of blood either into the retina itself (intraretinal), between the retina and the pigment epithelium (subretinal) or between the retina and the hyaloid face of the vitreous body (subhyaloid or preretinal).[23]

The causative mechanism for these haemorrhages is uncertain. They were thought to be a consequence of transmission of rapidly raised intracerebral pressure. However, they are found less commonly in subarachnoid than subdural haemorrhage where the rise in pressure is higher and more rapid. Other aetiological theories include: pressure waves set up in the vitreous by the oscillating lens, shearing forces within the eye from repetitive shaking, venous pressure transmitted from squeezing the chest (including resuscitation), epileptic seizure or valsalva.

Retinal haemorrhages were first reported in newborns by Jaeger in 1861.[24] Various studies since have stated varying incidence in neonates from 33–80%, the variation appears to be dependent upon the experience of the clinician and timing of examination. Like subdural haematoma, it may be that improvements in diagnostic aids or awareness has resulted in higher ascertainment. A higher incidence can be related to occipital presentation or prolonged labour which suggests an aetiological link with prolonged raised ocular venous pressure.[25] Neonatal retinal haemorrhages clear in the majority of infants within a few days.[26]

Between 20–32% of patients with subarachnoid haemorrhage have retinal haemorrhages.[23] Like neonatal retinal haemorrhages, the majority clear spontaneously. Mechanisms proposed for these haemorrhages include forcing of blood from the subarachnoid space along the optic sheath, retinal venous hypertension or raised central venous pressure secondary to epileptic seizures.

Zimmerman et al found retinal haemorrhages in over 80% of children with subdural haematomas.[27] These are more usually panretinal haemorrhages (through all layers of the retina) and can last for months or years. This creates forensic problems – can one confidently date an injury from the presence of retinal haemorrhages and be certain that the retinal haemorrhages did not antedate the events leading to the current presentation? Like many other areas in forensic paediatrics, specialist knowledge is creating subspecialists. It is unclear why these haemorrhages do not clear in the same way as bleeding in other sites. There may be another pathological mechanism beyond vessel rupture or it may be due to some intrinsic property of the retina. It has been suggested that centrifugal forces damage the orbital vessels beyond simple venous blowout. Differences in vessel flexibility, higher cardiac rate and lower intravessel pressures may affect cerebrovascular haemodynamic mechanisms more significantly in infants than in adults.[23] Panretinal haemorrhages were thought to occur in children who convulse or after resuscitation but prospective studies have questioned this unless they were already present as part of the prior traumatic condition.[28, 29]

It has been suggested that retinal haemorrhages (and especially panretinal haemorrhages) in children under 3 years of age were diagnostic of abusive aetiology.[30,31] However, like so many other areas of medicine, increasing experience teaches there is no simple or single diagnostic test. Retinal haemorrhages are seen in many non-abusive conditions including meningitis, vasculitis, endocarditis, generalised sepsis, coagulopathies (including aspirin and anticoagulant effect), sickle cell disease, hypertension and retinal diseases. Cause cannot be determined by fundal examination nor aetiology revealed by the morphology of the haemorrhage.

Presenting symptoms and signs

Older children who develop subdural haematoma usually present with acute signs of progressive drowsiness, vomiting, ataxia or other neurological dysfunction and often have focal signs or convulsions. In infants the signs are less specific and include increased irritability, poor feeding, lethargy or anaemia. Focal neurological signs such as delayed pupillary responses or asymmetric abnormality of tone may be absent even with extensive haematoma. Generalised or focal convulsions in a previously well infant often alerts the astute clinician. If the parents have a record of the child's head growth, rapid upward crossing of centiles may be identified.

Other signs of external trauma should be sought carefully with a complete external examination. There may be contusions or bruising to the scalp, tenderness of the neck, grip marks to the arms, chest, abdomen or grip marks at the ankle or feet indicating where the child has been grasped or thrown. Posterior rib fractures may be seen after squeezing injury. They are not seen with normal child care or clinical activity, including resuscitation. Metaphyseal fractures occur when growing bones are pulled or flailed.[1,32]

Skull fractures occur in accidental and non-accidental injuries but underlying brain damage indicates considerably more trauma than seen in normal toddler falls – when a history of significant accidental trauma is absent, the possibility of concealed history is raised. Persistent vomiting, impaired consciousness and headache were shown to be independent predictors of intracranial complications in retrospective studies of large numbers of children with head injury.[33,34] These neurological features are more valuable than skull x-ray in predicting intracranial injury.[10]

Chronic subdural haematoma/effusion may show the same symptoms and signs. Additionally, there may be failure to thrive, anaemia or developmental retardation.

Investigations

Advances in neuroimaging have greatly facilitated the diagnostic investigations in a child where brain injury is suspected. If the anterior fontanel is patent then cerebral ultrasound is usually the initial investigation because there is no radiation and no need for sedation. However, this can miss small frontal collections and may give poor imaging of the posterior fossa. High definition ultrasound can examine the interface between the grey and white matter.[35] Contusional or axonal injuries occur in this region especially at the frontal poles. They carry a graver prognosis irrespective of whether any subdural collection is evacuated. Jaspan and colleagues indicate such injuries are rarely seen in traffic accidents or simple impact,[35] there is increasing suspicion that they may be a pathognomonic marker of repetitive shaking which may be of assistance in differentiating between a frustrated carer and violent persistent shaking.

Because of similarity of the magnetic signal between fresh blood, CSF and brain, there may be diagnostic confusion in the first day or so after the haematoma collects and thus CT scan is preferred to MRI if there is clinical suspicion of an acute collection. MRI gives higher definition images and is, therefore, preferred after the acute phase for identification of subtle neuronal injuries which have prognostic implications. If there is suspicion of skull fracture, then plain x-rays are necessary. Such x-rays, however, do not replace a careful clinical examination and are of limited value in predicting underlying brain damage. Skeletal survey is indicated where there is suspicion of non-accidental injuries.

Clotting studies are recommended in all cases remembering that cerebral trauma may itself be associated with a degree of coagulopathy.[36] There are occasional reports of inborn errors of metabolism being associated with subdural haematoma, whether this is due to a bleeding diathesis or cerebral shrinkage or some other intrinsic factor is at present uncertain. Other investigations are indicated by the clinical condition and progress of the child.

Outcome

The outcome for children with shaken brain injury is entirely dependent upon the imposed forces. No treatment has yet been shown to be effective in rectifying axonal injury once incurred. Primate experiments show that increasing levels of rotational acceleration produce firstly concussion, then subdural haematoma, then axonal injury.[37,38]

Rotational head injuries have long been recognised to be among the highest risk groups for poor outcome.[39,40] The combination of the bony skull and CSF offers good protection to the brain from linear or translational injuries, but this gives poor protection against rotational injury. In the latter, there is not only high mortality, but also a high prevalence of severe handicap among survivors. This high morbidity is due to the nature of the brain injury rather than any pre-existing suboptimal environment. Compared with children who suffer accidental falls, rotational brain injury shows poor response to treatment. While the reasons for this high morbidity may relate to the immaturity of the injured brain and the high energy transfers involved, it is not possible to exclude cumulative repeated injury nor, in some cases, damage due to delay in seeking medical attention.

There have been limited studies of the long-term outcome of shaken baby. The available studies are of necessity selective, influenced by reporting of severe cases from specialist centres. The available studies show that if axonal injury is present, there is virtually always permanent impairment. Comparing children admitted to intensive care because of brain injury reveals much poorer outcome from presumed abuse than witnessed accidents. Cambridge paediatricians[41] described 15 cases of suspected non-accidental injury (6 with skull fractures) and compared their outcome with 10 children from witnessed accidents (7 had skull fractures). Among the presumed abuse group there is only one normal child, whereas 7 of the accidental injuries are fully normal. Of the abuse group 2 died, 9 have severe handicap and 3 have moderate handicap while among the accident group there was one death, one child with severe handicap and one with mild handicap. Bonnier et al[42] showed that longer term review reveals even worse outcome with only one child normal among a group of 13 shaken infants after a 6 year follow-up. They showed that the long-term influence of shaken brain is much more serious than the presenting symptoms would indicate: the reverse of children accidentally injured. They also showed there may be a deceptive symptom-free period. Prolonged follow up is necessary in cases of suspected shaken brain.

The gravity of these shaking injuries was recognised by the early authors. Both Guthkelch and Caffey described death and profound permanent handicap in cases where they obtained histories of infants shaken by a carer.[43,44] They and subsequent authors have stressed the paramount importance of preventing these injuries. Despite 30 years of advances in management, because of the nature of the injury, poor outcome remains the norm.

Timing of symptom onset

Although there is considerable literature on theoretical and experimental models, there is a paucity of literature on the length of time from reported shaking to the onset of symptoms. It has become received wisdom among many health care and social work professionals that there is only a very short interval between shaking and onset of symptoms. There is little to substantiate or refute this belief. Review of the English language literature[45] identifies only three case histories with sufficient information to allow evidential abstraction – and two of these cases come from Guthkelch[43] and Caffey.[44] All three cases were considered to be shaken infant with no signs or history to suggest impact injury. All three cases were fatal with death occurring between a few hours and 5 days after the confessed shaking.

Case 1

Guthkelch described a 6 month-old boy where the mother admitted that she feared the child was going to choke after several bouts of coughing. She held him up and shook him several times in order to clear his throat whereupon he began convulsing. On admission shortly afterwards the child was stuporous and breathing heavily with pronounced hyper-reflexia of all limbs and a tense fontanel. There were no external signs of injury. Despite draining bilateral subdural haematomas, the child died 3 days later. Necropsy identified torn bridging veins with underlying cerebral contusions and lacerations.

Case 2

Caffey reports the confession of the nanny who had shaken an 11 week-old girl because she refused to drink her bottle. This child was seized by the arms and shaken until the head bobbed and she became faint (presumed concussion). On admission to hospital there was no external sign of trauma to any part of the head and there were no fractured bones. She was semi-comatose, tachypnoeic with a bulging fontanel and increased reflexes. The CSF was blood stained and the ocular fundi were invisible. The infant died 2 hours after admission to hospital. Necropsy revealed bilateral subdural haematomas with subarachnoid haemorrhage and confirmed bleeding was from torn bridging veins.

Case 3

Lambert et al[46] reported a 13 month-old child who has been discovered unresponsive. A baby sitter admitted that she had shaken the child vigorously 4 days earlier. The child had vomited several times during the preceding 4 days but the parents had not noted any other symptom to suggest a neurological dysfunction. She was reported 'playful' earlier on the day of admission. On arrival at hospital she was unrouseable and unresponsive to pain with tonic/clonic seizures, no pupil response to light and bilateral retinal haemorrhages. There were no bone fractures, there were two ecchymoses on the sternum. CT scan revealed a right subdural haematoma. The child died the day after admission and necropsy confirmed the sternal contusions that were estimated to be 3–5 days old. There was a 50 ml right subdural haematoma with cerebral oedema and cerebellar tonsillar herniation.

Nashelsky and Dix[45] found 84 deaths among 268 reported cases of shaken baby but they concluded that the literature contains minimal data to substantiate or refute the contention that there is always a very short interval between shaking and onset of symptoms. Despite this, the belief is widespread. This has on occasion led to the carer who presents the child for medical attention being investigated as the sole possible perpetrator. Symptoms of brain injury may present early as seen in traffic accident or sporting injuries. However, these early signs are not always clear, specific or evident. Convulsions do not always occur in the immediate aftermath of traumatic brain injury. Feeding difficulties are not a good indicator of intracranial trauma – our neurosurgical nurses report that babies feed well after craniotomy.

Case 4

A 3 month-old male infant was brought to our hospital in the early hours of the morning by mother who said she was concerned because he was not himself. Thirty hours earlier she had gone out leaving the baby with her partner who was not the father. An 11 year-old half-sib subsequently related that 2 hours later the baby had been crying, dad had gone into him and he had stopped suddenly. Mother returned in the small hours and at some point was beaten up by the partner. The following morning she sought police and medical help for herself while her partner took the baby to the GP because of vomiting and lethargy. The doctor diagnosed mild gastroenteritis. The child was in the care of a friend for the rest of the day who reported he was still not himself. Mother collected him in the evening and as he continued to be non-specifically unwell, she brought him to hospital. Mother was noted to have a number of bruises, the baby had a pinch mark in the ear and probable finger tip bruises to his rib cage and legs. There were a few petechiae on the forehead but no other exterior marks of head injury. There was no focal neurological abnormality. He had bilateral retinal haemorrhages. Skeletal survey and clotting studies were normal, CT scan showed subdural haematoma. Eighteen hours after admission, during which he had been under close supervision, he developed focal left sided fits. These became generalised, frequent and difficult to control for 36 hours. At this time, a left hemiplegia developed and subsequently slowly almost completely resolved. The alleged trauma occurred 9 hours before an experienced GP found minimal non-specific signs; 27 hours before arrival at hospital and almost 48 hours before commencement of convulsions.

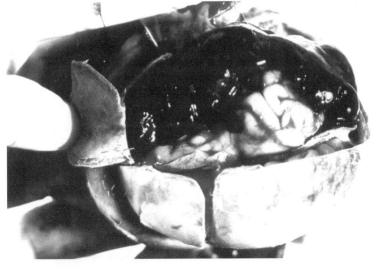

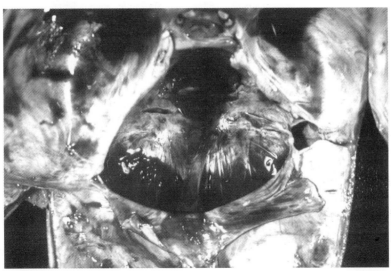

Fig. 3.4 Fresh subdural haematoma appears as a viscous clot (**A**). Chronic haematomas have a membrane and bulge under osmotic pressure (**B**). Note also the thin flexible skull plates and the poor structural support of the infant brain due to the relative lack of myelination. Courtesy of Dr F. Raafat.

Even had he been injured immediately before coming to hospital, 18 hours elapsed before the first fits.

Repeated imaging following operation or traffic accident has aided understanding of changing appearances which allows some estimation of timing of the initial insult. On CT, fresh blood is initially hyperdense to CSF and brain, becoming isodense then hypodense over approximately 3 weeks. MR detects methaemoglobin approximately 3 days after clot formation as a low intensity signal. As the red cells lyse, the haematoma becomes high intensity approximately a week after bleeding.[47] MR is also sensitive at

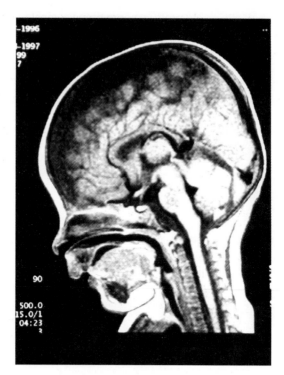

Fig. 3.5 MR image of a shaken brain showing old subdural haematoma (dark area over frontal and vertex) and re-bleed (white streaks at occiput) – child scanned lying on back. Courtesy of Dr S. Chapman.

identifying areas of increased water content – hence oedema or ischaemic areas. These CT and MR appearances however only allow approximation within a period of about 3 weeks. Once an intracerebral collection has become chronic, there is no imaging feature that allows a confident opinion that the collection is weeks, months or even years old.

The blood in a subdural haematoma is initially red, remaining dark red for the first 4 or 5 days; a brownish chocolate tinge increasingly develops over the next week then gradually changing to a straw coloured fluid as the red cells disintegrate. Towards the end of the first week after injury, a subdural membrane develops from the inner surface of the dura and eventually encapsulates the haematoma. Vascularisation of this capsule indicates a vital process that requires 4–14 days, which may be of assistance in dating the initial insult. Eventually, the haematoma becomes enclosed in the capsule and the collection may behave as an osmotic space occupying lesion (Fig. 3.4). Rebleeding around the margins of the encapsulated haematoma often precipitates requests for medical attention. The presence of old and fresh blood can confound attempts at dating the injury (Fig. 3.5).

Engineering explanations

The skull and CSF protect the brain from linear deceleration. To mechanical engineers, the design of the brain surrounded by CSF contained within a protective bony skull effectively protects nerve tissue against injury following a blow or fall. Unfortunately, this is less effective in protecting against rotational movements. A broad generalisation would divide these rotational movements into either fore and aft or side to side. Alternating rotational movements will result in the brain impacting the falx or parietal bone in side to side movements or the orbital roof and tentorium cerebelli in fore and aft movements.

The mechanical differences between blows and shaking have been expressed in homely analogies. Shaking a glass bowl containing blancmange and jelly will produce shearing strains at their interface with far less force than will shatter the bowl. Similarly an egg yolk and white in the bowl will homogenise more fully under gentle shaking than by striking, even to smashing the bowl.

Repetitive shaking accentuates inertial brain movements (Fig. 3.2). An initial backwards movement of the head will cause the frontal lobe of the brain to approximate the orbital roof until the brain starts moving. It then effectively hinges on the brain stem, producing a rotational movement. Once moving, it will continue until the occipital lobe approaches the tentorium cerebelli. As the head is jerked forwards, the brain will continue travelling backwards for a finite time before reversing. During this period, attachments between the brain and the skull will become increasingly stretched. The only attachments over the vault are the bridging veins – all nerves emerge from the base. These bridging veins run obliquely forwards to enter the sagittal sinus against the direction of blood flow. Veins are distensible but not significantly extensible. The backward and forward oscillation places increasing strain on the bridging veins which eventually rupture leading to subdural haematoma. It was at one time suggested that blood in the inter-hemispheric fissure was a pointer to non-accidental injuries. The bridging veins run in this fissure. Some of the blood sinks to the base of the skull, especially into the middle fossa, and some flows backwards, which is why blood is usually seen in these sites, irrespective of cause of injury.

The brain itself is not homogenous. Because the shear modulus of brain tissue is low, brain will deform more easily when subjected to rotational loads. Individual axons can sustain only tensile loads. The interface between grey and white matter is vulnerable to shearing by the same oscillating inertial forces described above. As the frontal poles are furthest from the brain's centre of mass, centrifugal forces result in tearing and shearing there. The frontal lobes have a lower threshold for acceleration injury than temporal lobes, possibly related to the anatomy of the base of the skull as well as the greater centrifugal forces.[48] The majority of subdural haematoma and DAI in infants are seen in the frontal area.

Shaking or impact?

One of the difficulties in dealing with abusive injury has been a tendency to seek a unifying hypothetical explanation for what are uniquely individual injuries. After Guthkelch[43] suggested whiplash shaking as a non-impact mechanism for infant brain injury, it became widely accepted as a mechanism for at least some of the brain and eye injuries. Latterly, there has been an unhelpful discussion as to whether all injuries attributed to shaking require some impact to produce the damage seen. Such causative distinctions may not be medically important but can have far-reaching legal implications. Such differences of opinion have done little to protect children or prevent injury.

Alexander and colleagues[49] searched for signs of external head trauma in 24 cases of severe intracranial injury. They found evidence of scalp contusion, subgaleal injury or fracture in 12. They considered the retinal haemorrhages and some of the shearing injuries could not be caused by impact alone. Evidence of external trauma was not predictive of fatal outcome. They considered the argument that impact need only be onto a padded surface but queried whether forces sufficient to cause severe internal head trauma would leave no sign on the scalp and no subgaleal injury. The burden of proof remained with those who would claim that impact must be present in all cases of severe intracranial injury. They concluded that the shaken baby syndrome reflected a spectrum of abuse that may include shaking, direct injury or both.

The minimal levels of force necessary for skull and brain injuries have been calculated from a number of studies. Postulated mechanisms for subdural haematoma and DAI cannot be tested experimentally in humans. Extrapolations from observed incidents are dependent upon a number of variables, any one of which could distort conclusions. There have been a number of experiments using primates which have shown that nothing need strike the head in order for brain damage to occur.[50] These experiments confirm that rotational movements produce a given brain injury more easily than linear acceleration. The accelerations needed to cause subdural haematoma in human adults have been estimated at 200 G or 1500 m/s^2 or 1600 radians/s^2.[51,52] Concussion is caused in monkeys at about 10 000 radians/s^2, subdural haematoma at 35 000 radians/s^2 and DAI at 40 000 radians/s^2.[52,53]

Extrapolations made from primates to infants require cautious interpretation. The Pennsylvania group[53] attempted to extrapolate this primate work to human experience by using an infant sized doll where the head had been packed tight with wet cotton waste and contained an accelerometer. A number of alternative neck mechanisms were used from a frictionless hinge to a dense rubber block. By vigorously shaking the doll, they attempted to generate the level of forces identified as causing concussion, subdural haematoma or DAI. In the primate work, a monkey had been securely fixed into a rigid seat and the head was fitted into a helmet. The helmet was then either rapidly jolted or connected through a cam to an electric motor which vibrated at between 100–1000 radians/s (up to 110 cycles/s). Forces greater than 14 G or 1140 radians/s^2 could not be produced by shaking the doll but 300 G or 52 500 radians/s^2 were achieved if the head was struck against even a soft mattress. Rather than querying the analogy or the model, it was concluded that some form of impact was necessary to generate sufficient energy transfer to cause vessel or axonal shearing.

This apparently small point has serious sociological and medicolegal implications. Instead of dealing with a child where a frustrated carer seizes and shakes the child in a despairing attempt to console or silence, the shaken **impact** theory indicates that the child is not only shaken violently but also flung away or struck, sustaining serious injury.

The doll model was limited in a number of areas: (i) experiments on adult monkeys cannot be directly transferred to infant humans because of differences in scale, anatomy and cerebral maturity; (ii) the frequency of vibration is unrealistic – it is difficult to shake an infant sized doll at more then 4–6 cycles/s; (iii) the unmyelinated infant brain is more distensible than adult brain (likened more to wet jelly rather than cold porridge); and (iv) the relatively large head, weak neck, open sutures, calvarium flexibility and the large CSF space in infants (up to 1 cm) were all ignored, yet all contribute to the potential for nerve damage. These inertial movements will produce impaction of the brain against the anterior cranial fossa. Perhaps this is the missing and potentially unifying factor. If the work on adult monkeys can be transferred to humans there has to be greater deceleration than shaking a solid doll's head could generate. External impact produced this – internal impact produced by inertial rotational forces could also suffice.

Adult experience

The first cases which suggested that the mechanism for subdural haematoma was different from direct head trauma were reported by Guthkelch.[43] One of these was a professor of neurosurgery (taking anticoagulants) who had come down a fairground ride. He gave no report of any impact. Ommaya and Yarnell[54] described two adult patients who sustained delayed subdural haematoma after vehicular whiplash injuries. Allied pilots captured during the Gulf War report being gripped by the shirt front and shaken vigorously to unconsciousness. They have no recollection of any blow to the head. A 30 year-old Palestinian man collapsed and died after being shaken violently under Israeli interrogation. Necropsy showed an acute subdural haemorrhage and bruising of the chest and shoulders.[55] It does not appear to be necessary for there to be external head impact for adult subdural haematoma and DAI. The infant brain may not be unique in its response to rapid rotational decelerations.

These adult experiences support the current consensus view that shaking requires forces beyond the actions of a reasonable carer or the type of accidents that occur in normal homes.

CONCLUSIONS

Acquired brain injury is emerging as an increasingly important cause of preventable handicap in infancy. There is little objective evidence of definitive differences between accidental and non-accidental injuries, they are separated by forensic questioning and matching history against injury. There is a dearth of appropriate biomechanical research to identify and understand the factors operating in children. There is also a disappointing absence of effective treatment for these injuries once sustained. Further preventive efforts are required.

There has been an unfortunate tendency to fill the vacuum of evidence by speculative extrapolation. Those who adhere to the shaken impact theory need to appreciate the weaknesses in the model and the absence of scalp trauma in many cases. The 'accidental backward fall' proposition cannot explain rib or limb injuries. The shaken infant model was expanded by Caffey to include 'vibrations induced by radio, television, hifi sets, air-conditioners, telephones, vacuum cleaners, blenders, garbage disposal and dishwashers...repeated convulsions in tetanus, epilepsy, meningo-encephalitis or lead poisoning may induce traumatic whiplash-brain damage'. In the absence of evidence there are no absolutes. All of us, whichever view we hold, would do well to remember:

It is the nature of an hypothesis, when once a man has conceived it, that it assimilates every thing to itself as proper nourishment, and, from the first moment of your begetting it, it generally grows the stronger by every thing you see hear read or understand.

Laurence Stern, *Tristram Shandy.*

Key points for clinical practice

- The prevalence of infant brain injury is unknown. One can expect identification to increase as imaging becomes safer and more available.

- The spectrum of brain injuries ranges from concussion and cerebral oedema, to subdural haematoma and diffuse axonal injury.

- Rotational injuries (including shaking) are more dangerous than linear ones.

- Severe intracranial injury can occur in the absence of skull fracture.

- Skull fracture can arise from short falls if impact is directly on the head.

- If there are no backward protective reflexes, then such falls may account for fractures and brain injury.

- Clinical neurological abnormalities (persistent vomiting, altered consciousness, headache) are good predictors of intracranial injury. The time from injury to symptoms may be seconds or days.

- Diffuse axonal injury is currently untreatable and has a high incidence of handicap or death.

- This is potentially the most serious form of child abuse.

- Further strategies for prevention are needed.

References

1 Chapman S. Recent advances in the radiology of child abuse. In: Hobbs CJ, Wynne J. (eds) Child Abuse. London: Ballière Tindall, 1993: 211–233
2 Bracewell J. Manchester City Council v B. Family Law Rep 1996; 1: 324–333
3 Taylor AS. Medical Jurisprudence. Philadelphia: Blanchard and Lee, 1856; 368
4 Weber W. Experimentelle Untersuchungen zu Schadelbruchverletzungen des Sauglings. Z Rechtsmed 1984; 92: 87–94
5 Weber W. Zur biomechanischen Fragilitat des Sauglingsschadels [Biomechanical fragility of skull fractures in infants] German with English abstract. Z Rechtsmed 1985; 94: 93–101

6 Lyons TJ, Oates RK. Falling out of bed: a relatively benign occurrence. Pediatrics 1993; 92: 125–127

7 Gurdijian ES, Webster JE, Lissner HR. Studies on skull fracture, with particular reference to engineering factors. Am J Surg 1949; 78: 736–742

8 Root I. Head injuries from short distance falls. Am J Forensic Med Pathol 1992; 13: 85–87

9 Wilkins B. Infant brain injury, abuse or accident? Arch Dis Child 1997; 76: 395–396.

10 Lloyd DA, Carty H, Patterson M, Butcher CK, Roe D. Predictive value of skull radiography for intracranial injury in children with blunt head injury. Lancet 1997; 349: 821–824

11 Last RJ. Anatomy Regional and Applied. Edinburgh: Churchill Livingstone, 1973: 802–803

12 Howard MA, Bell BA, Uttley D. Pathophysiology of infant subdural haematomas. Br J Neurosurg 1993; 7: 355–365

13 Aoki N, Masuzawa H. Infantile acute subdural haematoma: clinical analysis of 26 cases. J Neurosurg 1984; 61: 273–280

14 Ikeda A, Sato O, Tsugane R et al. Infantile acute subdural haematoma. Childs Nerv Syst 1987; 3: 19–22

15 Caffey J. Multiple fractures in the long bones of infants suffering from subdural haematoma. Am J Roentgen, 1946; 56: 163–173

16 Kempe CH, Silverman FN, Steele BF et al. The battered child syndrome. JAMA 1962; 181: 17–24

17. Merten DF, Osborne DRS, Radkowski MA, Leonidas JC. Cranial, cerebral trauma in the child abuse syndrome: radiological observation. Pediatr Radiol 1984; 14: 272–277

18 Berney J, Froidevaux AC, Favier J. Pediatric head trauma: influence of age and sex. I Epidemiology. Childs Nerv Syst 1994; 10: 509–516

19 Kasim MS, Cheah I, Shafie HM. Childhood deaths from physical abuse. Child Abuse Negl 1995; 19: 847–854

20 Hendrick EB, Harwood-Hash DCF, Hudson AR. Head injuries in children: a survey of 4465 consecutive cases at the Hospital for Sick Children Toronto, Canada. Clin Neurosurg 1964; 11: 46–65

21 Levene MI, deVries LS. Haemorrhagic and ischaemic lesions. Fetal and neonatal neurology and neurosurgery. In: Levene MI, Lifford RJ. (eds) Edinburgh: Churchill Livingstone, 1995: 350–353

22 Newton RW. Intracranial injury and non-accidental injury. Arch Dis Child 1989; 64: 188–190

23 Kaur B, Taylor D. Retinal haemorrhages. Arch Dis Child 1990: 65: 1369–1372

24 Jaeger E. Uber die Einstellung des Dioptrischen Apparates im menschlichen Auge (originally published in 1861). In: Giles CL. (ed). Vienna: LW Siedel, 1960

25 Kauffman ML. Retinal haemorrhages in the newborn. Arch Ophthalmol 1958; 46: 658–660

26 Baum JD, Bulpitt CJ. Retinal and congenital haemorrhage in the newborn. Arch Dis Child 1970; 45: 344–349

27 Zimmerman RW, Bilaniuk LT, Bruce D et al. Computed tomography of craniocerebral injury in the abused child. Radiology 1970; 130: 687–690

28 Sandramouli S, Robinson R, Tsaloumas M, Willshaw HE. Retinal haemorrhages and convulsions. Arch Dis Child 1997; 76: 449–451

29 Goetting MG, Sowa B. Retinal haemorrhage after cardiopulmonary resuscitation in children: an aetiologic reevaluation. Pediatrics 1990; 85: 585–588

30 Levin AV. Ocular manifestations of child abuse. Ophthalmol Clin North Am 1990; 3: 249–264

31 Eisenbrey AB. Retinal haemorrhage in the battered child. Childs Brain 1979; 5: 40–44

32 Caffey J. On the theory and practice of shaking infants. Its potential residual effects of permanent brain damage and mental retardation. Am J Dis Child 1972; 124: 161–169

33 Chan KW, Yue CP, Mann KS. The risk of intracranial complications in pediatric head injury. Childs Nerv Syst 1990; 6: 27–29

34 Rosenthal BW, Bergman I. Intracranial injury after moderate head trauma in children. J Pediatr 1989; 115: 346–350

35 Jaspan T, Narborough G, Punt JAG et al. Cerebral contusional tears as a marker of child abuse – detection by cranial sonography. Pediatr Radiol 1992; 22: 237–245

36 Hymel KP, Abshire TC, Luckey DW et al. Coagulopathy in pediatric abusive head

trauma. Pediatrics 1997; 99: 371–375

37 Gennarelli TS, Thibault LE. Biomechanics of acute subdural haematoma. J Trauma 1982; 22: 680–686

38 Gennarelli TS, Thibault LE, Adams JH et al. Diffuse axonal injury and traumatic coma in the primate. Ann Neurol 1982; 12: 564–574

39 Ryan GA, McLean AJ, Vilenius ATS et al. Brain injury patterns in fatally injured pedestrians. J Trauma 1994; 36: 469–476

40 Hanigan WC, Peterson RA, Njus G. Pediatrics 1987; 80: 618–622

41 Haviland J, Ross-Russell RI. Outcome after severe non-accidental head injury. Arch Dis Child 1997; 77: 504–507

42 Bonnier C, Nassogne M, Evrard P. Outcome and prognosis of whiplash shaken infant syndrome: late consequences after a symptom-free interval. Dev Med Child Neurol 1995; 37: 943–956

43 Guthkelch AN. Infantile subdural haematoma and its relationship to whiplash injuries. BMJ 1971; ii: 430–431

44 Caffey J. The whiplash shaken infant syndrome: manual shaking by the extremities with whiplash-induced intracranial and intraocular bleedings, linked with residual permanent brain damage and mental retardation. Pediatrics 1974; 54: 396–403

45 Nashelsky MB, Dix JD. The time interval between lethal infant shaking and onset of symptoms. A review of the shaken baby syndrome literature. Am J Forensic Med Pathol 1995; 16: 154–157

46 Lambert SR, Johnson TE, Hoyt CS. Optic nerve sheath and fetinal haemorrhages associated with the shaken baby syndrome. Arch Ophthalmol 1986; 104: 1509–1512

47 Bruce DA, Zimmerman RA. Shaken impact syndrome. Pediatr Ann 1989; 18: 482–494

48 Marguiles SS, Thiebault LE. An analytical model of traumatic brain injury. J Biomech Eng 1989; 111: 241–249

49 Alexander R, Sato Y, Smith W et al. Incidence of impact trauma with cranial injuries ascribed to trauma. Am J Dis Child 1990; 144: 724–726

50 Ommaya AK, Gennarelli TA. Cerebral concussion and traumatic unconsciousness. Correlation of experimental and clinical observations on blunt head injuries. Brain 1974; 97: 633–654

51 Ryan GA, McLean AJ, Vilenus ATS et al. Brain injury patterns in fatally injured pedestrians. J Trauma 1994; 36: 469–476

52 Hanigan WC, Peterson RA, Njus G. Tin ear syndrome: rotational acceleration in pediatric head injuries. Pediatrics 1987; 80: 618–620

53 Duhaime AC, Gennarelli TA, Thibault LE et al. The shaken baby syndrome. A clinical pathological and biomechanical study. J Neurosurg 1987; 66: 409–415

54 Ommaya AK, Yarnell P, Subdural haematoma after whiplash injury. Lancet 1969; 169: 237–239

55 Pounder DJ. Shaken adult syndrome. Am J Forensic Med Pathol 1997; 18: 321–324

David P. H. Jones Christopher N. Bools

CHAPTER 4

Factitious illness by proxy

This chapter discusses advances in the areas of epidemiology, the debate regarding terminology and classification, the development of hypotheses regarding aetiological factors, and treatments within a family context.

ORIGINS AND PREFERRED TERMINOLOGY

In 1977, Meadow[1] reported 2 children who suffered from illnesses which had been fabricated by their mothers; calling the situation Munchausen's syndrome by proxy (MSP). The term was derived from the adult Munchausen's syndrome, as described and named by Asher.[2] Further individual case reports followed, and an extensive range of fabricated illnesses were described.

In this chapter, we use the term factitious illness by proxy, rather than Munchausen's syndrome by proxy, to refer to the **situation** which is composed of a complex set of phenomena which are discussed below. We agree with Fisher and Mitchell[3] that the term is descriptive without aetiological assumptions. The term factitious disorder by proxy has been proposed in the American Psychiatry Association's *Diagnostic and Statistical Manual* (DSM-IV)[4] as research criteria for a psychiatric diagnosis applicable to the fabricator. The proposed criteria are presented and discussed below. In this chapter, we address only the situation of fabrication of illness by a parent in her/his own child, which only in a minority of cases has been the father,[5] whilst recognizing that other carers have been reported to have fabricated illness.

David P. H. Jones MB ChB FRCPsych DCH D(Obst) RCOG, Consultant Child and Family Psychiatrist and Honorary Senior Lecturer, Park Hospital for Children, Old Road, Oxford OX3 7LQ, UK

Christopher N. Bools MB ChB MMedSc MRCPsych, Consultant Child and Family Psychiatrist, Royal United Hospital, Combe Park, Bath BA1 3NG, UK

REPORTS OF SERIES OF CASES

In the UK, early reports came from Meadow[6] and from Southall's group.[7] Both of these series were probably unrepresentative of all examples of factitious illness by proxy, the former being a heterogeneous group of a range of subtypes of factitious illness by proxy, probably of greater than average severity, and the latter a more homogenous group of infants who had been smothered to induce physical signs. A third international series was by review and meta-analysis of the literature up to 1987 which identified 116 examples and added reports of three.[8] This review presented factitious illness by proxy as a syndrome cluster, which the author indicated may have multiple, or different, aetiologies. The Great Ormond Street Hospital series[9] will be presented later, as the study described aspects of therapeutic work by a psychiatry/paediatric liaison team.

The Leeds/Cardiff group with The British Paediatric Association Surveillance Unit[10] looked at the epidemiology over a 2 year period across the UK. Paediatricians in the UK were requested to report examples of factitious illness by proxy, smothering and deliberate poisoning as individual categories which were not mutually exclusive. The main findings of the study were the identification of 128 cases, of which 55 were factitious illness by proxy alone, 15 poisoning alone and 15 suffocation alone; 43 suffered more than one category of abuse. Of the 55 examples of factitious illness by proxy, 53 children suffered actual physical harm as a result of the fabrications, indicating that the reported cases were almost all at the severe end of the spectrum. The fabricator was the child's mother in 85% of cases. The combined annual incidence of the conditions in children was calculated to be 0.5/100 000, and for those under the age of 1 year at least 2.8/100 000.

In the USA, there have been 2 surveys of the smothering variety of factitious illness by proxy. Rosen et al[11] analysed data from 81 infants evaluated and monitored at home. The authors concluded that the behaviour of the parents of 6 infants was compatible with descriptions of factitious illness by proxy. A postal survey of 127 apnoea monitoring programmes across the USA[12] revealed that 51 programmes reported 54 examples of factitious illness by proxy amongst their 20,090 patients, an incidence of 0.27%. All of these surveys probably exclude a number of less serious examples of fabrication, and children not seen by a paediatrician.

A FRAMEWORK FOR ASSESSMENT

The elements of factitious illness by proxy

The term factitious illness by proxy has been used to refer to a complex set of phenomena, the main elements of which are: (i) the fabrication of an illness (with a range of subtypes and severities); (ii) the mental state of the fabricator (with putative psychological processes, psychiatric diagnoses, and effects on parent-child attachment or interaction); and (iii) the effects on the child's development (with consideration of physical and/or emotional effects).

Fabrication of illness in the child

The subtypes are based on presentation[13] and may be considered under three main groups: (i) verbal fabrications – most commonly of seizures;[14] (ii) verbal fabrications plus the falsification of specimens or charts; and (iii) illness induction by administering substances, smothering, withholding nutrients and medicines, and other means, e.g. introducing infectious material into the gut or bloodstream.

We previously drew attention to three 'special situations', which include elements of the above three: fabrication of psychiatric disorder,[15] factitious disorder in pregnancy,[16] and fabrication in the presence of genuine physical illness.[17]

An approach to initial assessment

The first stage in the assessment of factitious illness by proxy is almost always the process of paediatric diagnosis.[18] If the diagnosis of fabrication is confirmed, in a second stage a psychiatrist may contribute by assessing the behaviour of the perpetrator and the emotional effects on the child and siblings. In a few circumstances, the psychiatrist may be directly involved in stage one, notably when there is the question of psychiatric disorder in a child.[15] We have found the algorithm proposed by Waring[19] to be helpful when considering factitious illness by proxy as one of a number of differential diagnoses, including the vulnerable child syndrome, extreme exaggeration, malingering, symptom overemphasis, and maternal anxiety.[13]

Classification of psychiatric disorders

At present, the World Health Organization's *The ICD-10 Classification of Mental and Behavioural Disorders* (Chapter V: *Clinical Descriptions and Diagnostic Guidelines*)[20] does not have a category into which to place factitious illness by proxy as a specific diagnosis applicable to a fabricator. However, the proposal is made in the DSM-IV (in Appendix B: *Criteria Sets and Axes Provided for Further Study*) for 'research criteria for factitious disorder by proxy' to be applicable to the fabricator.[4] Both systems are multi-axial and allow for additional psychiatric diagnoses, for example relating to abnormalities of personality and learning difficulties, for general medical conditions, and for psychosocial and environmental problems. In addition, separate diagnoses relating to the child, for example recognizing physical abuse of a child, or one of the behavioural or emotional disorders, may be made.

The DSM-IV[4] research criteria for factitious disorder by proxy are:

A.   Intentional production or feigning of physical or psychological signs or symptoms in another person who is under the individual's care.

B.   The motivation for the perpetrator's behaviour is to assume the sick role by proxy.

C.   External incentives for the behaviour (such as economic gain) are absent.

D.   The behaviour is not better accounted for by another mental disorder.

Attention is also drawn to the possible role of life stressors as a trigger for the behaviour. The criteria may evolve as hypotheses develop regarding the mental state of the fabricator. A number of hypotheses are discussed below. However, it is our view that, at this stage, there is evidence to regard cautiously factitious disorder by proxy as a psychiatric disorder for research purposes (as defined by the DSM-IV research criteria) which will usually be one of a number of diagnoses applicable to the fabricator. Difficulties with the proposal could relate to the wide spectrum of fabricating behaviours, especially the spectrum of potential physical and emotional harm.

Effects on the child's health and development – the resulting harm

When physical signs are produced ('illness induction' subtype) this is highly dangerous to the child, with a risk of mortality. Rosenberg[8] calculated the mortality to be 9% from her review of the literature. McClure et al[10] reported that 8/128 index children had died from the abuse. In addition to mortality, child victims have suffered from permanent physical damage leading to scarring and contractures of limbs, epilepsy and severe learning difficulties.

The risk of emotional harm being suffered by a child subject to factitious illness by proxy, with or without physical harm, is less clear. A child could suffer as a consequence of being brought up in a fabricated, sick role, which may continue to result in lack of opportunity and a range of psychosocial disabilities. Perhaps another consequence is emotional harm as a result of other abnormal aspects of the relationship with the mother, and disturbed family relationships. Although this has not been systematically studied, there is evidence from clinical reports suggesting that, without successful treatment, emotional harm does occur. Meadow[6] reported early on that children were continuing to live in a fabricated sick role and this was examined in a follow-up study of 56 of the index children.[21] The latter study also identified a variety of emotional and behaviour disorders evident in child victims, including school non-attendance, excessive complaints of somatic symptoms, concentration difficulties, and conduct disorder. McGuire and Feldman[22] reported the occurrence of psychological morbidity in the form of a range of disorders, depending on the age of the child; feeding disorders in infants, withdrawal and hyperactivity in pre-school children, hysterical disorders and personal adoption of Munchausen's syndrome behaviour in adolescents.

Co-morbidity

Further evidence for the risk of other difficulties was reported in a descriptive study of what was termed 'co-morbidity'.[23] The sample was of an unusual and particularly severe group of factitious illness by proxy, studied prior to more widespread knowledge of factitious illness by proxy. However, 29% of index children had a history of failure to thrive (not necessarily as a direct result of the fabrication), and 29% had a history of non-accidental injury, inappropriate medication, or neglect. Other fabrications, in addition to the index fabrications, were also common, occurring in 64%. Overall, 73% of the index children had been affected by one of the above additional problems at the time when fabrications were first identified.

PREDISPOSING RISK FACTORS AND EXPLANATORY HYPOTHESES

Providing appropriate care during childhood sickness and obtaining necessary medicines are fundamental competencies for human parents. Rules and rituals surround this health seeking behaviour which parents typically undertake for their children. To render deliberately one's child sick, or appear to be sick, is a parental activity in the very opposite direction to that pursued by the majority. Paediatricians deal daily with the majority of parents who seek help for their unwell, diseased or distressed children, in the normal ways of the culture. Parents who harm their children through factitious illness by proxy, therefore, break a fundamental series of rules and patterns of normal behaviour. What is known about the background or circumstances which predispose to this phenomenon?

Factitious illness by proxy is clearly a form of child abuse. There is little reason to suppose that the predisposing risk factors for other forms of neglect and abuse[24] are not equally applicable to cases of factitious illness by proxy. Below, we will consider additional risk factors which have emerged from studies of factitious illness by proxy. It is important to consider all risk factors or hypotheses together rather than in isolation.

Psychiatric risk factors

Somatizing disorders

In a study of 47 mothers of cases of factitious illness by proxy, 79% had a history of a 'somatizing disorder', a term within which were included the somatoform disorders (conversion disorder, hypochondriasis and somatization disorder) and factitious disorders.[25] The general descriptive term, somatizing disorder, was chosen because of the difficulties in discriminating between the precise diagnostic categories. A similar situation exists regarding the rarer, male fabricator.[5] A history of somatizing disorder may not be obvious until, with hindsight, the past medical history is pieced together, when all the medical records are scrutinized. Even though the fabricator's somatization disorder may not have been diagnosed as such, the family is likely to be well known to the primary healthcare team, through frequent surgery attendance of the index child, siblings, or the mother.

Other psychiatric diagnoses in the fabricator

In a study of psychopathology, commonly carried out some time after the discovery of fabrication, it was reported that more than half of fabricators had a personality disorder. This was typically histrionic or borderline in type, especially amongst fabricators who actively induced symptoms. Dependent and avoidant personality disorders were also identified. Less common are personality disorders involving overt sociopathy, aggressive behaviour and criminality, although in the above study a small number of fabricators had a history of theft, fraud and arson.[25] We consider that these latter disorders are potentially especially dangerous. The personality difficulties usually present are unlikely to lead to legal or overt social difficulties, but are more likely to result in increased health care use. Fabricators were more likely to have seen a psychiatrist, either following an episode of self harm, or for other non-psychotic disorders.[25–27] The mothers involved may well have had a connection with health or caring professions in the past.[1,6]

Family patterns

Classical descriptions of family dynamics in factitious illness by proxy have emphasized the relatively closed style of functioning.[28] Typically, the family keeps themselves to themselves, and neighbours usually have few concerns about parenting. In 40% of cases serious marital problems were identified.[9]

Fathers have been described as relatively unassertive, tending to accede to their wife's perspective on child welfare and health issues and, in a small number of cases, being frankly collusive with their partner's falsehoods. Most, however, express surprise once their own denial is breached, and they appreciate the degree and extent of their wife's fabrications. Typically, some remain unrepentant on their partner's behalf, adamantly joining the cause of protest against the accusation of factitious illness by proxy. While typical cases undoubtedly occur, there have been no systematic surveys of family functioning, or the attitudes and beliefs of different adults involved in cases where factitious illness by proxy has occurred. Thus our understanding is based on highly unrepresentative and selected case series. While this is inevitable in the early stages of understanding any new disorder, there is now a real need to obtain some more objective and representative data.

The situation with factitious illness by proxy is mirrored by early exploration of the phenomenon of child sexual abuse. Here too, there were stereotypical descriptions offered of typical family interaction patterns, the roles of mothers, and the roles of perpetrating fathers. Indeed, with reversal of gender, there are remarkable similarities in the descriptions of early investigators concerning sexually abusing families and those in which factitious illness by proxy has occurred. As in the field of sexual abuse, it is likely that there will be less reliance on stereotype and greater appreciation of varieties of family situations and pathologies, personality characteristics and routes to factitious illness by proxy abuse as a final common pathway, as recognition, referral and assessment of cases increases.

The development of hypotheses

It appears that there are aspects of the fabricator's psychological status and family functioning which appear to predispose to factitious illness by proxy. However, these factors alone are insufficient to explain the phenomenon. There have been two predominant strands to the explanatory hypotheses which have been proposed by investigators. One has considered the behaviour to be an extension of the concept of the sick role, as an example of 'abnormal illness behaviour'. The other derives from seeing factitious illness by proxy behaviour by parents as a distortion of the transference relationship between mothers and their doctors. Some explanatory models have drawn these two themes together, but all agree that, once established, the abnormal behaviour can be self-perpetuating. We consider these hypotheses and others, below.

Social learning models

A set of hypotheses derive from Parsons' notion of the sick role and the relative benefits, as well as duties and responsibilities, which this confers.[29] This led to Mechanic's[30] influential views concerning 'abnormal illness behaviour' as a model for understanding the motivation of those adults who either somatize or grossly exaggerate symptoms and signs. In this model, parental needs, perhaps for attention and interest in their personal situation, are met via abnormal health seeking behaviours on behalf of their children. A social learning based model predicts that initial reward for such behaviour leads to further abnormal illness behaviour by parents, on behalf of their children. This model, therefore, will also predict gradually escalating severity of fabrication behaviour, from minimal exaggeration through to overt deception and eventual induction of ill health in the child.

Eminson and Postlethwaite[31] have elaborated these notions. They posit a continuum ranging from relative neglect of symptoms on the one hand, through normal health seeking behaviour, via exaggeration, to eventual fabrication of symptoms at the other extreme. In this model, both neglect of healthcare needs and, at the other extreme, gross exaggeration and factitious production of symptoms are abnormal, and potentially harmful to children. Gray and Bentovim[9] draw attention to the parent's developing belief that their child is unwell, based on an earlier perception that their child is different or unhealthy, combined with insecure parent/infant attachment. They emphasize that others in the immediate family may similarly be infected with this erroneous belief, and that it may extend to health care professionals.

Psychodynamic hypotheses

Hypotheses have been put forward regarding the psychological development of women, and the psychology of the 'imposter' when factitious illness by proxy is occurring. Subtypes of presentation based on the psychology of the fabricator were also suggested as being the 'help seeker', the 'active inducer' and the 'doctor addict'.[32] Transference hypotheses consider that the doctor is in a position of great power and influence in society and may become the focus of parental feelings derived from unresolved childhood conflicts. The child then becomes the instrument through which the parent can play out complex, disturbed dynamics with the doctor or other health professionals.

Attachment disorders

Disturbance of parent child attachment is a central element in cases of child abuse and neglect,[24] and is also crucial in factitious illness by proxy. Attachment difficulties arise through various mechanisms including lifelong parental deprivation and abuse, parental personality difficulties, functional illnesses such as postnatal depression, and sometimes severe personality disorder. Depression in the antenatal and postnatal period deserves special mention because of its frequency and marked association with attachment difficulties.[33] In our view, the attachment difficulties predating factitious illness by proxy have been underestimated, however, it is perhaps through recent attempts by psychiatric teams to provide treatment for selected cases that their full importance has been revealed. We hypothesize that the attachment difficulties may be intergenerational, as indicated by the parental histories of emotional deprivation or emotional neglect experienced, sometimes with added physical and sexual abuse.[9,25]

Diminishing coping strategies

We hypothesize that another significant influence which can lead to factitious illness by proxy is the specifically vulnerable parent's progressive perception of diminishing alternative coping strategies under stress, finally leading to a desperate attempt to have personal needs indirectly met through the child's factitious illness.

Summary

We have considered hypotheses concerned with the fabricator's individual development and psychopathology, those which attempt to explain the relationship between fabricators and the healthcare system, and those which incorporate attachment. These hypotheses are not mutually exclusive,[34] neither are they exhaustive. At this point in our understanding, we think it can be helpful for assessment and treatment planning to consider to what extent elements of each hypothesis fit the individual case.

TREATMENT

Early impressions

Early clinical impressions[35,36] were that family re-unification was unlikely to be successful, or may be frankly dangerous after factitious illness by proxy. Management was principally described in terms of managing the diagnostic conundrum in the paediatric setting, handling the delicate issue of confrontation and imparting the diagnosis, along with subsequent child protection measures.[35] The severity of the abuse uncovered in early cases, and the extent of the deception and sometimes repeated, apparently callous, abuse, accompanied by severe personality disorder in perpetrating parents,[7] did not auger well for successful intervention. Several paediatricians described the difficulties they had had persuading their psychiatric colleagues and other professionals, of the occurrence, let alone the severity, of the abuse which the paediatric team had painstakingly uncovered.[22,35] Furthermore, Rosenberg's review[8] emphasized the severity of the condition with respect to the harm actually inflicted on children, the persistence of cases and the fact that so much abuse and harm occurred within the confines of the hospital, under the watchful eye of staff. Added to this, 10 of the child victims in her meta-analysis (9% of the total) died. With this background, it is hardly surprising that treatment efforts aimed at family re-unification have proceeded with caution. As Parnell and Day[37] aptly put it, the question for many clinicians is not **when** the mother and child should be re-united, but **if** they should be re-united.

Single case reports

Single case reports of efforts in the direction of re-unification have appeared.[38-41] Successful interventions have usually focused on cases where the parent has gradually been able to take responsibility,[38-41] and is assessed to be amenable to psychological treatment. While most of the treatments offered have been psychoanalytically orientated psychotherapy for the abusing parent,[38,39,41] one report emphasizes a systematic approach to couple work, and to improving the father's level of understanding and assertiveness.[40] Another study is notable because initial admission of responsibility was not forthcoming.[39] Despite this, the mental health team strove to provide support to the mother through their home visiting programme, combined with benign, yet regular paediatric care. Despite periods of worsening child care, their persistence had some success, but the children had developed psychiatric problems at follow-up.

Case series

The Great Ormond Street team describe the hospital based management and the arrangements for child protection in a series of 41 cases.[9,42] Treatment towards re-unification was not part of the team's remit, though their meticulous approach to liaison with locally based services is stressed. Six points are stressed regarding the likelihood of successful outcomes; notably, the balanced combination of the use of the child protection process with therapeutic work for the mother and family.[42]

The Park Hospital group has described its experience of child and family psychiatric intervention.[43,44] The treatment concentrated on parents individually, families, and the parent/child dyad. This approach encourages acknowledgment of what has happened to the child and being able to accept responsibility for the abuse and its effect upon the children and family members. The group works at improving parenting sensitivity and competence as well as providing treatment for each parent individually, as in other types of child abuse.[24] In addition, therapy aimed at managing the abuser's inclination to somatize has been increasingly used (for a recent summary see Guthrie[45]).

The Park group has described the outcome of intervention with a consecutive series of 17 children and their families who were admitted to its inpatient Family Unit, subsequent to discovery of factitious illness by proxy.[46] Four of these 17 were essentially assessments, however, 13 were cases where treatment work had been directed towards whether family re-unification was viable. The cases were selected to admit those who had the best prospects for psychiatric treatment. Of the 13, 10 children were united with their biological parents, but 3 were considered insufficiently safe and alternative care was recommended. All recommendations were followed and the cases were followed up at an average of 27 months after discharge from the unit. Overall, the children had done well in terms of their overall development, growth, and adjustment. One child had been re-abused by her mother, fortunately causing relatively mild harm and leading to protective action and swift separation from her mother and leading to sole care subsequently by her father. Berg and Jones[46] cautiously conclude that family re-unification is reasonable to attempt for a selected sub group of cases of factitious illness by proxy but, where this is attempted, long-term follow-up is necessary in order to assure that psychological maltreatment does not occur and that the parent's mental health is monitored.

OVERVIEW OF PROGNOSIS

The effect of factitious illness by proxy upon the child's health and development has been reviewed, above. However, there has been little investigation of the longer term outlook for the child victims of factitious illness by proxy. Studies controlled for risk factors and standard outcome measures are almost impossible to carry out. In the follow-up study of the Leeds' group, it was considered that there were inadequate data to report, in detail, on the development of a large proportion of original potential cohort, more so in those children continuing to reside with the mother. Keeping in mind these methodological problems, the findings were that 54 children were identified an average of 5.6 years after fabrication of illness had been identified.[21] The majority of these children had not received systematic intervention from a psychiatric point of view, after the initial child protection response. Thirty of these 54 were living in the families where the parent had been the abuser. The other 24 were in alternative care, either with family members or in substitute families. Among the 30 living with the original abuser, there had been further fabrications in a third, and significant other concerns in a further third. No children had died during the follow-up period, however, half the 54 children had unacceptable outcomes, including conduct and emotional disorders, and difficulties at school including non-attendance, in addition to re-abuse. There was some indication that cases which had received active management, as indicated by a period of short-term foster care, did better than those which did not. Children who were younger at the time of discovery seemed to do better. In addition, a number of children with better outcomes had continued to be cared for by father or were with the small number of mothers who had been able to make positive changes in their lives. Both these findings give some cautious encouragement to the benefit of a therapeutic intervention and of continuity of care by a parent, if this is assessed to be safe.

Data from the British Paediatric Surveillance Unit have provided an insight into the outcome of a population based group of children subjected to factitious illness by proxy.[47] These authors followed up cases of factitious illness by proxy which had been ascertained within the UK and Republic of Ireland between 1992 and 1994. The authors obtained outcome data for 92% of the 128 index cases in the original cohort, with a mean duration of follow-up of 24 months. Of 119 children, 46 were at home without major conditions, at follow-up. Cases which had involved suffocation, and non-accidental poisoning

Table 4.1 Prognostic factors in factitious illness by proxy

Domain	Poor prognosis	Better prognosis
Abuse	Induced harm Sadistic element Accompanying child sexual abuse or PA Deaths of earlier children Harm to animals	Fabrication Shorter duration of factitious illness by proxy
Child	Developmental delay Physical sequelae of factitious illness by proxy Development of somatising behaviour	Absence of delay or sequelae of abuse
Parent	Personality disorder Denial Lack of compliance Alcohol/substance abuse Abuse in childhood – unresolved	Personality strengths Acknowledgement of abuse Compliance Treatment responsive mental illness Adapted to childhood abuse
Parenting and parent–child interaction	Disordered attachment Lack of empathy for child Own needs before child	Normal attachment Empathy for child
Family	Domestic violence Multigenerational abuse	Non-abusive partner Supportive extended family
Professional	Lack of informed resources	Partnership with parents Long-term psychological treatment and social casework
Social setting	Violent, unsupportive neighbourhood Isolation	Local child support facilities Social support

and those involving direct induced harm, as well as those children aged under 5 years were much less likely to be at home. 24% of the original children were still experiencing symptoms or signs of the original abuse at follow-up. The re-abuse rate among the 46 children remaining with their birth parent(s) was 20%. Of these 9 children, 2 had been abused through the mechanism of factitious illness by proxy, 4 were emotionally abused, 2 physically, and 1 through a combination of emotional abuse and neglect. In addition, 10% of the siblings of these children had suffered further abuse since the initial study. These authors note that when the re-abuse rate at follow-up is combined with the information on siblings and deaths from their first survey,[10] the abuse rate approached 50% for all the children in a family, during a childhood.

There is increasing recognition of the salience of personality disorder in relation to severe and persistent child abuse.[25,27,48] Berg and Jones' follow-up study[46] underlines the concern about enduring personality disorder in those cases of factitious illness by proxy which did less well. The warning from Southall et al[27] about the apparently caring and attentive nature of the perpetrators of some of the most severe acts of abuse captured through covert video surveillance, lends further weight to the importance of detecting severe personality disorder in child abuse, and in factitious illness by proxy in particular. Schreier and Libow[49] warn would be interveners of the snare of plausibility in those who have perpetrated factitious illness by proxy.

Table 4.1 draws together factors which have been associated with a poor or, alternatively, better prognosis. The approach is based on that applied to child abuse and neglect generally,[24,50,51] and examines prognosis via domains, or groups of factors which can be linked to aetiology and outcome of cases.

An approach to case management

We conclude by summarizing an approach to case management which is informed by the above observations on prognosis, and the data on treatment outcome. The child protection conference is necessary for all cases. Initially, separation of the child from the fabricating adult will probably be the safest action for all but the mildest cases, while the question of prognosis is fairly assessed. Early involvement of the local child psychiatry team is recommended in order to assist with the second stage of assessment and maximise the opportunities for therapeutic work to be undertaken with the fabricator, partner and other family members.[52] Treatment aimed at family re-unification is worth trying in cases with better prognosis, and where there is an indication of the beginnings of parental acknowledgment that abuse has occurred. If treatment aimed towards family re-unification is embarked upon, a clear treatment plan with explicit criteria for success is necessary, and will need to be shared by all professionals involved.[24,51] The time frame has to be sensitive to the developmental needs of the child, and as most cases of factitious illness by proxy involve young children, often infants, the time scale for change in parents and in parent-child relationships is necessarily shorter than that for older children.[24,50,51,53]

The primary healthcare team and one paediatrician are central to the long term management plan. The GP and Health Visitor will need to be fully appraised and informed about factitious illness by proxy and know where to obtain back-up help if they are concerned about health presentations of any of the children in the family. Equally, it is recommended[47] that one paediatrician, working closely with a child psychiatry team, takes responsibility for continuing monitoring of the child's development, growth and welfare, so that management is thoroughly integrated. Whilst acknowledging the substantial methodological difficulties of follow-up studies and the need for longer term follow-up, at the present time the indications are that long-term follow-up is necessary in all cases, for it is not only the risk of subsequent factitious illness by proxy to which professionals need to be alert, but also the continuing risk of significant parenting problems, parent–child relationships and psycho-logical maltreatment. We consider this to be high risk work, however, in selected situations intervention has led to good child outcomes.

References

1 Meadow R. Munchausen syndrome by proxy: the hinterland of child abuse. Lancet 1977; 2: 343–345

2 Asher R. Munchausen's syndrome. Lancet 1951; 1: 339–341

Key points for clinical practice

- At present. factitious illness by proxy is used to describe the **situation**. Factitious disorder by proxy is proposed for the psychiatric diagnosis applicable to fabricator.

- Factitious illness by proxy consists of three elements; illness fabrication, fabricator psychopathology, and potential physical and emotional harm to the child.

- There are three main types of factitious illness by proxy: verbal fabrication; tampering with charts and specimens; and producing physical signs (inducing illness).

- Diagnostic evaluation is a two stage process of: (i) paediatric diagnosis – is it fabrication? (ii) psychiatric assessment, look for aetiological factors in fabricator and effects on child, with focus on opportunities for treatment of psychiatric disorders.

- The annual incidence across the UK and Republic of Ireland in all children is 0.5/100,000. The condition is commonest in infancy, when the annual incidence is at least 2.8/100 000.

- Untreated factitious illness by proxy leads to serious effects on the emotional health of child, in addition to physical effects if fabrication involves production of physical signs.

- The outcome is likely to be poor if the problem is both untreated and not monitored

- These has been some success with treatment of selected, good prognosis cases.

- There are several possible pathways to factitious illness by proxy, with a number of risk factors and a range of explanatory hypotheses.

- The importance of parent–child attachment disorders is emerging.

- Long-term follow-up is necessary, both for the individual child and family, and for research purposes.

3 Fisher GC, Mitchell I. Munchausen's syndrome by proxy (factitious illness by proxy). Curr Opin Psychiatry 1992; 5: 224–227

4 American Psychiatric Association. Diagnostic and Statistical Manual of Mental Disorders, 4th Edn DSM-IV. Washington, DC: APA, 1994

5 Meadow SR. Munchausen syndrome by proxy abuse perpetrated by men. Arch Dis Child 1998; 78: 210–216

6 Meadow SR. Munchausen's syndrome by proxy. Arch Dis Child 1982; 57: 92–98

7 Samuels MP, McLaughlin W, Jacobson RR, Poets CF, Southall DP. Fourteen cases of upper airway obstruction. Arch Dis Child 1992; 67: 162–170

8 Rosenberg D. Web of deceit: a literature review of Munchausen syndrome by proxy. Child Abuse Negl 1987; 11: 547–563

9 Gray J, Bentovim A. Illness induction syndrome; paper 1 – a series of 41 children from 37 families identified at Great Ormond Street Hospital for Children. Child Abuse Negl 1996; 20: 655–673

10 McClure RJ, Davis P, Meadow RS et al. Epidemiology of Munchausen syndrome by proxy. Arch Dis Child 1996; 75: 57–61

11 Rosen CL, Frost JD, Glaze DG. Child abuse and recurrent apnoea. J Pediatr 1986; 109: 1065-1067

12 Light MJ, Sheridan MS. Munchausen syndrome by proxy and apnea (MBPA). A survey of apnea programs. Clin Pediatr 1990; 29: 162–168

13 Bools C. Factitious illness by proxy: Munchausen syndrome by proxy. Br J Psychiatry 1996; 169: 268–275

14 Meadow R. Fictitious epilepsy. Lancet 1984; ii: 25–28

15 Fisher G, Mitchell I, Murdoch D. Munchausen's syndrome by proxy. The question of psychiatric illness in a child. Br J Psychiatry 1993; 162: 701–703

16 Jureidini J. Obstetric factitious disorder and Munchausen syndrome by proxy. J Nervous Mental Dis 1993; 181: 135–137

17 Masterson J, Dunworth R, Williams N. Extreme illness exaggeration in pediatric patients: a variant of Munchausen's by proxy? Am J Orthopsychiatry 1988; 58: 188–195

18 Meadow R. What is, and what is not, Munchausen syndrome by proxy? Arch Dis Child 1995; 72: 534–538

19 Waring WW. The persistent parent. Am J Dis Child 1992; 146: 753–756

20 World Health Organization. The ICD-10 Classification of Mental and Behavioural Disorders. Geneva: WHO, 1992

21 Bools CN, Neale BA, Meadow SR. Follow-up of victims of fabricated illness (MSBP). Arch Dis Child 1993; 69: 625–630

22 McGuire TL, Feldman ND. Psychological morbidity of children subjected to Munchausen syndrome by proxy. Pediatrics 1989; 83: 289–292

23 Bools CN, Neale BA, Meadow SR. Co-morbidity associated with fabricated illness (Munchausen syndrome by proxy). Arch Dis Child 1992; 67: 77–79

24 Jones DPH. Treatment of the child and the family where child abuse or neglect has occurred. In: Helfer ME, Kempe RS, Krugman RD. (eds). The battered child. London: University of Chicago Press, 1997: 521–542

25 Bools CN, Neale B, Meadow R. Munchausen syndrome by proxy: a study of psychopathology. Child Abuse Negl 1994; 18: 773–788

26 Palmer AJ, Yoshimura GJ. Munchausen syndrome by proxy. J Am Acad Child Adolesc Psychiatry 1984; 23: 503–508

27 Southall DP, Plunkett MC, Banks MW et al. Covert video recordings of life-threatening child abuse: lessons for child protection. Pediatrics 1997; 100: 735–760

28 Griffith JL. The family systems of Munchausen syndrome by proxy. Fam Process 1988; 27: 423–437

29 Parsons T. The Social System. Glencoe: Free Press, 1951

30 Mechanic D. Medical Sociology. Glencoe: Free Press, 1978

31 Eminson D, Postlethwaite R. Factitious illness: recognition and management. Arch Dis Child 1992; 67: 1510–1526

32 Schreier H, Libow J. Hurting for Love; Munchausen by Proxy Syndrome. London: Guildford Press, 1993

33 Murray L. The impact of post natal depression on infant development. J Child Psychol Psychiatry 1992; 33: 543–561

34 Fisher GC. Etiological speculations. In: Levin AV, Sheridan MS. (eds) MSBP; Issues in Diagnosis and Treatment. New York: Lexington Books, 1995; 39–57

35 Meadow SR. Management of Munchausen syndrome by proxy. Arch Dis Child 1985; 60: 385–393

36 Kempe RS, Kempe CH. The untreatable family. In: Kempe RS, Kempe CH. (eds) Child Abuse. London: Open Books, 1978; 128–131

37 Parnell TF, Day DO. Munchausen by Proxy Syndrome; Misunderstood Child Abuse. London: Sage, 1998

38 Nicol R, Eccles M. Psychotherapy for Munchausen syndrome by proxy. Arch Dis Child 1985; 60: 344–348

39 Lyons-Ruth K, Kaufman M, Masters N et al. Issues in identification and long term management of Munchausen by proxy syndrome within a clinical infant service. Infant Mental Health J 1991; 12: 309–330

40 Black D, Hollis P. Treatment of a case of factitious illness by proxy. Clin Child Psychol Psychiatry 1996; 1: 89–98

41 Coombe P. The in-patient psychotherapy of a mother and child at the Cassel Hospital: a case of Munchausen syndrome by proxy. Br J Psychother 1995; 12: 195–207

42 Gray J, Bentovim A, Milla P. The treatment of children and their families where induced illness has been identified. In: Horwath J, Lawson B. (eds) Trust Betrayed; Munchausen Syndrome by Proxy, Interagency Child Protection and Partnership with Families. London: National Children's Bureau, 1995; 149–162

43 Newbold C, Byrne G, Jones DPH. Assessment of cases of factitious illness by proxy. In: Adshead G, Brook D. (eds) Munchausen Syndrome by Proxy. London: Imperial College Press, 1998; In press

44 Jones DPH, Byrne G, Newbold C. Management, treatment and outcomes. In: Eminson M, Postlethwaite RJ. (eds) Munchausen Syndrome by Proxy: a fabricated illness. A handbook for professionals. London: Butterworth Heinemann, 1998; In press

45 Guthrie E. Psychotherapy of somatisation disorders. Curr Opin Psychiatry 1996; 9: 182–187

46 Berg B, Jones DPH. Outcome of psychiatric intervention in factitious illness by proxy (Munchausen syndrome by proxy). Submitted for publication

47 Davis P, McClure RJ, Rolfe K et al. Procedures, placement and risks of further abuse following Munchausen syndrome by proxy, non-accidental poisoning, and non-accidental suffocation. Arch Dis Child 1998; 78: 217–221

48 Famularo R, Kinscherff R, Fenton T. Psychiatric diagnoses of abusive mothers; a preliminary report. J Nerv Ment Dis 1992; 180: 658–661

49 Schreier H, Libow J. Munchausen syndrome by proxy; a clinical fable of our times. J Am Acad Child Adolesc Psychiatry 1994; 33: 904–905

50 Jones DPH. The effectiveness of intervention. In: Adcock M, White R, Hollows A. (eds) Significant Harm. Croydon: Significant Publications, 1991; 61–84

51 Jones DPH. The effectiveness of intervention. In: Adcock M, White R. (eds) Significant Harm. Croydon: Significant Publications, 1998; 91–119

52 Fisher GC. The role of psychiatry. In: Levin AV, Sheridan MS. (eds) Munchausen Syndrome by Proxy; Issues in Diagnosis and Treatment. New York: Lexington Books, 1995; 369–397

53 Wolkind S. Legal aspects of child care. In: Rutter M, Taylor E, Hersor L (eds) Child and Adolescent Psychiatry: Modern approaches, 3rd edn. Oxford: Blackwell, 1994; 1089–1102

Sara Levene

Home safety for children

Accidental injury in the home kills about 200 children every year[1] and leads to about one million accident and emergency department attendances. This makes accidental injury a major problem for public health. This article will give more details about injuries to children at home and how they happen, and will seek to demonstrate that their epidemiology enables them to be understood and predicted. The many ways in which these injuries can be prevented will also be discussed. There will be a special emphasis on recent changes in the field, and how the paediatric practitioner can contribute to improving child safety.

NATURE AND EXTENT OF THE PROBLEM

The term 'accident' carries many connotations of an event that is totally unpredictable and unpremeditated, an act of God that could never have been predicted. A better definition is given by Ambrose Bierce:[2] *accident – an inevitable occurrence due to the action of immutable natural laws.*

Many so called accidents could readily have been predicted and prevented. Therefore ,the term 'injury' is to be preferred. 'Accidental injury' may be used to draw a specific distinction from abuse.

Sources of information

The most important source of general data is the Department of Trade and Industry's *Home Accident Surveillance System* (HASS).[1] This is an ongoing survey of patients presenting to a rolling sample of large 24 hour accident and emergency departments, in all parts of the UK. A detailed questionnaire about

Dr Sara Levene MA MRCP FRCPCH, Medical Adviser, Child Accident Prevention Trust, 18–20 Farringdon Lane, London EC1R 3AU, UK

the injury circumstances is completed by a dedicated clerk. Ideally information is taken directly from patients or parents but, in practice, it is often obtained from the casualty cards. HASS contains a mass of information and this is stored in a readily accessible computerised form. Tables or listings of brief incident histories can be obtained rapidly and free of charge. On the other hand, HASS does not ask many questions that might be of interest, such as was the child supervised or alone at home when injured. Products are identified as involved in the incident even when they did not cause it, for example falling off a chair onto a toy car and cutting the head would be identified both as a chair and a toy accident.

Information on fires is collected by the Home Office,[3] and fatal fires, in particular, are investigated in great detail.

Coroners investigate all accidental deaths at inquest. Their records are rich in information[4] and many coroners are agreeable to releasing records to researchers.

In many cases, research questions can only be answered by special studies. This may include in depth investigation of injury circumstances, reviews of the effects of interventions and the interviewing of children and families to gain understanding of their attitudes.

THE PATTERN OF INJURIES

As with any other health problem, the occurrence of injuries is amenable to epidemiological analysis. The following features are closely related to the occurrence of childhood injuries:

Sex of child

Study after study (see Pless[5] for review) has shown that, after the first few months of life, male children are more likely to be accidentally injured than female children. This is true for any accident type in which the child actively participates. The explanation is not clear. It may be due to the more adventurous behaviour of boys or to their injuries being viewed as macho. However, it may simply result from boys being allowed more personal freedom. For example, a study of cycling injuries[6] found that boys were injured twice as often as girls but that the boys were allowed to cycle twice as far as the girls, giving the same injury rate per mile travelled.

Social class

The incidence of injury both fatal and non fatal is higher in children from lower socio-economic groups.[7] This does not reflect either lack of care or ignorance of safety measures by the parents in these families,[10,11] but reflects the combination of a number of factors including: (i) poorer housing conditions[8] which increase children's exposure to dangerous settings, such as kitchens which have through routes past the cooker and where no storage is available for cleaning materials or medicines and where families living in poor accommodation may be unable to afford safety measures, nor to obtain the landlord's permission to make changes to increase safety; and (ii) stress factors in the family,[9] including factors such as depression or illness.

Intellectual and physical development

A child's physical development and intellectual skills at any stage of development will determine how they are injured.[12] For example, a newborn infant is unlikely to be injured by falling unless held by an adult who falls or drops the child. Within a few weeks, the infant will have the mobility to gradually rock a bouncing cradle off a work surface. As soon as they can crawl or shuffle, children can climb onto, and fall off, furniture or stairs. A walking infant will fall repeatedly and may fall onto sharp furniture or through glass. An older child with increased manual dexterity may climb onto a window sill then open the window and fall out. Still later, the child will be allowed to explore the outside environment and so may fall from walls or trees.

Viewing the link between development and injury from another perspective, children at a particular developmental level may use the same skills to injure themselves in different ways. For example, a child who has successfully learnt to unscrew something may unscrew a bottle top and ingest the contents or turn on a tap to be scalded by hot water or drown in water collecting in the bath.

The pattern of development is similar for every child though its timing may vary. Knowledge of the next developmental milestone to be expected enables potential accidents to be predicted. This means that they can be anticipated by setting safety measures in place before they become necessary. For example, once children can sit unaided, they will soon crawl or shuffle. This is the time to install a stairgate, before children have any mobility and are able to injure themselves on stairs.

The normal behaviour of children is not that of adults. Children are less experienced than adults and are liable to be impulsive and experimental.[13] Development of social and intellectual skills must also be considered.

Exposure

Recently, more attention has been given to exposure as a factor explaining why certain groups of people are injured. This work has mainly been carried out in the field of road safety. However, it can be shown in a general way that exposure is a factor in home accidents. For example, the main age group injured[1] is children under 5 years, who spend much of their time at home. The rooms in which they are injured are the living room and the kitchen; this simply reflects where they spend their time. Exposure can be an important factor where product safety is considered. If an item causes an injury and sales are small, this indicates a greater degree of hazard than where an injury is caused and several million have been sold.

WAYS OF PROTECTING CHILDREN FROM INJURY

There are three levels at which children can be protected from injury.[14] These are termed **primary**, **secondary** and **tertiary** prevention. Primary prevention is the prevention of an incident which could lead to injury. An example in the home is the use of a stair gate to prevent a toddler from falling down stairs. Secondary prevention is the prevention of serious injury even though the incident has taken place. An example is the use of a smoke detector to alert a family to a house fire. The fire may still happen, but the consequences are mitigated. Tertiary prevention is the use of medical management to minimise the eventual consequences of an injury. A simple example is the use of cold water on a burnt area as first aid.

There are three principal routes which are used to prevent accidental injury. These are usually termed **education, engineering** and **enforcement.** Education is giving people information which can prevent injury. It is absolutely not telling people to be careful or giving people information which is so obvious and basic that it is rejected. For parents, useful education can involve: (i) giving safety advice which is tailored to the age and abilities of the child, so that it is directly relevant to the family; (ii) backing the advice with practical information which enables it to be put into action, for example the price and availability of safety equipment;[15] (iii) developing the advice in conjunction with parents and by learning what they have already done to keep their children safe; and (iv) using discussion and group sessions to overcome the barriers (practical and intellectual) which prevent the parents putting into practice the safety actions that they know they should carry out.

Education directed towards children does not only mean that children should be told to keep off things and not touch things. It needs to be developed with a knowledge of the intellectual and physical abilities of the child. The role of education in the youngest children is limited. Infants and toddlers may only be protected by barrier methods of child safety, though they can soon learn concepts such as 'sharp', 'hot' and 'hurt'. Young children cannot be relied on to avoid doing things that they know they should not do. Older children, certainly once they have reached junior school level, can start to learn more sophisticated concepts. They can identify hazards for themselves. They can assess the risks involved in carrying out activities and decide whether to carry them out.[16] They can learn the physical skills that adults employ to deal with every day dangers. They can use sharp knives, boil kettles and strike matches. If children are to become competent safe adults, they are best trained in such activities rather than picking them up haphazardly as they get older.

Supervision

Supervision does play an important part in the safety strategy of some families, and many of the family stresses which are linked to accident may be related to a lower level of effective supervision. Different levels of supervision are appropriate in different circumstances. Older children can be listened to in another room, a toddler can be monitored by a carer in the same room, a child cutting paper or cooking needs an adult standing close at hand. The wrong level of supervision may be selected, as with the toddler playing in the garden who was watched through the kitchen window. Unfortunately a river ran through the garden and the child fell in, but was rescued downstream. Supervision may play a part in injury prevention but cannot be expected to be completely effective especially if delegated to one person.[17,18]

Safety equipment

Many people view safety equipment as the be all and end all of prevention of home injuries. Unfortunately this is not the case. Safety equipment will only be of value if an item is: (i) appropriate to the development of the child for whom it is purchased, for example a stairgate is irrelevant to a 4 year-old who will have no difficulty climbing over it; (ii) the correct model and size for the family home, for example stairgates come in a variety of widths and levels of adjustability; (iii) removed from the packet and fitted correctly; and (iv) used on every occasion, for example a stairgate will be totally ineffective if left undone.

Furthermore, there have been few studies in which items of safety equipment have been evaluated in case control or even before and after studies. It is, therefore, impossible to recommend many such items on firm scientific grounds.

Demonstrated to work

The following items of safety equipment have been demonstrated to be effective and can clearly be recommended for use in the home: (i) child resistant closures,[19] especially on solid dose aspirin and paracetamol; (ii) barriers to prevent window falls;[20] (iii) smoke detectors;[21] and (iv) reduction in the temperature of domestic hot water.[22]

Items to be avoided

Baby walkers[23] have been repeatedly shown to be involved in more injuries that any other item of nursery equipment. They give children the ability to move unexpectedly fast especially for their young age and limited development. They may fall over obstacles, into fires or down stairs. They may collide with ovens which have the door open, or where there is a chip pan on the hob. They may move around and reach for sharp objects, hot objects or toxins. There are also concerns that far from promoting early walking they encourage children to use abnormal leg muscle patterns. The Child Accident Prevention Trust does not recommend the use of baby walkers.

Cooker and hob guards are expensive items of equipment which do little to prevent the spillage of hobs from pans. Pans must be lifted over the guards; this is heavy and awkward so that the cook is injured by spills. The guards become hot and many designs have gaps through which children can reach the cooker rings. The children may, therefore, be burnt either on the cooker or the guard. The guards are difficult to remove for cleaning purposes, posing a potential problem with hygiene.

Items that are simply gimmicks

Manufacturers have a limitless imagination and are continually coming up with innovative ideas to solve problems that are not very important or to find safety solutions that are not very efficacious. Examples are toilet lid locks to counteract the non existent problem of drowning in the toilet and video barriers which are intended to prevent children putting their hands into the

Table 5.1 Recommended safety equipment at different ages

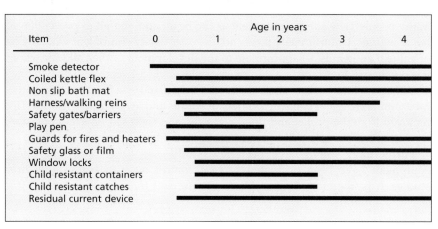

video. This may be damaging to the video recorder but poses little threat to the child. Fridge locks are readily removed by children. Adhesive corner protectors do not last long unless attached by superglue.

Practical safety advice

Some safety products may be recommended (Table 5.1) though not all have been conclusively demonstrated to be effective. The items required are dependent on the developmental stage of the child. They can be bought as the child grows and do not need to be installed at birth. However, their installation does need to anticipate the child's skills. For example, a stairgate is needed before the child can crawl.

There are many potential low cost or no cost safety measures (Table 5.2) which can replace safety equipment.

Table 5.2 Low cost safety measures

- Keep the floor and the stairs tidy
- Store plastic bags away from children
- Do not overload electrical sockets
- Choose the right toy for the child's age and ability; keep toys for older children away from little ones
- Store medicines high up and out of sight, preferable in a cupboard with a child resistant catch
- Never leave babies or toddlers alone in the bath
- Fit at least one smoke detector and check it regularly
- Turn the hot water thermostat to 54°C (130°F) or less
- Use the rear hobs of the cooker and keep pan handles turned to the back
- Do not buy a baby walker
- Keep matches, cigarettes and lighters well away from children
- Keep the front door shut so children do not get out of the house

The most common types of incident leading to children being injured in the home are listed in Table 5.3.[1]

Uncommon incidents

Electrocution is perceived by the public as a frequent cause of serious child injury and much effort is made to protect children especially from electrical sockets. However, electrical injury is very infrequent. The design of UK sockets requires something to be inserted into the upper hole to open the shutters to the live contacts and this cannot be done just by pushing a finger into the socket.

Toy injuries receive considerable publicity especially in the pre-Christmas period. However, safety regulation through the European Toy Safety Directive and the European Standard EN 71 Safety of Toys[24] ensures that toys that can cause injury are illegal. In the UK this is enforced by the Trading Standards service as well as by reputable manufacturers and suppliers. The number of incidents where a design fault with the toy causes injury is extremely small.

Table 5.3 Mechanism of home accidents to children by age and sex

| Mechanism | Age in years | | | | | |
| | 0–4 | | | 5–14 | | |
	Male	Female	Unknown	Male	Female	Unknown
Fall on same level	2166	1409	1	1275	1050	1
Fall on/from stairs	1227	1020	2	573	777	3
Fall on/from ladder	19	13	0	28	15	0
Fall from building	69	37	0	128	46	0
Other fall	3828	2799	6	2076	1782	0
Struck – explosion	2	1	0	7	4	0
Struck – moving object	818	503	2	1067	632	1
Struck – static object	2306	1462	1	1793	1327	0
Struck – other	550	430	1	843	613	0
Pinch/crush (blunt)	733	619	1	544	529	0
Cut/tear (sharp)	720	437	1	1156	674	0
Puncture	143	116	0	340	261	0
Bite/sting	352	283	0	375	359	0
Foreign body	1049	961	2	504	397	2
Suffocation	88	55	0	64	52	0
(Suspected) poisoning	985	787	0	104	116	0
Chemical effect	44	29	0	20	13	0
Thermal effect	961	734	0	314	347	0
Electric/radiation	18	7	0	11	11	0
Acute overexertion	122	157	0	65	92	0
Other	949	858	7	770	785	6
Column totals	**17149**	**12717**	**24**	**12057**	**9882**	**13**
%	12.5	9.3	0	8.8	7.2	0
National estimate (000s)	313	232		230	181	238

Figures in table are actual numbers reported at the HASS hospitals, which are a sample of UK hospitals.
National estimates are calculations of total numbers of injuries obtained by statistical analysis of HASS data.
Source: Department of Trade and Industry.[1]

Most toy accidents happen when people fall over a toy or when a toy is supplied to a child too young to manage it, usually in contravention of warnings and guidelines on the packaging.

Fires in the home and other thermal injuries

House fires are the leading cause of death to children in the home. They cause proportionately more deaths to young children. This is because young children are more dependent on adults for rescue. There is currently a steady fall in the number of child deaths in fires. Poor housing conditions, single families and families with children as opposed to those without are all at increased risk of house fire.[3] Many house fires begin in the kitchen and chip pans are a frequent cause. All families should know how to tackle a chip pan fire. The purchase of an electric deep fat fryer and a fire blanket for the kitchen can be considered. Children may also start fires, particularly if they gain access to smokers' materials. Children may be able to strike a match from the age of 18 months. Cigarette lighters may also be operated by children, and the USA, Canada and Australia require lighters to be of child resistant designs.

Fire deaths often result from the fumes released by burning foam in furniture rather than direct injury by flame. Regulations in the UK[25] ban the use of the more dangerous types of foam and there is evidence that this is leading to a fall in the number of fire deaths where furniture is mainly responsible.[3]

The increased used of smoke detectors may also be contributing to a fall in fire deaths. Like any other product, they can only be efficacious where they are properly installed and batteries are fitted and functioning correctly. They remain one item of safety equipment which is cheap, easy to use and valuable for all age groups including adults.

Other thermal injuries are scalds, principally from kettles and hot drinks, or bathwater, and burns from hot appliances such as cookers or ovens. The use of a thermostat to control hot water temperatures has been proven to be effective.[22] The use of coiled kettle flexes, which do not fall over the work surface, seems useful. Simple no cost measures are pouring away unused hot water that remains in the kettle, using mugs not cups and replacing tablecloths with mats. Highchairs should be placed away from the table so that the child cannot reach anything hot.

Falls

Falls are serious when they are from a height. Falls from low levels, such as out of bed, do not lead to severe injuries and if this is reported by carers it should be viewed with suspicion.[26] Falls on stairs can be reduced by good house design without open treads, bannisters that can be climbed and small steps without adequate landings. Stairgates in Europe are designed to prevent a child of under 24 months from reaching the stairs, though research suggests[27] that children of up to 48 months may be injured falling on the stairs. It would seem sensible to remove stairgates when children reach the age of 2 years as they may be hurt trying to climb over the gate.

Severe injuries may also follow falls from windows. The use of window bars in New York[20] was shown to prevent child deaths and is now mandatory. In the

UK, the use of window locks may be helpful, and these can be fitted to most window designs. The need to escape by the window in case of fire must also be considered. Furniture should not be placed directly under the window in children's rooms if possible, to discourage climbing up to the window.

Glass injuries

Falls onto glass are potentially fatal. Ordinary annealed glass can break into dagger like fragments. Low lying glass in the home is a feature of poor house design. Current building regulations no longer permit it. Glass can be replaced by safety glass, either laminated which is difficult to break, or tempered which smashes into small fragments which are not very sharp. A special plastic film can also be used to retain glass fragments after breakage. Young people of all ages are at risk from injury by glass but the nature of the incidents differs. Toddlers tend to fall through doors or windows but teenagers tend to push their hands through next to the handle as they rush from room to room.

Drowning

Drowning in the home strongly reflects the development of the child.[28] Infants are drowned in the bath, often when they have been left in the care of an older, but still very young, sibling. Toddlers tend to drown in the pond, often in the house next door. Older children are less likely to be drowned in the home. Preventive measures include removing convenient bodies of water such as full buckets or paddling pools filled by rain. Adequate supervision at bathtime is also essential. Drowning is a rapid, silent incident and, if water is sufficiently deep to cover the nose and mouth, it is deep enough to drown in.

Poisoning

Suspected poisoning is a very frequent cause of attendance at accident and emergency departments but only about 10 children die of poison ingestion every year. This is because many household products ingested by children are of very low toxicity and many medicines are taken in very small amounts. Many poisoning incidents are scares rather than medical emergencies. The UK differs from many countries, such the USA and Australia, in not having public access to poisons information. This means that, after a poisoning incident, carers cannot obtain rapid reliable free telephone advice and are forced to attend hospital with an increase in psychological and physical trauma to the child and the family as well as a financial burden to the health services.

Access to medicines can be prevented by the use of child resistant containers which have been demonstrated to be effective.[19] Bottles with child resistant closures are the most difficult for children to open. Low cost measures include checking the home for unwanted medicines, returning all unused medicines to the pharmacist, storing medicines out of reach and out of sight, keeping them in the kitchen rather than the bathroom, and using imaginative alternatives for storage of medicines, such as a locked suitcase, as lockable medicine cabinets, which are usually recommended, are not normally sold by major furniture retailers.

Choking, entrapment and strangulation

Normal infants up to the age of 3–4 years will use their mouths to explore their surroundings. This means that they are at risk from choking on small items. Toys for children under 3 years of age exclude parts small enough to fit entirely within a test device set in the Toy Safety Standard.[24] Other household items such as coins and food items, particularly peanuts, are a frequent cause of asphyxiation.[29]

Entrapment is a particular hazard to infants who may be fatally asphyxiated if trapped in settings such as between the mattress and the cot.

Strangulation is an accidental injury in children up to the age of 9 years. For infants, causes such as clothing and blind cords are prominent. Poorly designed bunk bed rails have led to several deaths of older children.

RECENT ADVANCES IN INJURY PREVENTION

The field of injury prevention has made considerable progress over the last 10 years. There has been recognition both by practitioners and the government of the importance of this field. Reduction in injury to children is a *Health of the Nation*[30] target. Though this initiative did not carry funding with it, it did lead to the establishment of many accident prevention groups, accident prevention units and individuals with a responsibility for accident prevention. Directors of Public Health report on accident statistics within their area. Activities such as the Child Accident Prevention Trust's Child Safety Week seek to support the workers in this field.

The subject has become academically more respectable. The number of units carrying out research into injury prevention in particular in the UK remains small, but many other workers are now contributing to the field. The International Society of Child and Adolescent Injury Prevention has been established and its journal, *Injury Prevention*, is now published by BMJ publishing. The scientific basis for injury prevention advice has been examined in great detail in a number of reviews,[6,31,32] enabling the subject to be set on a secure scientific footing. This work has also identified priority areas for further research.

The value of listening to parents and learning from what they have to say has been widely accepted. Not only do many parents know much basic information about child safety, they have ways of dealing with difficult social and environmental circumstances which can educate practitioners. On the other hand, where it is important to educate parents, better understanding of their needs enables appropriate information to be put across in appropriate ways.

DISAPPOINTMENTS

Child injury prevention has not become a topic of general interest and its importance has not reached the general public. Child murders receive massive media attention; parents worry about abduction if their child goes out alone; schools are reinforced against lunatic killers. This combines to deprive children of their personal freedom in a way which would not happen if parents were able to combine a realistic risk assessment with training for their child on managing rather than avoiding risk.[33]

Social class continues to predominate as an underlying cause of injury and the evidence suggests that there is no improvement in the lot of the poorest sections of the population. The inequalities in child health related to social deprivation have recently become more, not less, marked.[7]

The moves towards European harmonisation have impaired the ability of the UK to maintain safety measures. The product safety standards developed by the British Standards Institution are being replaced by standards produced at European level. Rather than chosing the best of each national standard, these show a worrying levelling down towards the lowest common denominator.

THE FUTURE

It is likely that the *Health of the Nation* targets will be achieved as they were estimated from existing trends. It is to be hoped that more rigorous examination of safety advice and better attention to understanding and communicating with families will enable the reduction in accidents to reach all sections of the population.

Key points for clinical practice

- Be aware:
  (i) know that home injury is a major cause of child morbidity
  watch for trends in injuries that may present themselves to you as a clinician
  (ii) contribute to the making of local and national policy which can contribute to child safety

- Be positive:
  (i) statistics indicate a fall in injuries, and many injuries are preventable
  (ii) do not assume that because health visitors take on most of the responsibility for injury prevention there is no role for other health workers

- Set an example:
  (i) follow good safety practices in your own household
  (ii) avoid being judgemental — if you think about your own home, you will have danger spots that you will know about but do nothing about for a variety of excuses

- Remind and inform:
  (i) do use contacts with parents for any cause to remind them of the importance of child safety
  (ii) do give advice related to the child's development and to family circumstances
  (iii) be aware of relevant safety measures
  (iv) know of low cost safety measures

- Do not underestimate parents

References

1 Department of Trade and Industry. Home Accident Surveillance System Annual Report (1995). London: Department of Trade and Industry, 1997
2 Ambrose Bierce. The Devil's Dictionary. Dover Publications, 1993
3 Home Office. Fire Statistics United Kingdom 1996. London: Home Office, 1998
4 Levene S. Coroner's records of accidental deaths. Arch Dis Child 1991; 66: 1239–1244
5 Pless IB. The scientific basis of injury prevention. London: CAPT, 1993
6 Towner E, Jarvis S, Walsh D et al. Measuring exposure to risk in schoolchildren aged 11–14. BMJ 1994; 308: 449–452
7 Roberts I, Power C. Does the decline in childhood injury mortality vary by social class? A comparison of class specific mortality in 1981 and 1991. BMJ 1996; 313: 784–786
8 Lowry S. Housing and Health. London: BMJ Publications, 1991
9 Sibert JR. Stress in families of children who have ingested poisons. BMJ 1987; 275: 87–89.
10 Combes G. You can't watch them twenty four hours a day: parents' and children's perceptions, understanding and experience of accidents and accident prevention. London: Child Accident Prevention Trust, 1991
11 Roberts H, Smith SJ, Bryce C. Children at risk? Safety as a social value. Buckingham: Open University Press, 1995
12 Jackson RH. Setting the scene. In: Jackson RH. (ed) The Environment and Accidents. Tunbridge: Pittman Medical, 1977: 1–4
13 Berfenstam R. The work of the Swedish joint committee for accident prevention. In: Jackson RH. (ed) The Environment and Accidents. Tunbridge: Pittman Medical, 1977: 141–142
14. Child Accident Prevention Trust. Basic Principles of Child Accident Prevention. London: CAPT, 1989
15 Colver A, Hutchinson P, Judson E. Promoting children's home safety. BMJ 1982; 285: 1177–1180
16 Wooley A. The Risk Pack. London: Child Accident Prevention Trust 1996
17 Levene S. Is there more to parental supervision than political incorrectness? Injury Prevention 1996;2:10-11.
18. Roberts I. Parental supervision, a popular myth. Injury Prevent 1996; 2: 9–10
19 Sibert JR, Craft AW, Jackson RH. Child resistant packaging and accidental child poisoning. Lancet 1977; ii: 289–290
20 Speigel C, Lindaman F. Children can't fly: a program to prevent childhood morbidity and mortality from window falls. Am J Public Health 1977; 67: 1143–1147.
21 Mallonee S, Istree GR, Rosenberg M et al. Surveillance and prevention of residential fire injuries. N Engl J Med 1996; 335: 27–31
22 Erdmann T, Feldman K, Rivara F et al. Tap water burn prevention: the effect of legislation. Pediatrics 1991; 88: 572–577
23 Kavanagh CA, Banco L. The infant walker: a previously unrecognized health hazard. Am J Dis Child 1982; 136: 205–206.
24 British Standards Institute. BS EN 71 Safety of Toys. London: BSI, 1988
25 Department of Trade and Industry. Furniture and furnishings (Fire safety) regulations. London: HMSO, 1988
26 Helfer RE, Slovis TL, Black M. Injuries resulting when small children fall out of bed. Pediatrics 1977; 60: 533–535
27 Nixon J, Jackson RH, Hayes HRM. An analysis of childhood falls involving stairs and banisters. London: Department of Trade and Industry, 1987
28 Kemp A, Sibert J. Drowning and near drowning in the United Kingdom, lessons for prevention. BMJ 1992; 304: 1143–1146
29 Altmann AE, Ozanne-Smith J. Non fatal asphyxiation and foreign body ingestion in children aged 10–14 years. Injury Prevent 1997; 3: 176–182
30 Department of Health. The Health of the Nation: key area handbook Accidents. London: Department of Health, 1993
31 Towner EML, Dowswell T, Simpson G et al. Health promotion in childhood and adolescence for the prevention of unintentional injuries. London: Health Education Authority, 1996
32 Aynsley-Green A, Jarvis SN, Roberts I, Towner EML. (eds) Unintentional Injury in Childhood and Adolescence. London: Ballière Tindall, 1997
33 Hillman M, Adams J, Whitelegg J. One false move: a study of children's independent mobility. London: Policy Studies Institute, 1990

Joseph Britto   Parviz Habibi

Stabilisation and transport of critically ill children

Critically ill children managed in tertiary centre paediatric intensive care units (PICU) have improved outcomes when compared to children managed in non-tertiary care facilities.[1] Despite the lack of randomised controlled trials, there is a growing body of professional opinion that critically ill children are more safely cared for and have the best chance of survival if looked after in designated and centralised PICUs that are appropriately staffed and equipped.[2-4]

Between October 1993 and February 1998, our specialised paediatric transfer team transferred 817 critically ill children to our PICU from 72 different referring hospitals in the south east of England. In this article, in addition to reviewing certain important aspects of paediatric transport medicine, we have incorporated data based on the first 263 consecutive interhospital transfers by our specialised paediatric transfer team. The median age for our group of patients was 23.4 months (8 days to 17.3 years). The diagnostic groups are listed in Table 6.1.

In order to assess the severity of illness of the patients transferred, we used the paediatric risk of mortality (PRISM) score which is an objective scoring system used to predict the probability of death of critically ill children. It assigns an integer value to 14 routinely measured physiological variables (Fig. 6.1).[5] The sum of the integer values constitutes the PRISM score. The PRISM score may then be used in a logistic regression equation to determine the probability of death.

The pretransport PRISM score has been validated as an accurate predictor of hospital mortality.[6] The median (range) pretransport PRISM score for our group of 263 patients was 11 (0–48) and the predicted mortality was 34.5 deaths.

This chapter deals with the stabilisation and transfer of critically ill children in the paediatric age group. The reader interested in neonatal transport medicine is referred to a comprehensive review.[7]

Dr Joseph Britto MBBS MD, Consultant in Paediatric Intensive Care, Department of Paediatrics, Imperial College School of Medicine and Science at St Mary's, South Wharf Rd, London W2 1NY, UK

Dr Parviz Habibi FRCP PhD FRCPCH, Director of Paediatric Intensive Care, Dept of Paediatrics, Imperial College School of Medicine and Science at St Mary's, South Wharf Rd, London W2 1NY, UK

Table 6.1   Diagnostic groups

Diagnostic groups	Number	(%)
Meningococcal disease	320	(40)
Other causes of sepsis/septic shock	74	(9)
Other meningitis/encephalitis/ status epilepticus	72	(9)
Bronchiolitis	117	(14)
Croup/status asthmaticus/pneumonia/others	156	(20)
Accidental overdose	19	(2)
Trauma	18	(2)
Near drowning	4	
Acute life threatening episode	4	
Non accidental injury	3	
Others	30	(4)
TOTAL	**817**	

PRINCIPLES

In the UK, a standard of practice for the transport of critically ill children has been set by the Paediatric Intensive Care Society.[8] This should involve specialised paediatric transfer teams which are usually based at paediatric intensive care units and can be contacted in the event of requests for transfer to that unit or to a specialised facility such as a neurosurgical or burns unit. The ethos of such transfers are based on the principle of mobile intensive care.

Critically ill children frequently need to be moved from one location in the hospital to another. If the morbidity during intrahospital transfers is to be minimised then the ethos of mobile intensive care needs to be extended to transfers within the hospital, however short the distance.

Recognition of the critically ill child at the referring hospital and involvement of appropriately skilled personnel to deliver life saving therapeutic interventions is crucial to outcome while awaiting the arrival of the specialised paediatric transport team. This initial role is and must remain the responsibility of the referring hospital and should be provided at senior level in conjunction with advice given by the specialised paediatric transport team.

One major advantage of specialised paediatric transport teams is that advice can be given regarding appropriate step-up in therapy at the moment of referral. Intensive care is initiated at the referring hospital and is continued until the patient is delivered to the paediatric intensive care or other specialised unit.

THEORETICAL AND PRACTICAL ASPECTS OF TRANSFER

The ethos of mobile intensive care

The belief that the patient should be transported to the PICU as quickly as possible ('swoop and scoop') is no longer appropriate.[9,10] The ethos of mobile

Variable	Age Restriction & Ranges		Score
	Infants	**Children**	
Systolic BP (mm Hg)	130 - 160	150 - 200	2
	55 - 65	65 - 75	2
	> 160	> 200	6
	40 - 54	50 - 64	6
	< 40	< 50	7
Diastolic BP (mm Hg)	**All Ages**		
	> 110		6
Heart rate (beat / min)	**Infants**	**Children**	
	> 160	> 150	4
	< 90	< 80	4
Respiratory rate (breath / min)	61 - 90	51 - 70	1
	> 90	> 70	5
	Apnoea	Apnoea	5
Arterial oxygen tension (Kpa): Fractional inspired oxygen ratio[a]	**All Ages**		
	26.6 – 40		2
	< 26.60		3
Arterial CO_2 tension (kPa)[b]	6.80 - 8.66		1
	> 8.66		5
Glasgow Coma Score[c]	< 8		6
Pupillary reactions	unequal or dilated		4
	fixed and dilated		10
Prothrombin time : partial thromboplastin time ratio	> 1.50 X control		2
Total bilirubin (μmol / 1)	**> 1 month**		
	> 60		6
Potassium (mmol / 1)	**All Ages**		
	3.00 - 3.50		1
	6.50 - 7.50		1
	< 3.00		5
	> 7.50		5
Calcium (mmol / 1)	1.75 - 2.00		2
	3.00 - 3.74		2
	< 1.75		6
	> 3.74		6
Glucose (mmol / 1)	2.20 -3.30		4
	13.90 - 22.20		4
	< 2.20		8
	> 22.20		8
Measured bicarbonate (mmol / 1)	< 16		3
	> 32		3

Fig. 6.1 The paediatric risk of mortality (PRISM) score.

intensive care implies that intensive care is established by the specialised paediatric transport team at the referring hospital. The level of therapy and monitoring that the child receives at the referring hospital during the period of stabilisation and transport should be comparable to that received by the child had he or she been admitted directly to the PICU.[11] The need to anticipate and pre-empt clinical problems is more imperative during interhospital transfer than on a PICU. Major therapeutic interventions such as endotracheal intubation and vascular access, besides being hazardous are extremely difficult to accomplish within the confines of a moving ambulance or a helicopter.

Stabilisation and transport of critically ill children

In our series, the median stabilisation time (interval from arrival of the specialised paediatric transport team at the referring hospital to departure from the referring hospital) was 165 minutes Table 6.2.

The mean stabilisation time in other studies vary from 75 to 156 minutes.[11,12] The major benefit of instituting intensive care at the referring hospital is that appropriate therapeutic interventions and monitoring by the specialised paediatric transport team could lead not only to a decrease in the morbidity, but also to a reduction in the severity of illness during stabilisation and transport.[48]

Composition of the transport team

The composition of a specialised paediatric transport team is dictated by an accurate assessment of the nature and severity of illness of the child at the time of referral to the PICU and the anticipated need for major therapeutic interventions during stabilisation prior to transport. The accuracy of information given on the telephone is usually dependent on the paediatric critical care experience of the observer and, therefore, is variable. In our experience, the use of a questionnaire in the form of a transfer log ensures that the right questions are asked and this can improve the accuracy of assessments over the telephone (Table 6.3).

Although the pretransport PRISM score has been validated as an accurate predictor of hospital mortality, it does not perform adequately as a triage tool in trying to decide transport team composition and the need for major therapeutic interventions during stabilisation.[6,13–15] In the transport situation, children with low PRISM scores remain at risk of morbidity and mortality and often need major therapeutic interventions prior to transport.[13]

The problem of assessing severity of illness and the need for major therapeutic interventions on the telephone is compounded by the fact that the condition of the child could rapidly change at any stage of the transfer. Several studies have addressed the question of the need for a physician on transport teams and, despite a lack of consensus, the majority of specialised paediatric transfer teams in the USA include a physician.[16]

We believe that, to ensure quality of care, all interhospital transfers of children admitted to a PICU should be performed by a specialised paediatric transport team.[15] Members of the specialised paediatric transport team should be adequately trained and equipped with appropriate expertise in paediatric transport medicine. Such a team should be under the direct supervision of a specialist in paediatric transport medicine and should include a career paediatric intensivist, a paediatric intensive care nurse and medical and nursing trainees in paediatric transport medicine.

Communication

Communication in transit between the specialised paediatric transport team, the PICU and the referring hospital are vital. Cellular telephones are convenient but could interfere with electronics on board aircraft and in medical equipment.[17]

Table 6.2 Operational time intervals

	Median (min)	Range (min)
Mobilization[a]	70	20–330
Journey out[b]	35	10–140
Response[c]	105	40–380
Stabilisation[d]	165	36–525
Journey in[e]	40	15–175
Retrieval[f]	310	130–615

[a]Time from referral to departure of specialised paediatric transport team (SPTT) from PICU.
[b]Time from departure of SPTT from PICU to arrival at patient's bedside.
[c]Time from referral to arrival of SPTT at patient's bedside.
[d]Time from arrival of SPTT at the patient's bedside to departure of patient from the referring hospital.
[e]Time from departure of patient from referring hospital to arrival at tertiary centre.
[f]Time from referral to arrival of the patient at PICU.

Utilising the response time

The time taken to deliver intensive care to the child awaiting transfer is crucial to patient outcome.[18] The median response time (interval from the initial referring phone call requesting transfer to the PICU until arrival of the specialised paediatric transport team at the referring hospital) for our urban based team was 105 minutes (Table 6.2). As a consequence of the inevitable length of the response time, the immediate institution of therapeutic measures by personnel at the referring hospital while awaiting arrival of the specialised paediatric transport team, becomes crucial to patient outcome.

Advanced Paediatric Life Support and the Paediatric Advanced Life Support courses among other factors have resulted in a rapidly growing number of health care personnel trained in the recognition, initial resuscitation and stabilisation of the seriously ill child. Early recognition of the seriously ill child at the referring hospital and involvement of appropriately skilled personnel to deliver life saving therapeutic interventions is crucial while awaiting the arrival of the specialised paediatric transport team.

When and what intervention to perform or how aggressive to be in the initial management can be difficult decisions even for those who care for critically ill children on a daily basis. Such decisions are understandably more difficult for the referring hospital staff, who may be called upon to resuscitate seriously ill children on an occasional basis. Detailed discussion with the specialised paediatric transport team can facilitate the decision making process. It is, therefore, very helpful if the specialised paediatric transport team is involved in the patient's management from the time of the initial request for transfer. Depending on the clinical situation, this would include advice over the telephone regarding the airway, ventilatory support, fluid resuscitation, vasoactive therapy, correction of metabolic derangements, haematological support, anti-infective therapy, anti-convulsants, measures to control raised intracranial pressure (ICP), the need for further investigations and, if appropriate, moving the child safely to a high dependency area or adult ICU while awaiting the specialised paediatric transport team.

Table 6.3 The transfer log

Referring hospital and physician data
Patient data
Provisional diagnosis and reasons for transfer
Brief history
Patients initial clinical status at referring hospital
Patients current clinical status at referring hospital
Most recent investigations at referring hospital

Recommendations:
      Intubation and ventilation
      Colloid and crystalloid therapy
      Vasoactive drugs
      Sedatives and muscle relaxants
      Management of raised ICP and seizures
      Acid base, glucose and electrolytes
      Anti-infective agents and haematological support
      Further investigations

Composition of specialised paediatric transport team (SPTT):
      Name of nurse
      Name of physician
Mode of transport
Patient's clinical status at referring hospital assessed by SPTT

Action taken by specialised paediatric transport team (SPTT):
      Endotracheal intubation/tube change
      Ventilatory support
      Central venous access
      Arterial access
      Nasogastric tube and bladder catheter
      Peritoneal dialysis/intercostal drain/others
      Colloid/crystalloid used
      Vasoactive drugs
      Metabolic corrections
      Anti-infective agents and haematological support
Investigations/blood gases/ventilator settings during transfer
Cardiorespiratory status and metabolic condition on arrival at PICU
Problems/remarks during transfer

In order to facilitate initiation of intensive care at the referring hospital while the specialised paediatric transport team is being mobilised, requests from hospitals referring children for intensive care should be directed immediately to the specialist at the tertiary centre directly supervising the specialised paediatric transport team. At the time of the initial phone call, clinical and laboratory data are recorded on the transfer log (Table 6.3). The transfer log accompanies the specialised paediatric transport team to enable documentation of morbidity, severity of illness and therapeutic interventions before, during and after stabilisation and transport. Besides serving as a medico-legal document, the transfer log facilitates audit and research.

Equipment and monitoring

The ethos of mobile intensive care implies that all the equipment essential for the resuscitation, stabilisation and monitoring of a critically ill child needs to be carried by the specialised paediatric transport team. The referring hospital should not be relied upon to make up for deficiencies in equipment. Equipment should not only be dedicated for use on transfer but must meet the specific requirements of the transport environment.

We use a portable monitoring system that allows the following parameters to be monitored continuously and stored for subsequent printing and analysis: heart and respiratory rate, invasive and non-invasive blood pressure, central venous pressure, percutaneous oxygen saturation, end tidal CO_2 and core and peripheral temperatures. In addition, urine output using a bladder catheter, neurological status including pupillary size and degree of muscle relaxation and blood sugars are also assessed periodically.

We are currently evaluating the impact of portable blood gas and electrolyte analysers on the therapeutic decision making time and the titration of therapy during stabilisation by the specialised paediatric transport team at the referring hospital and on the journey back to the PICU.

We believe tracheally intubated patients should be ventilated mechanically rather than manually. Portable mechanical ventilators (which function solely on pipe/cylinder oxygen and air) allow one to accurately set, deliver and measure peak inspiratory pressures and positive end expiratory pressure (PEEP), inspiratory and expiratory times (respiratory rate) and minute volume. In addition, fractional inspired oxygen concentration (FiO_2) and disconnect/low pressure alarms can also be altered. New models of portable ventilators also offer synchronised intermittent mandatory ventilation or continuous positive airway pressure modes of ventilation.

An oxygen cylinder to drive the portable ventilator with an attached flow meter capable of delivering up to 15 l/min is an essential part of the specialised paediatric transport team's equipment. One should always allow at least twice as much oxygen as the estimated journey time requires.

The required amount of oxygen for the journey is calculated as follows:

(PSI × 0.3)/flow rate l/min = minutes of oxygen available

For example   a size E cylinder reads 2000 PSI pressure and the oxygen flow rate range = 4 to 60 l/min

Then   (2000 × 0.3)/4 = 150 minutes of oxygen available.
              (2000 × 0.3)/60 = 10 minutes of oxygen available.

Battery powered syringe pumps capable of handling up to 50 ml syringes and of performing accurately at both slow rates (less than 1 ml/min) and fast rates (up to 99 ml/min) are vital on transfer.

Neonatal intensive care transport incubators are heavy, non-standardised and often incompatible with an ambulance's internal fixations. We have abandoned the use of such transport incubators. For the transfer of term neonates and infants up to 10 kg, purpose built, portable, time cycle pressure-limited ventilators capable of delivering a variable FiO_2 between 0.21 and 1 are used and hypothermia prevented by the use of heat packs in addition to standard space blankets and continuous core-peripheral temperature monitoring.

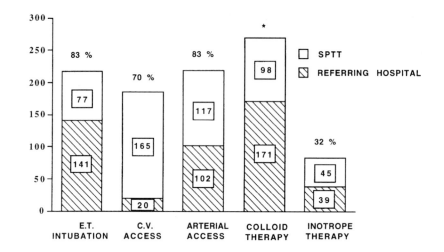

Fig. 6.2 Major therapeutic interventions by the referring hospital and the specialised paediatric transfer team (SPTT) in our series of 263 patients.
*Colloid therapy 20 ml/kg; 86 patients received this volume of colloid from both the referring hospital and the SPTT. [ET = endotracheal, CV = central venous access].

Direct blood pressure monitoring

In all critically ill, ventilated and/or, haemodynamically unstable patients, mean, systolic and diastolic arterial blood pressures should be monitored directly by pressure transduction of an indwelling intra-arterial catheter, as well as indirectly by oscillometry. Besides facilitating repeated steady state blood sampling, direct blood pressure monitoring also provides a continuous pulse-pressure wave form and an alternative source for measurement of the heart rate. Direct monitoring of heart rate and blood pressure during transfer is more accurate, reliable and practical than palpatory and auscultatory methods.[19] Two hundred and nineteen (83%) patients underwent intra-arterial catheterization and direct blood pressure monitoring and on one occasion loss of distal pulses necessitated removal of the catheter (Fig. 6.2).

Mode of transport

Ground versus air transport

The choice of the most appropriate mode of transport depends on the nature and severity of illness of the child (e.g. trauma needing definitive surgical management), the distance to and geographical location of the referring hospital (e.g. urban or rural based), the proximity of the referring and receiving hospitals to a helipad or an airport, weather and flying conditions and the number of personnel in the specialised paediatric transport team.

Ground ambulances are effective in transporting critical or unstable patients up to 50 km and stable patients up to 150 km.[20] The majority of tertiary centre PICUs are urban based and the obvious disadvantage of ground based transport is the length of time spent on the road negotiating traffic congestion.

Table 6.4 Relative stresses during ground and air transport

	Ground ambulance	Helicopter	Fixed-wing	Pressurised cabin
Acceleration	–	–	+/-	+/-
Vibration	+	++	+	+/-
Noise	+	++	+	+/-
Thermal	–	+/-	–	+/-
Hypoxia	–	+/-	+	+/-
Gas expansion	–	+/-	+	+/-
Electromagnetic interference	+/-	+	+	+

A negative (–) sign means there may be no problem in that mode of transport, while a positive sign (+) suggests specific problems of varying degrees of severity may be encountered.

Helicopters are effective for transporting patients up to a 150 km radius; for distances greater than that, fixed-wing aircraft are preferred.[20] The absence of a helipad in close proximity to the hospital results in multiple transfers of the child between the referring hospital, ambulance, aircraft and PICU. Whichever mode of transport is used, the most important consideration is the ability of the team travelling in the vehicle or aircraft to care for the child.[10] Familiarisation with helicopter and fixed-wing aircraft, training in aviation physiology and safety and the use of aircraft compatible monitoring equipment are essential for the safe and effective transfer of critically ill children by air.

Air medical physiology

Depending on the type of aircraft used, changes in altitude, acceleration and deceleration forces, temperature, humidity, noise and vibration, could have significant physiological effects (Table 6.4).[21]

In fixed-wing aircraft with increasing altitudes, there is a decrease in the partial pressure of oxygen at the alveolus which could result in a fall in arterial oxygenation. The partial pressure of oxygen decreases by approximately 30% at an altitude of 2000 metres. Patients with pulmonary problems and an increased alveolar-arterial gradient are at increased risk of developing hypoxia and will require increasing FiO_2 with increasing altitude (Fig. 6.3).[21] Children breathing spontaneously and requiring an FiO_2 of 1 on the ground will require a change in ventilatory support prior to air transport.[20] The problems of hypoxia during air transport could be further compounded by a decrease in the haemoglobin and the oxygen carrying capacity of blood.[21]

According to Boyle's law, if temperature is constant, the volume of a gas varies inversely with the pressure. In fixed-wing aircraft with increasing altitude, as the pressure of gas in a closed space decreases the volume increases (dysbarism). There are several important clinical implications of this phenomenon that need to be borne in mind. The cuff on endotracheal tubes needs to be minimally inflated to allow for expansion. Small asymptomatic pneumothoraces or pneumatocoeles at sea level could expand by approximately 30% at an altitude of 7000–8000 feet and, therefore, should be drained

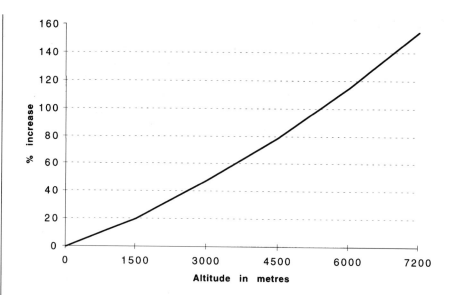

Fig. 6.3 Percentage increase in oxygen required at altitude.

(and connected to Heimlich valves) prior to transport. Gastric distension and bowel gas should be treated prophylactically with gastric and rectal tubes. Air trapped in other closed spaces like the intracranial sinuses and ventricles (head injury) or bowel wall air (necrotizing enterocolitis) is likely to expand and cause morbidity at high altitudes. Special precautions are, therefore, necessary before transporting such patients by air.

Acceleration and deceleration forces could alter blood flow and cerebral perfusion during take off and landing in fixed-wing aircraft. These factors need to be considered when transferring haemodynamically unstable patients and patients with raised ICP.[20]

There are a few situations which constitute a contra-indication to air transport. Neurosurgical patients with residual intracranial air, or who have had recent pneumo-encephalograms, or patients with gas behind the globe of the eye from trauma or surgery should not be transported by air. Patients following recent abdominal surgery and with significant ileus should have air transport delayed for about 48 hours. The significant risk of decompression sickness must be born in mind prior to air transport of a sick or injured recreational SCUBA diver. A suitable time lapse at sea level to blow off excess nitrogen is therefore mandatory. Help should be sought from personnel experienced in diving medicine.

Airway and ventilatory management

Airway and ventilatory intervention is often the earliest and most important task the specialised paediatric transport team is called upon to perform. It is, therefore, mandatory for members of the specialised paediatric transport team to be skilled in airway management, ventilatory techniques, and the use sedatives and muscle relaxants.

Endotracheal intubation

In keeping with the principles of paediatric resuscitation, the first priority of a specialised paediatric transport team on arrival at the referring hospital is assessment and management of the airway and breathing. Studies indicate that up to 43% of critically ill children require some form of airway management or respiratory support by the specialised paediatric transport team on arrival at the referring hospital.[22] In our series of 263 patients, airway intervention by the specialised paediatric transport team was required in 158 (60%) patients.

Rapid sequence tracheal intubation

The vast majority of children who present with an acute life threatening condition are at risk of regurgitating and aspirating stomach contents. The abolition of the protective airway reflexes by anaesthetic induction agents and muscle relaxants involved in the rapid sequence tracheal intubation further increases the risk of pulmonary aspiration. This risk can be significantly reduced if pressure is maintained over the cricoid just prior to administration of the drugs and until intubation is confirmed to be successful. The essence of the rapid sequence tracheal intubation technique is to keep to a minimum the duration of time between administration of the drugs and ideal intubating conditions by administering the drugs in rapid sequence. The need for bag-mask ventilation is decreased by preoxygenation for 2–3 minutes with 100% oxygen. To prevent gastric distension, gentle bag-mask ventilation is used while continuing to maintain cricoid pressure only in the event of rapid oxygen desaturation.[23] Depending on the clinical situation, the drugs we use for rapid sequence tracheal intubations are a combination of anti-cholinergics (atropine), sedatives (thiopentone or ketamine) and muscle relaxants (suxamethonium or vecuronium). For tracheal intubation in the presence of upper airway obstruction, we use the inhalational agent sevoflurane.

Of patients transferred by our specialised paediatric transport team, 218 (83%) were endotracheally intubated and mechanically ventilated (Fig. 6.2). In 77 (35%) of these patients, rapid sequence tracheal intubation was performed by our specialised paediatric transport team immediately on arrival at the referring hospital. The indications for endotracheal intubation included shock,[24] a Glasgow Coma Scale score of < 9,[25] and respiratory failure/upper airway obstruction. Early elective intubation and ventilation in shock states protects the airway, ensures adequate oxygenation and ventilation, eliminates the work of breathing which is often increased in shock and the fraction of cardiac output used by respiratory muscles is made available for perfusion of other organs.[24]

Reintubation of the trachea by specialised paediatric transport team is frequently necessary. In our series, 81 of the 141 (57%) patients that underwent endotracheal intubation by referring hospital personnel, were reintubated by the specialised paediatric transport team. The reasons for reintubation of the trachea include the need to replace an oral endotracheal tube for a nasal one (unless contra-indicated) or to change to an endotracheal tube of a more appropriate diameter and/or length.

Route of endotracheal intubation

Of the 218 intubated patients in our series, 152 (70%) were transferred with nasotracheal tubes which were secured using either metal or a disposable Tunstall connector. Although there are no published studies comparing the incidence of accidental extubation in children with orotracheal as opposed to nasotracheal tubes during paediatric transfer, it is generally considered that nasotracheal tubes are secured more easily and safely in children and are preferable for long-term use.[26] It is our policy to change an oral endotracheal tube for a nasal one unless the patient is suspected to have a fracture of the cribriform plate with cerebrospinal fluid leak, has a nasal deformity, has clinical evidence of a bleeding diathesis or if the initial oral intubation was a complicated one.[27]

Endotracheal tube blockage

The incidence of endotracheal tube blockage has been reported to be as high as 8% for intubated patients during transfer by non-specialised paediatric teams.[28] To counter the effects of the cold dry gas that is used to ventilate patients during transfer, we perform frequent suction with saline and use an in-line thermal condenser with a humidifier filter. There was one instance of endotracheal tube blockage in our series of 218 intubated patients.

Accidental extubation

The incidence of accidental extubation for all intubated paediatric patients has been reported to vary between 3–13%.[26] Inadequate sedation or muscle relaxants were implicated as common risk factors in these and the appropriate use of sedatives or muscle relaxants has been shown to decrease the incidence of accidental extubation.[26,29] All intubated patients in our series were mechanically ventilated and maintained on continuous infusions of sedatives and analgesics (one, or a combination of: fentanyl or morphine and midazolam) and muscle relaxants (atracurium or vecuronium) during transfer. There were no instances of accidental extubation in our group of patients.

Ventilatory intervention

In our series, the specialised paediatric transport team initiated mechanical ventilation in 66 of the 141 (47%) patients already intubated by the referring hospital. In addition, controlled hyperventilation was used to treat raised ICP in 21 (15%), we applied positive end expiratory pressure (PEEP) in 35 (25%) of patients and withdrew PEEP in 7 (5%) of patients with raised ICP and normal lungs.

Fluid and drug therapy

Central venous access

Studies have shown that the incidence of loss or lack of intravenous access during transfer by non-specialised teams to be as high as 10%.[30] We believe that central venous access should be obtained in any patient with established or potential haemodynamic instability especially in the context of transfer. Large bore (5 Fr) multi-lumen central venous catheters facilitate measurement of central venous pressure, rapid administration of colloid that is often not possible through peripheral venous lines,[31] administration of vasoactive drugs and hypertonic or irritant solutions (bicarbonate/potassium/calcium) into the central circulation, and safe, sutured and secure venous access for the administration of multiple infusions, i.e. dextrose, sedation and muscle relaxants.

There were no instances of loss of intravenous access in our study. Central venous catheters were inserted in 185 (70%) patients in our series (Fig. 6.2). In one instance, catheterisation of the femoral vein resulted temporary venous congestion of the distal limb. In the majority of instances, we catheterise either the subclavian or internal jugular veins. Catheterisation of the subclavian vein should be avoided in the presence of a bleeding diathesis.

The aim of treatment of shock states in children is to optimise the perfusion of critical vascular beds and to prevent or correct metabolic abnormalities arising from cellular hypoperfusion.[32] To this end, besides airway and ventilatory intervention and achieving vascular access, among other major therapeutic measures that specialised paediatric transport team will undertake are fluid resuscitation, institution or modification of vasoactive drug therapy and correction of metabolic derangements.

In our series, half of the patients suffered from meningococcal or other forms of septic shock and, therefore, colloid and inotrope therapy and correction of metabolic derangements were required in many of them. 98 (37%) received ≥ 20 ml/kg of colloid from specialised paediatric transport team and, in 45 (17%) patients, a vasoactive drug was started by the specialised paediatric transport team. During stabilisation and transport, low plasma levels of potassium, bicarbonate and calcium were corrected in 90 (34%), 59 (22%) and 51 (19%) patients, respectively, by the specialised paediatric transport team.

Intrahospital transfers

Critically ill children frequently need to be moved from one location in the hospital to another. This could include transfers from a general ward or the accident and emergency department to the PICU or two-way transfers from the PICU to a nonportable diagnostic facility or the operating theatre.

Intrahospital transfers are associated with a surprisingly high incidence of serious transport related adverse events. In a study on intrahospital transfer of critically ill children, Wallen et al showed significant physiological deterioration in up to 72% of children and equipment related mishaps in up to 19% of children: 14% of children needed at least one major therapeutic intervention during transfer.[33] Studies such as this suggest that, prior to every intrahospital transfer, the benefits of the planned diagnostic test or surgery need to be weighed against the potential risks of the transfer.

If the morbidity during intrahospital transfers is to be minimised, then the ethos of mobile intensive care needs to be extended to transfers within the hospital, however short the distance. The principles, philosophy, personnel and equipment that make up the interhospital specialised paediatric transport team, place the latter in an ideal situation to perform transfers within the hospital.

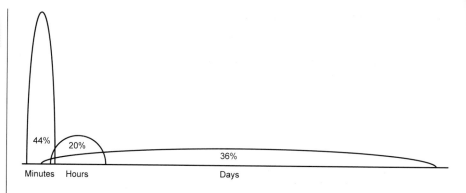

Fig. 6.4 Trimodal distribution of deaths from trauma.

Special disease-specific requirements

A complete list of such medical conditions and situations is beyond the scope of this chapter and the reader is referred to a manual of *Paediatric Transport Medicine*.[34]

Transfer of trauma patients

As shown in Figure 6.4, the first group (44%) die very quickly from overwhelming damage at the time of the injury. Those in the second group (20%) die because of progressive respiratory failure, circulatory insufficiency or raised intracranial pressure secondary to the effects of injury. Death occurs within hours if no treatment is administered. The immediate resuscitation and stabilisation of these injured children is crucial to outcome even if transfer is being arranged to an intensive care unit. The third group (36%) die from complications such as raised intracranial pressure, infection and multi-organ system failure. Appropriate management in the first few hours will decrease mortality in this group.[35]

The relative sensitivity of the central nervous system to hypoxia and ischaemia following trauma renders it a prime target for secondary insults during stabilisation and transport.

In a study by Sharples et al, 121 potentially avoidable factors that possibly or probably contributed to death were identified in 255 fatal head injuries in children.[36] Eleven (9%) of these factors occurred during 68 interhospital transfers to a regional neurosurgical centre. 15 of these 68 children (22%) were described as being in a critical condition at the end of the transfer. The concept of the 'golden hour' in trauma does not preclude appropriate stabilisation of patients by specialised paediatric transport team prior to transport. Studies on pretransport stabilisation of trauma patients have shown improved outcomes in patients with a higher rate of therapeutic interventions such as endotracheal intubation, fluid resuscitation, blood transfusion and thoracic decompression.[9,16] A child with a life threatening subdural/epidural haematoma or a penetrating injury of the chest or abdomen needs rapid transfer by specialised paediatric transport team to a centre offering definitive surgery. A favourable outcome in such patients will ensue only if the principles of A (airway), B (breathing), C

Table 6.5 Causes of non-traumatic central neurological failure

- **Hypoxic-ischaemic brain injury**
  Following respiratory or circulatory failure
- **Status epilepticus**
- **Non-accidental injury**
  Intracranial haemorrhage, brain swelling
- **Infections**
  Meningoencephalitis
- **Poisons**
- **Metabolic**
  Renal, hepatic, failure, Reye's syndrome, hypoglycaemia,
  hypothermia, hypercapnia
- **Vascular lesion**
- **Hypertension**

(circulation) of paediatric resuscitation have been attended to. Depending on the clinical situation, appropriate pre-transport stabilisation in such children could include endotracheal intubation, controlled hyperventilation, the use of sedatives and muscle relaxants, diuretics, fluid and inotrope therapy.

Non-traumatic central neurological failure

The majority of cases of coma in childhood (95%) are caused by a diffuse metabolic insult including cerebral hypoxia and ischaemia, the remainder (5%) are caused by structural lesions (Table 6.5).

Assessment: Neurological signs in childhood coma may be diffuse, incomplete and asymmetrical, early signs may be subtle and the conscious level quite variable. Rapid assessment of conscious level may be performed using the AVPU score or, more formally, by the Glasgow coma scale score modified for children.[37]

The AVPU score
Consists of placing the child in one of four categories according to the level of consciousness:

> **A** alert
> **V** responds to voice
> **P** responds to pain
> **U** unresponsive

Raised intracranial pressure: In a previously well, unconscious child (Glasgow coma scale ≤ 8) who is not post-ictal, the following are suggestive of raised ICP:

- Cushing's triad: hypertension, bradycardia, abnormal breathing patterns (hyperventilation, Cheyne-Stokes or apnoea)

- Abnormal pupils: unilateral or bilateral

- Abnormal oculocephalic reflexes; test with caution in cases of suspected neck injury

- Abnormal posture: decorticate, decerebrate

Absolute signs of raised ICP: papilloedema, bulging fontanelle and absence of venous pulsation in retinal vessels may all be absent in the acute stage. A CT scan of the brain is an insensitive test for detection of acutely raised intracranial pressure.[38,39]

Management: Lumbar puncture is contra-indicated in a child with decreased level of consciousness or haemodynamic instability.[40] The results of lumbar puncture are not necessary for initiating antimicrobial treatment; diagnosis of meningoencephalitis can be confirmed or refuted at a later stage once the child's condition has stabilised.

In cases of coma:

- Give high flow oxygen

- Head up, (30° with horizontal) midline position

- Avoid insertion of central venous lines in the neck

- If Glasgow coma scale ≤ 8, rapid sequence intubation using thiopentone (see airway and ventilatory management):
  ventilate ($PaCO_2$ low normal range);
  sedate (midazolam and morphine/fentanyl); and/or
  consider muscle relaxants for the duration of transport (vercuronium)

- Consider anticonvulsant therapy in muscle relaxed patients with seizures

- In cases of suspected raised ICP, give manitol 0.5 g/kg by rapid intravenous bolus, (or frusemide 1 mg/kg if doubt about kidney function) catheterise as the bladder may be very full

Treat the treatable, e.g.

- Metabolic derangements: glucose, calcium, sodium, acidosis etc.

- Poisoning: opiates, tricyclic antidepressants, paracetamol, salycylates etc.

- Infection: meningococcal, pneumococcal, herpes simplex etc.

Monitoring of vital signs, coma score, fluid balance and blood gases should commence as soon as possible together with early investigation.

Prior to transfer for definitive care, further neurological assessment and examination may reveal the need to plan other investigations and imaging, particularly in the presence of focal neurology:

- Toxicology screen

- Liver enzymes, blood ammonia, lactate

- Blood/urine metabolic screen

- Blood film

- Chest x-ray
- Cranial CT/MR

Suspected meningoencephalitis

Bacterial meningitis and herpes simplex encephalitis remain the important therapeutic diagnoses in the immediate period prior to transfer of a comatose child. Emergency peritransport treatment as for comatosed child; priority is attention to **ABC** of life support, anticipate/treat raised ICP and convulsions. In cases of suspected meningoencephalitis:

- Avoid lumbar puncture
- Start immediate empirical treatment:
    ceftriaxone (80 mg/kg i.v.), acyclovir 500 (mg/m^2 i.v.)
- Consider: erythromycin (25 mg/kg i.v., to cover *Mycoplasma* infection), ampicillin 50 mg/kg i.v., to cover *Listeria* in the neonatal period) and dexamethasone (0.15 mg/kg i.v., prior to antibiotic administration if bacterial meningitis is likely)

Child abuse

Non-accidental injury may occasionally present as an acute emergency with a spectrum of clinical features. These include status epilepticus, coma, hypothermia, poisoning or shock. Initial management will, therefore, be directed by the clinical presentation, with resuscitation and stabilisation of **ABC** and attention to **D** disability. These children will invariably need transfer to a paediatric intensive care unit. Prior to transfer for definitive care, further neurological assessment and examination may reveal the need to plan other investigations and imaging:

- Detailed fundoscopic examination
- Toxicology screen
- Serum saved for future screening
- Blood/urine metabolic screen
- Skeletal survey
- Cranial CT/MRI

As soon as the diagnosis of non-accidental injury is suspected, the transport team should follow established protocols for the management of suspected child abuse. All those engaged in the transport of critically ill children must be familiar with the medico-legal aspects of child abuse cases. The urgency of the resuscitation scenario and the demands of the child protection agencies add further stress to those involved in the transfer. Involvement of a senior paediatrician and the local team to share these tasks is very important. However, members of the specialised paediatric transfer team will often be called upon to give statements and discuss evidence.

Respiratory emergencies

Disorders of the respiratory tract are the most common illnesses of childhood. Although most are self-limiting, some present as potentially life threatening emergencies. Such patients are often referred to a paediatric intensive care facility and, therefore, in most cases will need to be transferred. Accurate diagnosis and prompt initiation of appropriate treatment are essential to avoid preventable morbidity and mortality, and should proceed along Advanced Paediatric Life Support (APLS) protocols. Early contact with the specialised paediatric transfer team will allow the best utilisation of the response time.

Childhood respiratory illnesses presenting as emergencies:

- Acute upper airway obstruction:
    croup, tracheitis, and epiglottitis account for 98% of cases;
    other causes include acquired subglottic stenosis, diphtheria (only seen in non-immunised children), infectious mononucleosis, retropharyngeal abscess, or foreign body in the larynx or trachea

- Lower airway obstruction:
    asthma and bronchiolitis account for most cases

- Pneumonias:
    pneumococcal, staphylococcal, *Pneumocyctis carinii* pneumonia

Acute upper airway obstruction: Croup is the most common cause, although an increasing number of children with subglottic stenosis following neonatal intensive care are presenting with acute upper airway obstruction. The decision to intubate is a clinical one when there are signs of impending respiratory failure. Usually, the patient will already be intubated by the time the specialised paediatric transfer team arrive. Occasionally, the patient has suddenly deteriorated following initial response to medical treatment and will need urgent intubation. Ideally, the procedure should be performed under general anaesthesia (we use the inhalational agent sevoflourane) by an experienced paediatric anaesthetist or intensivist. A smaller endotracheal tube than usual is often required. If a difficult intubation is anticipated, an ENT surgeon capable of performing a tracheostomy should be present. Anyone contemplating intubation in the case of a difficult airway must be confident in their technique and be able to perform an emergency needle cricothyroidotomy, which should always be regarded as a technique of failure.

In some cases pulmonary oedema may occur after relief of airway obstruction and usually responds to ventilation and the application of PEEP.[41]

Although much less common, epiglottitis may mimic croup. In countries where there is routine immunisation with the conjugate vaccine against HiB, there has been a dramatic reduction of the incidence of epiglottis. This means that medical staff will be much less experienced in the early recognition and management of this life threatening paediatric respiratory emergency.

Although intubated children with croup and epiglottitis may be managed without muscle paralysis and minimal sedation while on a paediatric intensive care unit, they are often sedated and muscle relaxed for transfer in order to protect against accidental extubation.

In severe croup:

- Nebulised adrenaline 0.5 ml/kg of 1:1000 (5 ml maximum) given with oxygen and close monitoring produces only transient improvement for 20–30 minutes

- Steroids are beneficial:
  (i) nebulised budesonide 2 mg, dexamethasone 0.6 mg/kg i.v. or prednisolone 1 mg/kg oral; (ii) the effects start within hours, last for up to 24 hours and may reduce the need and the duration of intubation; and (iii) reduces the need for reintubation

- Intubation under inhalational anaesthesia (sevoflourane)

- The endotracheal tube needs meticulous care to avoid blockage from secretions and accidental displacement.

- Consider antibiotic therapy

In suspected epiglottitis:

- Avoid lateral neck x-ray, or painful/distressing procedures

- Nebulised adrenaline or steroids are of no benefit

- Intubation may be difficult due to intense swelling and inflammation of the 'cherry red epiglottis'

- Intubation should be performed following inhalational induction of anaesthesia (sevoflourane)

- Blood should be sent for culture and intravenous cefotaxime 50 mg/kg commenced

Bacterial tracheitis: This is an uncommon but potentially life threatening infection of the trachea, distinct from both epiglottitis and viral laryngo-tracheobronchitis (croup). Bacterial infection of the trachea is thought to occur secondary to a primary viral infection. Clinical presentation of bacterial tracheitis may be similar to both croup and epiglottitis, but is characterised at endoscopy by the presence of a normal epiglottis, marked subglottic narrowing and copious purulent secretions in the trachea. Uncomplicated viral croup similarly may produce purulent tracheal secretions, but bacterial tracheitis is suggested by the persistence of high fever and toxicity after passage of an endotracheal tube. The toxic shock syndrome, septic shock, pulmonary oedema and the acute respiratory distress syndrome have been recognised in children with bacterial tracheitis.[42]

Acute lower airway obstruction: Bronchiolitis is the most common serious respiratory infection of childhood. About 2% of those hospitalised will require advanced respiratory support which will often need transfer to a paediatric intensive care unit. Infants with chronic lung disease of prematurity and congenital heart defects are particularly at risk and difficult to treat. Asthma is the most common reason for hospital admission in the UK. Most patients with asthma will not require mechanical ventilation if given intensive medical therapy. However, these patients are at risk of severe respiratory failure and will, therefore, need to be transferred to a paediatric intensive care facility.

In severe bronchiolitis:

- Bronchodilator therapy, especially ipratropium, may be beneficial

- Nebulised adrenaline 0.5 ml/kg 1:1000 (5 ml maximum) may be helpful

- CPAP via face mask or nasal prong improves respiratory failure and may avoid the need for intubation

- Mechanical ventilation for apnoea, exhaustion, respiratory failure

- Mechanical ventilation is complicated due to underlying lower airway disease

- Intermittent saline tracheobronchial lavage will improve respiratory compliance in ventilated patients

- Nebulised ribavirin therapy has no place in the immediate treatment period

In severe/life-threatening asthma:

- Intravenous hydrocortisone (5 mg/kg, 6 hourly)

- Half hourly or continuous β_2 bronchodilator therapy

- Addition of ipratropium to maximal β_2 therapy is beneficial

- Intravenous salbutamol 5 mcg/kg over 10 min then 1–5 mcg/kg/min. Use with caution – risk of serious hypokalaemia, potentiated by theophylline

- Intravenous magnesium sulphate 25 mg/kg infused over 30 minutes may be helpful

- Need for mechanical ventilation – a clinical decision based on:

    (i) increasing $PaCO_2$, hypoxia, acidosis;
    (ii) exhaustion.
    (iii) requires experienced paediatric intensivist/anaesthetist;
    (iv) meticulous attention to tracheobronchial toilet will improve respiratory compliance.
    (v) obstructive airway ventilator settings (slow rates, adequate expiratory time, minimal PEEP)
    (vi) permissive hypercapnia

- Sedation and muscle relaxants:

    (i) sedative/analgesic agents like sevoflourane or intravenous ketamine are useful as they have bronchodilator properties;
    (ii) fentanyl is preferred for sedation/analgesia to morphine which may cause release of histamine; and
    (iii) full sedation and muscle paralysis is preferred during transport
    (iv) isoflurane for refractory status asthmaticus

Circulatory failure – shock

Shock follows acute failure of the circulatory function, resulting in inadequate delivery of nutrients and oxygen to body tissues and accumulation of waste products. Shock is a progressive syndrome and can be divided into three phases:

1. *Compensated*: Vital organ function is preserved by normal physiological compensatory mechanisms and the patient is normotensive but tachycardic, pale with cool peripheries and may be slightly agitated/combative/confused. The clinical signs are subtle, but it is important to recognise this early and treatable phase of shock.

2. *Uncompensated*: A progression from early shock, the failure of the normal compensatory mechanisms lead to hypotension and a depressed level of consciousness and other organ dysfunction such as oligoanuria.

3. *Irreversible*: End stage shock where the damage to vital organs is of such a magnitude that death is inevitable.

Early recognition and aggressive treatment of shock before decompensation is, therefore, crucial for a good outcome. Rapid assessment of circulatory status may be done following APLS protocols.[43] Classification of the causes of shock are summarised in Table 6.6.

Table 6.6 Classification of causes of shock (common causes in bold)

• Hypovolaemic
haemorrhage
diarrhoea, vomiting
burns
peritonitis
• Distributive
septicaemia
anaphylaxis
anaesthetic drugs, vasodilators
spinal cord injury
• Cardiogenic
arrhythmias
cardiomyopathy, heart failure
myocardial contusion
• Obstructive
tension pneumothorax
haemopneumothorax
cardiac tamponade
flail chest
pulmonary embolism
hypertension (coarctation of the aorta)
• Dissociative
profound anaemia
carbon monoxide poisoning
methaemoglobinaemia

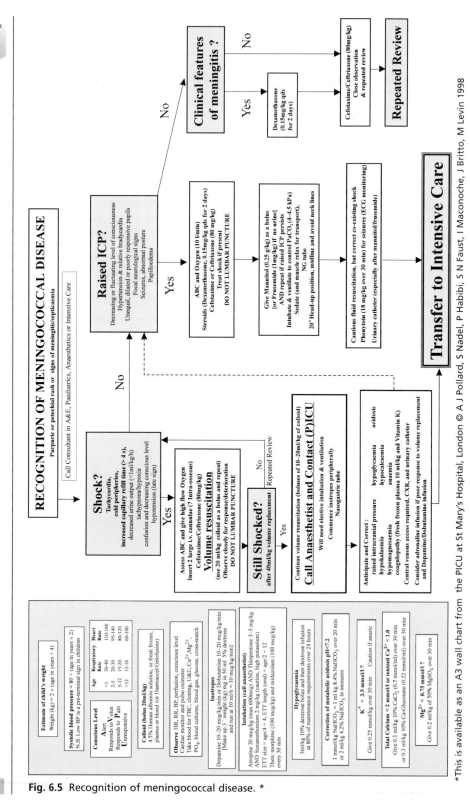

Fig. 6.5 Recognition of meningococcal disease. *

*This is available as an A3 wall chart from the PICU at St Mary's Hospital, London © A J Pollard, S Nadel, P Habibi, S N Faust, I Maconochie, J Britto, M Levin 1998

In meningococcal shock the cardiac output may be low, normal or raised. The pathogenesis of shock in meningococcal septicaemia is mutifactorial:

- Severe capillary leak resulting in loss of circulating volume
- Vasodilatation of some vascular beds co-existing with vasoconstriction of others
- Intravascular thrombosis
- Severe depression of myocardial function

There may be rapid deterioration and death from overwhelming shock and multiple organ system failure. For a more detailed review on the pathophysiology and management of meningococcal disease the reader is referred to the algorism in Figure 6.5 and to a recent review.[44]

Rapid assessment of cardiovascular status is possible by checking heart rate, pulse volume, capillary refill time and toe-cone temperature gradient. The effects of circulatory inadequacy on other organs is assessed by checking respiratory rate and pattern of breathing, skin appearance and temperature, mental status, urine output and acid base status. The blood pressure may be preserved while in the phase of compensated shock. Hypotension is a preterminal sign in the context of circulatory failure.

Shock management: Urgent attention to ABC: **the work of breathing is increased in shock**[24]

- Ensure a patent, protected airway
- Support breathing with 100% oxygen
- Consider early, elective ventilation (> 40 ml/kg fluid resuscitation)
- Immediate treatment of hypovolaemia
- Anticipate/prevent hypotension
- Rapid vascular access: intra osseous needle or central venous access
- Give 20 ml/kg fluid immediately

Re-assess and repeat fluid bolus if necessary

- Check and perform metabolic corrections:
  acidosis, glucose, potassium, calcium, magnesium and phosphate
- Consider inotropic drugs after adequate fluid resuscitation:
  dobutamine 5–20 mcg/kg/min by intravenous infusion;
  adrenaline 0.1–2 mcg/kg/min by intravenous infusion

Choice of fluid for volume resuscitation:

- 4.5% albumin or plasma for septic shock and burns
- Blood in haemorrhagic shock
- Cystalloids (isotonic) in physiological dehydration

Near drowning and hypothermia

Near drowning is defined as recovery (however transient) following a submersion incident. There is hypoxic insult to the brain, the patients are often

Table 6.7 Prognostic factors in near drowning

Type of water whether fresh or salt has no bearing on outcome. Rectal temperature < 33°C increases chances of survival
Poor prognosis for recovery:
Time to first gasp > 40 minutes
Persisting coma
Arterial blood gases despite treatment: pH < 7.0, PaO_2 < 8.0
CPR not commenced at waterside

hypothermic and possibility of cervical spine injury should be considered in situations where there was diving. Children who present with near drowning, therefore, require assessment and treatment of all the above problems. Hypothermia and other associated injuries should be actively sought and treated. Whether sea or fresh water has no bearing in prognosis. Early involvement of a specialised paediatric transfer team is essential.

Basic measures:

•   Attention to ABC and cervical spine immobilisation

•   Gastric decompression to protect from aspiration

Hypothermia is common and adversely affects resuscitation attempts unless adequately treated.

    External rewarming is sufficient if core temperature is > 32°C:

•   Remove cold, wet clothes

•   Apply warm blankets/heating blanket

•   Radiant heaters

Active core rewarming is required if core temperature is < 32°C:

•   Use warm intravenous fluids to 39°C

•   Warm ventilator gas to 42°C

•   Gastric, peritoneal N/saline lavage at 42°C

•   Pleural or pericardial lavage

•   Extracorporial blood warming may be necessary

•   Rewarming may result in shock/hypovolaemia

    Prognostic factors in near drowning are summarised in Table 6.7.

Burns

The most common cause of death, within the first few hours following a burn injury, is from smoke inhalation. Indications of inhalation injury are from the history of exposure to smoke in a confined space, the presence of deposits around the mouth and nose, and carbonaceous sputum. Therefore, attention to airway and breathing is of paramount importance. Significant early circulatory compromise is usually not due to losses from the burn area and other causes such as bleeding from associated injuries should be sought. Early contact with a specialised burns unit is essential for advice regarding initial management and transfer.

Accurate assessment of the burn is very important, including surface area, depth, special areas involved, e.g. mouth, face, hand, perineal areas.

Urgent attention to resuscitation of **ABC**:

- **A**irway may become compromised by inhalational injury and/or direct burns to face
- **B**reathing may be compromised by inhalational injury and/or circumferential burns restricting chest movement
- **C**irculation may be compromised by fluid loss proportional to percentage burn

Criteria for transfer to a burns unit: (i) 10% partial and/or full thickness burn; (ii) 5% full thickness burn; (iii) burns to special areas.

Give fluid replacement for burn + the amount for normal requirements. The additional fluid (ml/24 h) required is calculated from:

$$\text{\% burn} \times \text{weight (kg)} \times 4.$$

SPECIALISED AND NON-SPECIALISED TRANSPORT TEAMS

The transfer of an unstable, ill child is potentially hazardous. Besides the risk of deterioration from the primary illness, there are the added risks of complications of therapy and secondary insults of the transfer process itself.

The interhospital transfer of critically ill children by personnel not trained in paediatric transport medicine (non-specialised transfer teams) has been shown to be associated with unacceptable transfer related morbidity. In an observational study from Birmingham by Barry et al, 75% of 56 critically ill children transferred to a PICU by non-specialised referring hospital personnel suffered serious clinical complications, 23% of which were considered life threatening.[45,46] A study from the USA, by Kanter and Tompkins of 117 children transferred to a PICU by non-specialised referring hospital personnel showed that 24 patients (21%) suffered physiological deterioration or equipment related adverse events during transfer.[28] The two studies cited above lacked a control group: therefore, a direct correlation between transfer related morbidity and non specialised transfer teams, although suggestive, cannot be established.

There is evidence that teams trained in paediatric transport medicine (specialised paediatric transfer teams) can transfer critically ill children more safely than non-specialised teams. In a non-randomised retrospective study of 130 seriously ill or injured children transferred to a tertiary level intensive care unit in Vancouver, Macnab noted that 64 errors in management occurred in 34 transfers by untrained personnel compared to 25 errors in 96 transfers by personnel trained in paediatric transport medicine.[12] Using the criteria of Kanter and Tompkins, a study in the USA by Edge et al compared specialised ($n = 47$) and non-specialised ($n = 92$) paediatric transfers to two tertiary paediatric intensive care units, using two types of transport systems. This prospective, but non-randomised, study demonstrated that the specialised paediatric transfer team significantly reduced the occurrence of equipment related adverse events (from 20% to 2%) but not the occurrence of physiological deterioration (12% to 11%) during transport.[47]

Our own prospective study evaluated the morbidity and severity of illness during the transfer of 51 critically ill children to our PICU by our specialised paediatric transfer team. The severity of illness of our patient group was comparable to that in Edge's study. Using the same criteria of Kanter and Tompkins, we demonstrated that physiological deterioration during transport occurred in 4% of patients and there were no instances of equipment related adverse events. Further, there was a significant decrease in the severity of illness measured by the paediatric risk of mortality (PRISM) score, in the majority of patients during stabilisation and transport.[48,49]

CONCLUSIONS

The use of specialised paediatric transfer teams has been recommended in several countries including the USA,[50] Australia,[51] and the UK.[3,4,8,46] An increasing number of PICUs in the UK now provide a transfer service for children referred for intensive care. A centralised, specialised transfer team set up and dedicated to meet all the demands of the interhospital transfer of critically ill children in the region has several distinct advantages. A single phone call to the regional specialised paediatric transport team would give referring hospital personnel immediate and expert clinical advice on the initial resuscitation and stabilisation. The specialised paediatric transport team can be dispatched immediately ensuring that intensive care is rapidly delivered to the child at the referring hospital while the base unit of the regional specialised paediatric transport team finds a suitable bed on a PICU within or even outside the region. A regional specialised paediatric transport team would also prevent the duplication involved in the current model where each PICU provides a transfer service and would result in more efficient use of expensive resources in terms of both personnel and equipment.

The volume of work generated by a centralised, specialised transfer team would ensure that doctors and nurses interested in a career in paediatric intensive care and transport medicine are adequately supervised and optimally trained. Further, the data and the opportunities generated would be an invaluable resource for systematic research in paediatric intensive care and transport medicine.

References

1 Pollack MM, Alexander SR, Clark N, Ruttimann UE, Tesselaar HM, Bachulis AC. Improved outcomes from tertiary centre pediatric intensive care: a state-wide comparison of tertiary and nontertiary care facilities. Crit Care Med 1991; 19: 150–159

Key points for clinical practice

- The transfer of an unstable, ill child is potentially hazardous. Besides the risk of deterioration from the primary illness there are the added risks of complications of therapy and secondary insults of the transfer process itself.

- The interhospital transfer of critically ill children by non-specialised transfer teams may be associated with unacceptable and largely preventable transfer related morbidity.

- Specialised paediatric transport teams can transfer critically ill children with minimal transfer related morbidity and with a significant decrease in the severity of illness during stabilisation and transport.

- The ethos of mobile intensive care implies that the level of therapy and monitoring the child receives at the referring hospital during the period of stabilisation and transport should be comparable to that received by the child had it been admitted directly to the paediatric intensive care unit.

- Children with trauma often need rapid transfer by specialised paediatric transport team to a centre offering definitive surgery. A favourable outcome in trauma patients will ensue only if the **ABC** of paediatric resuscitation has been adhered to.

- The immediate institution of therapeutic measures by personnel at the referring hospital while awaiting arrival of the specialised paediatric transport team is crucial to patient outcome. It is, therefore, essential that the specialised paediatric transport team be involved in the patient's management from the time of the initial request for transfer.

- Up to 60% of critically ill children require some form of airway management or respiratory support by the specialised paediatric transport team on arrival at the referring hospital. It is, therefore, mandatory for members of the specialised paediatric transport team to be skilled in airway management, ventilatory techniques, and the use of sedatives and muscle relaxants.

- Central venous access should be obtained in any patient with established or potential haemodyanamic instability prior to transport.

- In all critically ill, ventilated and/or haemodynamically unstable patients, mean, systolic and diastolic blood pressures should be monitored directly by pressure transduction of an indwelling intra-arterial catheter as well as indirectly by oscillometry.

- Fluid resuscitation, institution or modification of vasoactive drug therapy and correction of metabolic derangements are among the major therapeutic measures that specialised paediatric transport team will need to perform.

- The ethos of mobile intensive care should apply to transfers within the hospital, however short the distance.

2 Audit Commission. Children first. A study of hospital services. London: HMSO, 1993; 17–28

3 British Paediatric Association. Transfer of critically ill children. In: The Care of Critically Ill Children. Report of the multidisciplinary working party on intensive care. London: British Paediatric Association, 1993; 7–17

4 NHS Centre for Review and Dissemination. Which way forward for the care of critically ill children? (CRD report No.1). York: University of York, 1995; 15–84

5 Pollack MM, Ruttimann UE, Getson PR. Pediatric risk of mortality (PRISM) score. Crit Care Med 1988; 16: 1110–1116

6 Pollack MM. Pediatric transport research: it is improving (finally). Crit Care Med 1994; 22: 1073–1074

7 Neonatal transport. In: McCloskey KA, Orr RA. (eds) Pediatric Transport Medicine. St Louis: Mosby, 1995; 404–462

8 Paediatric Intensive Care Society. Standards for Paediatric Intensive Care. Bishop's Stortford: Saldatore, 1996; 19–29

9 Krug SE. Principles and philosophy of transport stabilisation. In: McCloskey KA, Orr RA. (eds) Pediatric Transport Medicine. St Louis: Mosby, 1995; 132–142

10 Orr RA, McCloskey KA, Britten AG. Transportation of critically ill children. In: Rogers MC. (ed) Textbook of Pediatric Intensive Care. Baltimore: Williams & Wilkins, 1992; 1571–1587

11 Whitfield JM, Buser NNP. Transport stabilisation times for neonatal and pediatric patients prior to interfacility transfer. Pediatr Emerg Care 1993; 9: 69–71

12 Macnab A. Optimal escort for interhospital transport of pediatric emergencies. J Trauma 1991; 31: 205–209

13 Orr RA, Venkataraman ST, Cinoman MI, Hogue BL, Singleton CA, McCloskey KA. Pretransport pediatric risk of mortality (PRISM) score underestimates the requirement for intensive care or major interventions during interhospital transport. Crit Care Med 1994; 22: 101–107

14 Britto J, Nadel S, Habibi P, Levin M. Paediatric risk of mortality score underestimates the requirement for intensive care during interhospital transport. Crit Care Med 1994; 22: 2029–2030.

15 Britto J, Nadel S, Levin M, Habibi P. Severity of illness scores and risk of complication during transfer. Intensive Care Med 1996; 22: 1130–1131

16 Ramsey CB, Holbrook PR. Pediatric critical care transport. In: Holbrook PR. (ed) Textbook of Pediatric Critical Care. Philadelphia: Saunders, 1993; 1108–1116

17 Sperrin M, Davies A, Smith R, Burgess R. Protection of sensitive patient connected medical devices from the subversive use of mobile telecommunication equipment. Intensive Crit Care Nurs 1997; 13: 170–172

18 Black RA, Mayer T, Walker ML et al. Air transport of pediatric emergency cases. N Engl J Med 1982; 307: 1465–1468

19 Runcie CJ, Reeve W, Reidy J, Dougall JR. A comparison of measurements of blood pressure, heart rate and oxygenation during interhospital transport of the critically ill. Intensive Care Med 1990; 16: 317–322

20 Brink LW, Neuman B, Wynn J. Air transport. Pediatr Clin North Am 1993; 40: 439–456

21 Ackerman N. Aeromedical physiology. In: McCloskey KA, Orr RA. (eds) Pediatric Transport Medicine. St Louis: Mosby, 1995; 143–157

22 Fuller J, Frewen T, Lee R. Acute airway management in the critically ill child requiring transport. Can J Anaesth 1991; 38: 252–254

23 Houck CS. Access to the airway. In: Holbrook PR. (ed) Textbook of Pediatric Critical Care. Philadelphia: Saunders, 1993; 430–441

24 Hussain SNA, Roussos C. Distribution of respiratory muscle and organ blood flow during endotoxic shock in dogs. J Appl Physiol 1985; 59: 1802–1808

25 Vera FT, Dean MJ, Hanley DF. Evaluation of the comatose child. In: Rogers MC. (ed) Textbook of Pediatric Intensive Care. Baltimore: Williams & Wilkins, 1996; 733–745

26 Rivera R, Tibbals J. Complications of endotracheal intubation and mechanical ventilation in infants and children. Crit Care Med 1992; 20: 193–199

27 Backofen JE, Rogers MC. Emergency management of the airway. In: Rogers MC. (ed) Textbook of Pediatric Intensive Care. Baltimore: Williams & Wilkins, 1992; 52–74

28 Kanter RK, Tompkins JM. Adverse events during interhospital transport: physiological deterioration associated with pretransport severity of illness. Pediatrics 1989; 84: 43–48

29 Scott PH, Eigen H, Moye LA, Georgitis J, Laughin JJ. Predictability and consequences of spontaneous extubation in a pediatric ICU. Crit Care Med 1985; 13: 228–232

30 Henning R. Emergency transport of critically ill children: stabilisation before departure. Med J Aust 1992; 156: 117–124

31 Rosen KR, Rosen DA. Comparative flow rates for small bore peripheral intravenous catheters. Pediatr Emerg Care 1986; 2: 153–156

32 Wetzel RC, Tobin JR. Shock. In: Rogers MC. (ed) Textbook of Pediatric Intensive Care. Baltimore: Williams & Wilkins, 1992; 563–613

33 Wallen E, Venkataraman ST, Grosso MJ, Kiene K, Orr RA. Intrahospital transport of critically ill pediatric patients. Crit Care Med 1995; 23: 1588–1595

34 McCloskey KA, Orr RA. (ed) Pediatric Transport Medicine. St Louis: Mosby Year Book Company, 1995.

35 Causes of death in childhood. In: Advanced Paediatric Life Support, 2nd edn. London: BMJ, 1997; 3–5

36 Sharples PM, Storey A, Aynsley-Green A, Eyre JA. Avoidable factors contributing to the death in children with head injury. BMJ 1990; 300; 87–91

37 Rubenstein JS, Hageman JR. Monitoring of critically ill infants and children. Crit Care Clin 1988; 4: 621–639

38 Rennick G, Shann F, de Campo J. Cerebral herniation during bacterial meningitis in children. BMJ 1993; 306: 953–955

39 Archer BD. Computed tomography before lumbar puncture in acute meningitis: a review of the risks and benefits. Can Med Assoc J 1993; 148: 961–965

40 Berkowitz ID, Berkowitz FE, Newton C, Willoughby R, Ackerman AD. Meningitis, infectious encephalopathies and other central nervous system infections. In: Rogers MC. (ed) Textbook of Pediatric Intensive Care. Baltimore: Williams & Wilkins 1996; 1039–1090

41 Kanter RK. Watchko JF. Pulmonary oedema associated with upper airway obstruction. Am J Dis Child 1984; 138: 356–358

42 Britto J, Habibi P, Levin M, Nadel S. Systemic complications associated with bacterial tracheitis. Arch Dis Child 1996; 74: 249–250

43 Shock. In: Advanced Paediatric Life Support, 2nd edn. London: BMJ, 1997: 85–98

44 Nadel S, Habibi P, Levin M. Management of acute meningococcal disease in childhood. In: Meningococcal Disease. Cartwright K. (ed) New York: Wiley, 1995: 207–243

45 Barry PW, Ralston C. Adverse events occurring during interhospital transfer of the critically ill. Arch Dis Child 1994; 71: 8–11

46 Britto J, Nadel S, Habibi P, Levin M. Adverse events occurring during interhospital transfer of the critically ill. Arch Dis Child 1994; 71: 559

47 Edge WE, Kanter RK, Weigle CGM, Walsh RF. Reduction of morbidity in interhospital transport by specialised pediatric staff. Crit Care Med 1994; 22: 1186–1191

48 Britto J, Nadel S, Machonochie I, Levin M, Habibi P. Morbidity and severity of illness during interhospital transport: Impact of a specialised paediatric retrieval team. BMJ 1995; 311: 836–839

49 Britto J, Nadel S, Machonochie I, Levin M, Habibi P. Impact of specialised paediatric retrieval teams. BMJ 1996; 312: 121

50 McCloskey KA. Transport team training. In: McCloskey KA, Orr RA. (eds) Pediatric Transport Medicine. St Louis: Mosby, 1995: 100–107

51 Shann F. Should there be specialist paediatric transport services? NHS Centre for Review and Dissemination. Which way forward for care of critically ill children? (CRD report No.1). York: University of York, 1995; 49–50

John M. Bamford   Adrian Davis

CHAPTER 7

Hearing screening

About 840 children are born each year in the UK with a significant permanent hearing loss, the severity of which may vary from moderate to profound. A smaller number, about 160, **acquire** a permanent hearing loss in their early years. The majority of these children have a sensorineural hearing loss, and the effects on their development can be substantial. Early detection can offset some of these problems, and so hearing screening programmes aim to help secure the early identification of children with permanent childhood hearing impairment.

A much larger number of children encounter temporary and fluctuating hearing loss of a mild or moderate degree due to otitis media with effusion, with a point prevalence of perhaps 20% and a period prevalence (0–8 years) of some 90%.[1] The point prevalence of otitis media with effusion increases in the winter months, in the second 6 months of life, and at school entry. Some groups (e.g. children with Down's syndrome, cleft palate, and a history of neonatal special care) are particularly at risk for repeated bouts of otitis media with effusion.

The short and medium term effects of hearing impairment associated with otitis media with effusion are contentious, and are dependent upon the persistence and severity of the condition. It is likely that 1–5% of children will suffer repeated bouts of otitis media with effusion of severity and persistence sufficient to have measurable effects upon speech and language development, verbal and cognitive development, behaviour and early educational (including literacy) skills.[1] These effects may not be apparent in the long-term. Prediction of **which** children with transient effusions will suffer effects in the medium term is difficult, and their identification, therefore, depends on a process of 'watchful waiting' which to be efficient involves primary health services as well as community and tertiary (ENT and audiology) services, with good information

John M. Bamford BA PhD, Professor of Audiology and Education of the Deaf; Centre for Human Communication and Deafness, University of Manchester, Oxford Road, Manchester M13 9PL, UK

Adrian Davis BSc MSc PhD, Head of Epidemiology, Public Health and Clinical Section, MRC Institute of Hearing Research, Nottingham, UK

exchange. Since the condition is common, transient, and has variable effects depending upon severity and persistence, one-off screening tests of hearing as a way of identifying appropriate cases are difficult to justify on a universal basis; targeted screening for identified sub-populations at risk for otitis media with effusion awaits increased understanding of the condition, its causes, risk factors and natural history. Hearing screening tests are justifiable, however, for children with permanent hearing impairment, and such screens will adventitiously refer a number of cases with otitis media with effusion; this route provides, therefore, an opportunistic though non-optimal pathway for the identification of **some** of the effusion cases which turn out to have an associated hearing impairment of sufficient severity or persistence to warrant active intervention (advisory, therapeutic and/or surgical).

The impact of permanent hearing impairment upon child and family can, however, be substantial and long-term. It has been argued since the 1950s that the 'early detection and management of [permanent] hearing impairment will help to lessen the impact of the condition on the child's social, emotional, intellectual and linguistic development. The child and family will benefit from such early detection and management'.[2] While parental observation and good responsive services will identify some children relatively early, satisfactory identification rates will not be achieved without secondary intervention – that is to say, screening programmes. The opportunities for primary intervention (i.e. prevention) for permanent hearing impairment in the UK are still limited (despite notable exceptions, such as rubella immunisation) and await further research (e.g. in genetics).

These arguments underpin the long history in the UK of hearing screening for permanent hearing impairment, particularly the Health Visitor Distraction test and the School Entry Screen introduced universally in the 1950s and 1960s.[3] The UK's public health perspective on hearing screening for permanent hearing impairment has been founded upon beliefs and observations about its epidemiology, its effects, and the efficacy of hearing screening tests. In the last decade or so the evidence base on epidemiology, outcomes and screen performance has increased in quantity and quality; in addition, new tests with screening potential have been developed – particularly neonatal tests – and evidence on costs of screens has become available. This article summarises the main evidence on the epidemiology of permanent hearing impairment, outcomes, screen performance, and costs, and draws conclusions about the direction in which screening services might develop cost-effectively. For a more detailed review, the reader is referred to the authors' report to the Department of Health under the Health Technology Assessment programme.[4] As part of this review, a survey of current UK practice was carried out in order to provide the context for developments and recommendations, and the first of the following sections summarises key aspects of this survey.

CURRENT PRACTICE

The opportunities for hearing screening depend upon having suitable and developmentally-appropriate tests, and an accessible population. Table 7.1 summarises the details of the three hearing screening programmes which

Table 7.1 Hearing screening for Permanent Hearing Impairment: programmes, tests, target populations, and timing

Screening programme	Test(s)	Target population	Timing
Neonatal	Transient evoked oto-acoustic emissions Auditory brainstem response Portable auditory response cradle	All newborns or at-risk newborns	At or soon after birth
Health Visitor Distraction Test	Distraction test	All infants	7–8 months
School entry screen	Pure tone 'sweep' audiometry	All infants	School entry: 4–5 years

utilise (potentially) suitable tests and which could be (or are) applied to an accessible population in the UK. Otoacoustic emissions[5] reflect an active physiological process of the healthy cochlea, and involve presentation of rapid clicks to the neonate's ear via a small probe, and the measurement and averaging of the acoustic response picked up by a miniature microphone also in the probe assembly. Auditory brainstem response[6] also involves presentation of rapid clicks, via an earphone, and the measurement and averaging of the consequent electrical activity generated in the VIII nerve and auditory brainstem pathways, via electrodes attached to the baby's head. The Portable Auditory Response Cradle[7] monitors the behavioural response of the neonate (e.g. head/body movement) in response to high pass noise presented via headphone. All these tests can be completed in a matter of minutes, or even seconds, depending upon the baby's state and background noise levels. Rate of screening is determined more by other factors (availability of babies, time to collect and return, interaction with parent) than by test time.[8]

The infant Distraction Test Screen is a behavioural test of hearing involving parent, child and two testers, one of whom at least is a Health Visitor. A semi-automated version which might necessitate only one tester is being developed and will, in due course, be evaluated. Frequency-specific low-level (35 dB) sounds are presented to the child sitting on parent's knee, and localisation (head turn) responses noted. The School Entry Screen test involves frequency-specific pure tones (0.5, 1, 2, and 4 kHz usually) presented via headphones at 20 or 25 dB HL for an appropriate behavioural response from the child (e.g. button press, placing a brick in a box, etc.).

Table 7.2 summarises some of the main points from the survey of current practice[4] which are relevant to this chapter. The survey was based upon detailed questionnaires to all providers in the UK, with an eventual response rate in excess of 90%. Since the quality of information kept by respondents was not always as high as one would wish, some of the detailed data returned may be questionable; however, the main results are representative. Two Districts have universal neonatal screening in place (one using otoacoustic emissions, one the Portable Auditory Response Cradle); over half the UK Districts are implementing, often in a highly targeted or ad hoc way (i.e. not yet approaching full

Table 7.2 Summary of current UK screening practice

Screen	Implementation	Reported coverage (mean)	Reported referral rate (mean)	Average age of confirmation of Permanent Hearing Impairment for cases identified via this route	Reported yield for Permanent Hearing Impairment as % of expected total cases
Targeted (at risk) neonatal	Nearly two-thirds of all Districts[1,2]	30%[3]	5–8%	3 months	16%[4]
Universal neonatal	2 Districts	95%+	1%	3 months	85% or more
Health Visitor Distraction Test	Almost all Districts	90%	10%	18 months	27%
School Entry Screen	Almost all Districts	95%	10%	_[5]	_[5]

[1]We use the 'old' term District for ease of interpretation.
[2]This figure reflects much ad hoc practice, rather than true (at risk) population screening.
[3]Thus, coverage of the definable at-risk population is low.
[4]The tests have high sensitivity (see later sections); this figure is low largely because of the low coverage.
[5]The School Entry Screen will pick up late onset cases of Permanent Hearing Impairment, and any missed by earlier screens; thus entries here could be misleading.

coverage of all at-risk cases) neonatal screening targeted to at-risk cases. Nevertheless, the reported yield from neonatal screening for 1994 of cases with permanent childhood hearing impairment > 50 dB HL was 100 cases in 39 Districts, representing about 16% of the expected total cases born in the UK that year. The Health Visitor screen and the School Entry screen are implemented in almost all Districts, but the yield from the Health Visitor screen (even in Districts without neonatal screening) is low, reflecting concern which has been expressed previously (see below).

EPIDEMIOLOGY

Much of the epidemiological work on Permanent Hearing Impairment has been carried out with small populations using solely clinic-based lists or registers that were not uniformly ascertained across all levels of severity. The most recent and thorough study in the UK is reported by Fortnum and Davis.[9] This study ascertained children with bilateral Permanent Hearing Impairment of 40 dB or more born in Trent Region between 1985 and 1993 and resident in the Region in the study period (1994–1996). This Region has a population of 5 million, an ethnic minority population of about 5%, and an annual birth cohort of about 61 000. Ascertainment of cases was high, probably approaching 100%

Table 7.3 The discrete prevalence per 100 000 children of three broad severity categories of Permanent Hearing Impairment as a function of onset (congenital versus 'acquired') for the birth cohort 1985–1990 in Trent[4,9]

	Severity dB HL	Prevalence per 100 000	95% confidence intervals	
Congenital	40–69 Moderate	64	56	73
	70–94 Severe	23	19	29
	> 95 Profound	24	20	30
'Acquired'	40–69 Moderate	9	7	12
	70–94 Severe	5	3	8
	> 95 Profound	7	5	10

for the years 1985–1990, and the data presented here are based upon the 487 hearing-impaired children born in that period.

Table 7.3 summarises the discrete prevalence (per 100 000 children) of the three broad severity categories of Permanent Hearing Impairment as a function of onset (congenital versus 'acquired') in Trent. Congenital cases refer to those presumed to have had hearing impairment pre or perinatally. 'Acquired' cases are those thought to be late onset, progressive or truly acquired (e.g. from meningitis). There are about 112 per 100 000 children who have **congenital** Permanent Hearing Impairment of 40 dB or more in the better ear. The Trent study suggests that about 16% of all Permanent Hearing Impairment cases are late onset, progressive or acquired of which one-third are from meningitis; thus about 10% of all Permanent Hearing Impairment cases may be progressive or late onset, and would not be detected by a screen at birth nor possibly by a 7–8 month screen. (Some other studies have suggested a higher proportion of progressive or late onset cases.) If these prevalence figures are combined with the UK live births (for 1994), we might expect there to be just under 1000 hearing-impaired children (bilateral, moderate or greater) in the UK per annual birth cohort, 840 of whom would be congenitally impaired. This translates into about 11 000 school age children (5–15 years) of which about 2500 will have a profound hearing loss; and about 5000 pre-school children with Permanent Hearing Impairment. Thus the implications for Education Services are considerable (see below).

With regard to at-risk newborn screening, Fortnum and Davis[9] found that just under 30% of the hearing-impaired children have a Neonatal Intensive Care history, about 27% have a family history of Permanent Hearing Impairment and nearly 4% have a craniofacial abnormality (taken in precedence). Thus, in theory, about 60% of cases have a major risk factor. However, the actual yield of neonatal screening targeted at these three risk factors is likely to be no greater than 35–45% due to the difficulty of implementing the family history factor.

Age of referral, confirmation of hearing loss, prescription and fitting of hearing aids have been used in the past as useful if surrogate measures of screening outcome.[2] Fortnum and Davis[9] collected these data for their cohort born between 1985 and 1990, with presumed congenital onset and who were born in their district of residence ($n = 350$). Figure 7.1 shows the cumulative

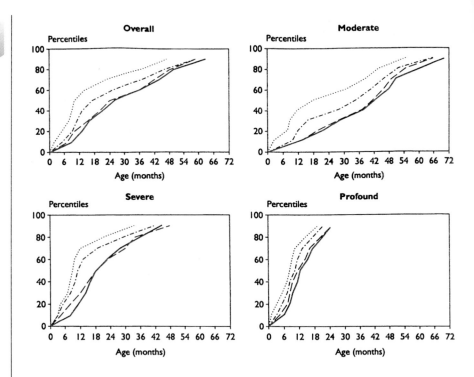

Fig. 7.1 Distribution of age at referral (*n* = 284), confirmation of permanent hearing impairment (*n* = 309), prescription of hearing aids (*n* = 223), and fitting of hearing aids (*n* = 336) for children born 1985–1990 with presumed congenital onset (*n* = 350) who were born in their district of residence, within Trent Region. The four panels show the overall data and separately for moderate, severe and profound hearing loss. (From Fortnum and Davis[9]).

distributions of the service indicators for the whole sample, and for the moderate, severe and profound degrees of hearing impairment separately.

The figure shows that for all hearing-impaired children the referral rate distribution is in two parts. The first part is fairly steep and is then followed by a shallower curve indicating a slowing of referrals. The age of confirmation of hearing impairment lags behind the age of referral by about 12 weeks at the lower quartile but the delay increases as the distribution gets more extreme. It is interesting to compare all three severities of hearing impairment. For the profound impairments the rate of referral is relatively high, with 75% of referral being completed by 11 months. There does not appear to be an obvious effect of the Health Visitor screen at 6–9 months on the referral pattern, suggesting that many of these children are identified by professional and parental concern in the early months of life. However, for severe impairments the upper quartile is only reached after 17 months, and for moderate impairments it is a very long 41.8 months. The change in slope of referral comes at about 70% for the severely impaired. This reflects the incremental yield from the Health Visitor screen, which is quite marked, ceasing at about 12 months. It is not until later when these children are noticed to have delayed language that the remaining thirty per cent start to trickle in for hearing assessment. There is a small change in the rate of referral for moderately impaired children due to the Health Visitor screen. However, the slope is much shallower than that for the severely and profoundly impaired, and is a trickle of referrals most of the time. The difference between referral, confirmation and hearing aid fitting is small for the profound, larger for the severe and very large for the moderate impairment groups. This reflects partly the urgency for profound cases, but also the difficulty some services find in assessing accurately the severely and moderately-impaired children. For children with a hearing impairment in excess of 50 dB HL the current wait for hearing aid fitting is longer than recommended.[10] It is not the impetus of screening that lies behind the incremental yield patterns, it is the severity of the hearing impairment, with the profound cases being similar to more adequate service provision and moderate cases being similar to poor service provision. The immediate challenge is to lift the severe and moderately impaired detection rate to be similar to that of the profoundly impaired, and to improve all detection rates to meet suggested targets. It should be recognised that the paediatric audiological services in Trent are regarded as being reasonably well developed, and the efforts put into making the Health Visitor screen effective have been quite large. Hence, these data can be thought of as being towards the better end of the quality distribution.

OUTCOMES

The evidence from epidemiological studies is that Permanent Hearing Impairment is a significant public health issue, with considerable implications for education services, and that services identify children at ages significantly later than current quality targets.[2] It is clear from our own focus groups[4] and from parent surveys[11,12] that parents want identification to be as early as possible. The ethical (and legal) arguments for very early identification – which implies neonatal screening – are now strong, if neonatal screens can be shown to be a practical proposition (see below). The evidence to support the view that early detection (and management) lessens the social, emotional, intellectual and linguistic impact of the hearing loss on the child and family is less clear. The evidence that early identification brings outcome benefits is reviewed in Davis et al.[4] However, the number of good quality studies which allow reasonably unequivocal data interpretation in the field of early identification of congenital Permanent Hearing Impairment is rather few. Many studies are marred by small samples, potential biases and lack of controls, variable definitions of 'early', lack of agreement of appropriate outcome measures, lack of specification of the details of the interventions used, and the failure to separate the effects of 'earlyness' from the effects of the interventions used.

Nevertheless, some studies provide useful and indicative data. Yoshinaga-Itano et al[13] compared the language abilities of hearing-impaired children identified before 6 months of age with those whose hearing loss was identified after 6 months, but who were enrolled in the same support programme. The early identified children showed significant benefits in vocabulary size, expressive and receptive language, and consonant and vowel production. Markides[14] showed more intelligible speech in hearing impaired children who had been fitted with hearing aids before 6 months of age, compared with groups fitted 6–12 months, 12–24 months, and 24+ months. Ramkalawan and Davis[15] studied a number of language metrics in a group of children with congenital hearing-impairment, and found that the lower the age of intervention, the better the language measures were found to be. Eilers and Oller[16] showed a significant relationship between the age of hearing aid fitting and the onset of canonical babbling. Robinshaw,[17,18] in a detailed study of the habilitative progress of a small group of children with congenital hearing impairment who were identified very early (3–6 months), has shown that it is possible for some deaf children to follow a normal pattern of communicative development provided that appropriate and timely intervention is carried out.

Thus, the hard experimental evidence from early intervention studies needed to conclude that very early identification and habilitation are better than at, say, 12 months is still emerging. A review of the evidence on early sensitive periods for language acquisition and on neural plasticity[4] points to: (i) early sensitive periods for aspects of language acquisition; and (ii) substantial and long-term detrimental effects of the lack of sensory input on neuronal pathways.

These two conclusions help to buttress the findings from the review of outcome evidence, namely that there is a potential for more successful language acquisition with early intervention; and that better short- and medium-term outcomes in the communication domain are achieved for children with moderate to profound impairments who are identified earlier.

PERFORMANCE OF HEARING SCREENS

There have been a relatively large number of published studies examining the efficacy and effectiveness of neonatal and Health Visitor screening in the UK. Again, for a detailed review see Davis et al.[4] The two existing universal neonatal screens as service in the UK,[7,8] and the one controlled study[19] show that high coverage for universal newborn screening (95%+) is possible despite current patterns of early maternity discharges. All neonatal methods show high screen specificity, generally well above 90%. However, coverage and specificity achieve acceptable levels only after a significant 'settling in' period (including explicit training) of up to 12 months. This, and other evidence, points to the very considerable implementation and planning issues, for both health and education services, that accompany the introduction of universal neonatal hearing screening.

Evidence on screen sensitivity for moderate and greater cases of congenital Permanent Hearing Impairment indicates figures in the range 80–100%.[20–22] Programme sensitivity, bearing in mind coverage loss, may be conservatively estimated to be nearer 70–80% than 100%; however, the necessary retrospective nature of sensitivity estimates, coupled with rapid technological improvements, may mean that the sensitivity of current neonatal screening programmes could be higher. Certainly, the two large cohort studies of universal hearing screening in the UK[8,19] produce yields of the expected order; and, furthermore, reduce the subsequent incremental yields of the Health Visitor screen to very low levels.

With regard to targeted (at risk) neonatal screens, the population to be screened consists of babies admitted to neonatal intensive care units for more than 48 hours, babies with craniofacial abnormalities, and babies with a family history of Permanent Hearing Impairment. This represents 5–10% of the total birth cohort but has a potential yield of 60% of congenital Permanent Hearing Impairment cases.[9] In current practice, however, this is lower, perhaps 35–45% at best, because of the system's difficulty of identifying and referring cases with a positive family history from antenatal appointments and postnatal wards.

For cases screened neonatally, the median age of identification is of the order of 2 months,[9,23] depending upon follow-up procedures and severity of impairment,[8] and is significantly earlier than cases not screened neonatally.[19]

Although the evidence was not published, it seems likely that the Health Visitor screen significantly improved the age of identification of Permanent Hearing Impairment when it was introduced in the 1950s. More recently, however, doubts have been expressed about its effectiveness.[24,25] Much recent effort has been put in to improve its sensitivity.[26] Since the screen cannot, for developmental reasons, be implemented before about 7 months, the identification age is necessarily later than for neonatal screening. However, because of the relatively high fail rate (5–10%) and consequent false positive rate (for Permanent Hearing Impairment, although not perhaps for cases of fluctuating otitis media with effusion), delays occur in achieving confirmation. The reported median identification age ranges from 12–20 months, depending upon severity of impairment.[27,28] Coverage of the Health Visitor screen can be high, 90%+, but some evidence indicates poor coverage in inner city areas.[29]

Sensitivity estimates for the Health Visitor screen vary widely from 18–88%. The recent large cohort study with high ascertainment indicated an overall sensitivity of only 65%, varying from 80% for profound cases to 54% for moderate.[9] Other large and good quality studies present similar figures,[30] and these are from areas where service provision and monitoring is likely to be quite good. Thus the yield may be at best 40–45%, falling to 20–25% or to near zero when at-risk or universal neonatal screening (respectively) is introduced.

With regard to the School Entry Screen, there is little or no published evidence on the aims and effectiveness of the screen. However, costs are probably low, coverage is high[4] and it probably serves to raise awareness of the importance of hearing at a key developmental and educational point. On balance, therefore, reviewers have been supportive of the screen,[1] although more service research and audit is needed.

COSTS

Stevens et al[31] designed a cost study to obtain systematic data on neonatal and Health Visitor screening in 10 provider units. Providers were chosen who: (i) had ongoing neonatal screens in place; or (ii) had the Health Visitor screen in place; and (iii) could identify staff costs and provide audit data. Details of the methodology can be found elsewhere.[4,31] Table 7.4 summarises key costing evidence from this study.

The data, using the three established UK screening programmes, suggest that universal neonatal hearing screening has lower costs per child screened than the Health Visitor screen. Note that variations in the associated costs should be expected due to the details of local organization and implementation. Since

Table 7.4 Estimated cost per thousand live births (not per 1000 children tested) for differing preschool hearing screening programmes.[4,31] Note that these estimates include follow-up costs to the point at which false positives are correctly identified as normally hearing

Screen programme	Cost per 1000 births (£)
Targeted neonatal	5100
Universal neonatal	13 900
Health Visitor Distraction Test	25 700

screen sensitivity is higher for neonatal screening, the cost per case found would be much lower with universal neonatal screening. Stevens et al investigated both the cost per child tested and the cost per 1000 birth cohort. The cost per hearing impaired child detected was examined to show the relative differences between screening programmes.[4] Under different sets of assumptions the relativities favoured the neonatal screening over the Health Visitor screen quite substantially.

This costs study examined costs of screens up to the point at which false positives would be correctly identified as normally hearing. It should be noted, however, that earlier identification itself brings extra costs in both the health and education sector. The extra health costs might be £2000 per annum per hearing impaired child (earmoulds, hearing aids earlier, assessments, extra reviews, etc.). The major impact is likely to be felt in the education sector, where extra home support and management from teachers of the deaf and educational audiologists would be required to a significant degree – we estimate that these could be in the region of £6000 per child per year. On the other hand, if indeed earlier intervention results in improved outcomes in communication, educational achievement, mental and family health, and employment then the later savings to education, health and social services could be substantial. This is an area in need of much further detailed research.

IMPLEMENTATION ISSUES

In reality, there is currently no national hearing screening programme in the UK for identifying children with permanent hearing impairment. Provider units offer a wide variety of systems, including: Health Visitor screening; Health Visitor screen and targeted neonatal screening; Health Visitor screen and universal neonatal screening; universal neonatal screening and Health Visitor surveillance; targeted neonatal screening and Health Visitor screening. Each area is at a different point in its development of screening and habilitative services, and development plans differ. The current purchaser/provider arrangements have probably exacerbated this variability of service, leading to what parents and professionals perceive[4] to be a fragmented and unsatisfactory service, from screening onwards. There is considerable support for the view that effective habilitation is crucially dependent upon not only early identification, but family-centred services in which collaboration

Table 7.5 Main screening options (from Davis et al[4])

Option	Details
O	No screen – responsive service only
HO	Universal health visitor screen
H1	Targeted neonatal screening plus universal health visitor screen
H2	As for H1, but with semi-automated health visitor screen
H3	As for H1, but replace health visitor screen with surveillance by questionnaire
T1	Targeted neonatal screen
T2	Targeted neonatal screen plus targeted infant distraction test
U1	Universal neonatal screen
U2	Universal neonatal screen plus targeted infant distraction test

between primary, community and hospital care, and between health and education, is 'seamless'. The review by Davis et al[4] suggests strongly that this is currently not the case. Whatever screening programme for identifying Permanent Hearing Impairment is in place, more effort is required to set up local monitoring procedures and multi-agency teams to implement policy changes, involving health, education and parents. Although challenging to achieve, joint commissioning might offer a mechanism for conceiving of hearing screening not as an end in itself, but as the start of a lifelong process from birth to adulthood of the hearing impaired child and family, involving health, education and social services.

With regard to the hearing screens, Davis et al[4] evaluated nine possible options for combinations of hearing screens on the basis of their review of the evidence and survey of current practice. Each option was appraised on the basis of running costs, yield, efficiency, responsiveness and equity.[32] The options are listed in Table 7.5 (note that option H1 is that suggested in the Hall Report recommendations[33]). While it is acknowledged that different Districts are at different stages in their hearing screening development, it is to be hoped that one of the effects of the Davis/Bamford report will be to encourage development plans to converge, such that there is significant movement towards uniformity of practice across the UK. Such policy convergence must be led by evidence, and the major points from the evidence are to be found in summary form in the Key Points for Clinical Practice (below). The main recommendation from the option appraisal is that purchasers and providers should be working (from different starting points) towards universal neonatal hearing screening. Such a screen will identify most (but not all) children with Permanent Hearing Impairment, at an earlier age than currently achieved, and at lower cost than at present; furthermore, later but cost-efficient surveillance procedures such as Health Visitor surveillance, and a **targeted** infant distraction test should be in place for those cases that missed the neonatal screen; and that very early intervention and family support will have implications for the services provided both by health and education.

These conclusions form the basis for recommendations made in the Health Technology Assessment report,[4] covering service development, implementation and research. The UK National Screening Committee will consider the report and recommendations during 1998. The outcome of their deliberations may be to convene a working group to define, amongst other things: (i) the quality standards that would define adequate screen performance; (ii) how to specify an information system that will allow performance to be measured; (iii) what should be done if screening falls below the required level of quality; and (iv) a recommended model for commissioners.

The recommendation that there be a national screening programme based on universal neonatal hearing screening, if adopted by the National Screening Committee, will take some time to evolve. The transition between current services and those envisaged in the recommendations will need careful multi-agency planning and will have cost implications. During the transition, the Health Visitor Screen will continue to play an important role. It is crucial to ensure adequate quality of such arrangements, in part by making use of existing training materials.

Hearing screening and consequent identification of Permanent Hearing Impairment is the start of a long process involving family, child, health and education. A multi-agency monitoring and policy-development body would be helpful to this process. Sharing information by way of a shared register between health and education of children with Permanent Hearing Impairment would be useful locally for monitoring service performance, and could be a start towards the development of a shared national register. Such a register would in time provide more detailed evidence on outstanding research questions, particularly in the areas of severity effects, and the effectiveness of different interventions and outcomes.

References

1 Haggard MP, Hughes E. Screening Children's Hearing. London: HMSO, 1991
2 NDCS. Quality standards in paediatric audiology, Vol I: Early identification of childhood hearing impairment. London: NDCS, 1994
3 Ewing AWG. (ed) Educational Guidance and the Deaf Child. Manchester: Manchester University Press, 1957
4 Davis A, Bamford J, Wilson I, Ramkalawan T, Forshaw M, Wright S. A critical review of the role of neonatal hearing screening in the detection of congenital hearing impairment. Health Technol Assess 1997; 10: 177
5 Kemp DT, Ryan S. Otoacoustic emission tests in neonatal screening programmes. Acta Otolaryngol Suppl 1991; 482: 73–84
6 Hyde ML, Malizia K, Riko K, Alberti PW. Audiometric estimation error with the ABR in high risk infants. Acta Otolaryngol Suppl 1991; 111: 212–219
7. Tucker SM, Bhattacharya J. Screening of hearing impairment in the newborn using the auditory response cradle. Arch Dis Child 1992; 67: 911–919
8 Watkin PM. Neonatal otoacoustic emission screening and the identification of deafness. Arch Dis Child 1996; 74: 16–25
9 Fortnum H, Davis AC. Epidemiology of permanent childhood hearing impairment in Trent Region 1985–1993. Br J Audiol 1997; 31: 409–446
10 NDCS Quality Standards in paediatric audiology, Vol II: Audiological management of the child with permanent hearing loss. London: NDCS, 1996
11 Watkin PM, Beckman A, Baldwin M. The views of parents of hearing impaired children on the need for neonatal hearing screening. Br J Audiol 1995; 29: 259–262
12 Watkin PM, Baldwin M, Dixon R, Beckman A. Maternal anxiety and attitudes to universal neonatal hearing screening. Br J Audiol; 1998; 32: 27–37

Key points for clinical practice

- The prevalence of congenital Permanent Hearing Impairment is about 112 per 100 000, and of late onset, progressive and acquired Permanent Hearing Impairment in children about 21 per 100 000 by age 5 years. About 1000 children per annual UK birth cohort have Permanent Hearing Impairment.

- About 60% of the congenital Permanent Hearing Impairment cases have a risk factor, not always identifiable at birth. Family history of Permanent Hearing Impairment is an important risk factor, as is neonatal intensive care admission.

- Evidence from parental surveys, animal studies, and outcome studies suggests that identification as early as possible of congenital Permanent Hearing Impairment gives the greatest potential for normal development.

- Current practice does not match service targets[2] for identification age.

- The School Entry Screen has been little researched, but is probably cost effective and fulfils a useful 'long stop' purpose.

- The Health Visitor Distraction Test screen has the disadvantage that it cannot be implemented before 7 months of age, for developmental reasons. It has a (relatively) high fail rate and a (relatively) poor sensitivity which is severity-dependent. Its performance is compromised by the high prevalence of otitis media with effusion in the second half of the first year of life. Its continuation as a universal screen is not a preferred option.

- The technology exists to screen neonates for auditory function using one (or more) of three tests. The evidence points to high yield, probable high test sensitivity, and low costs especially if implemented universally.

- Coverage of universal newborn hearing screening can be high, despite current birthing practice with short maternity stays, but the initial 'learning curve' may be up to 12 months or so.

- Implementation issues for neonatal hearing screening are not trivial. Parent information, tester training, database monitoring and case tracking, and interagency liaison are crucial.

13 Yoshinaga-Itano C, Sedey A, Coulter D, Mehl A. Language of early and later identified children with hearing loss. Paediatrics 1998: In Press

14 Markides A. Age at fitting of hearing aids and speech intelligibility. Br J Audiol 1986; 20: 165–167

15 Ramkalawan TW, Davis AC. The effects of hearing loss and age of intervention on some language metrics in young hearing-impaired children. Br J Audiol 1992; 26: 97–107

16 Eilers RE, Oller DK. Infant vocalisations and the early diagnosis of severe hearing impairment. J Pediatr 1994; 124: 199–203

17 Robinshaw H. Early intervention for hearing impairment: identifying and measuring differences in the timing of communication and language development. Br J Audiol 1995; 29: 315–334

18 Robinshaw H. The pattern of development from non-communicative behaviour to language by hearing impaired and hearing infants. Br J Audiol 1996; 30: 177–198

19 Kennedy CR, Kimm L. Early identification of permanent childhood hearing impairment: a controlled trial of universal neonatal screening. Lancet 1998: In press.

20 Lutman ME, Davis AC, Fortnum HM, Wood S. Field sensitivity of targeted neonatal hearing screening by transient-evoked otoacoustic emissions. Ear Hearing 1997; 18: 265–276

21 Mason S, Davis AC, Wood S, Farnsworth A. Field sensitivity of targeted neonatal hearing screening using the Nottingham ABR screener. Ear Hearing; 1998; 19: 91–102

22 Maxon AB, White KR, Behrens TR, Vohr BR. Referral routes and cost efficiency in a universal newborn hearing screening programme using transient evoked otoacoustic emissions. J Am Acad Audiol 1995; 6: 271–277

23 McClelland RJ, Watson DR, Lawless V. Houston HG, Adams D. Reliability and effectiveness of screening for hearing loss in high risk neonates. BMJ 1992; 304: 806–809

24 Boothman R, Orr N. Value of screening for deafness in the first year of life. Arch Dis Child 1978; 53: 570–573

25 Robinson K. The scandal of late diagnosis in children. Health Visitor 1983; 56: 452–453

26 McCormick B. Hearing screening by Health Visitors: a critical appraisal of the distraction test. Health Visitor 1983; 56: 449–451

27 Watkin PM. The age of identification of childhood deafness – improvements since the 1970s. Public Health 1991; 105: 303–312

28 Sutton G, Scanlon P. Health visitor screening versus vigilance for childhood hearing impairment in West Berkshire: a ten year review. Personal communication

29 Brown J, Watson E, Alberman E. Screening infants for hearing loss. Arch Dis Child. 1989; 64: 1488–1495

30 Wood S, Davis AC, McCormick B. Changing performance of the Health Visitor Distraction Test when targeted neonatal screening is introduced into a health district. Br J Audiol 1997; 31: 55–62

31 Stevens JC, Hall DMB, Davis AC, Davies CM, Dixon S. The costs of early hearing screening in England and Wales. Arch Dis Child 1998; 78: 14–19

32. NHS. Priorities and Planning Guidance for the NHS. London: NHS Executive, 1996

33 Hall DMB. (ed) Health for All Children, 3rd edn. Oxford: Oxford University Press, 1996

Michael F. Smith

Advances in the management of the cerebral palsies

This chapter reviews recent developments in cerebral palsy (CP) management including evaluation of the effectiveness of physical therapy, the improved understanding of feeding disorders in children with CP, the use of botulinum toxin, the use of baclofen by intrathecal infusion, selective dorsal rhizotomy, and the development and application of gait analysis as a prelude to the 'simultaneous event multi level' orthopaedic surgical approach.

FEEDING DISORDERS IN CEREBRAL PALSY

Feeding disorders are commonplace in children with CP and, in general, affect those children with the more severe physical disabilities. Up to 40% of children with moderate and severe CP are frequently undernourished,[1] poor nutrition being more common amongst the younger and more severely disabled children. The major problems in feeding include incoordinate deglutition, tracheal aspiration of food and liquid and reflux oesophagitis. Of a group of 16 children with CP who were slow, inefficient, eaters, tracheal aspiration was demonstrated in 5 children by barium videofluoroscopy.[2] Mirrett et al[3] reported 15 of 22 children with severe CP had silent tracheal aspiration during feeding. This can have an important effect on respiratory morbidity in these children, resulting in recurrent lung infection, repeated admission to hospital and contributing to the high early mortality in the more severely affected patients.[4] Additional problems include gastro-oesophageal reflux, observed commonly in the most severely affected children. Reyes et al[5] reported an incidence of significant gastro-oesophageal reflux in 70% of children with feeding difficulties, vomiting and recurrent chest infection. Management of such children presents significant difficulties and, increasingly, it is recognised

Michael F. Smith MBBS FRCP FRCPCH
Consultant Paediatrician, Ryegate Children's Centre, Tapton Crescent Road, Sheffield, S10 5DD, UK,

that resort to an alternative feeding technique is indicated for those children with recurrent pulmonary problems, symptomatic gastro-oesophageal reflux, marked reluctance to feed and failure to thrive. Early indications are that children treated by fundoplication and gastrostomy placement enjoy an improved quality of life, nutritional state and probably a reduction in pulmonary morbidity. Such intervention cannot be undertaken lightly, because of the perioperative and early postoperative morbidity. Surgical treatment is preceded by detailed evaluation including assessment of concurrent medical problems, videofluoroscopy assessment of deglutition and gastro-oesophageal reflux, oesophagogastroscopy and pH monitoring. Borgstein et al[6] reported 50 neurologically impaired children who underwent fundoplication and gastrostomy between 1976 and 1992. While the procedure was generally successful, 12 children needed re-operation. There were 9 deaths during the follow-up period and in two of these children the death was operation related. The authors concluded that the improvements in quality of life achieved by the majority of the patients out-weighed the risks. More recently, laparoscopic fundoplication has been described and seems to carry a low intra-operative and postoperative complication rate with good outcome (e.g. see Ramachandran et al[7]).

PHYSICAL THERAPY

The cerebral palsies are a group of conditions which share the features of central (i.e. brain) motor deficits which are non progressive and are caused in early life. These conditions are permanent impairments and growth and development and changing musculo-skeletal relationships will inevitably alter the manner in which the motor impairment manifests. The fundamental pathology cannot be altered and it is, perhaps, not surprising to find that a wide variety of treatments have developed. Different approaches (e.g. Peto, Bobath, Ayres) have, from time to time, attracted considerable interest and enthusiasm, as well as equally vociferous opposition. More recently, attempts have been made to study the relative merits in an objective way. Of the studies thus far reported, it has been difficult to show a convincing argument in favour of a particular approach.[8–10] The holistic educational system referred to as conductive education has attracted significant interest and debate in recent years. Conductive education developed at the National Motor Therapy Institute in Budapest, Hungary, by Andras Peto (1903–1967) has a number of characteristics: relatively little special equipment, activities for children are mainly group based, the method is applied by 'conductors' who are staff trained in the Institute, rhythmic intention is used widely (the child and group rehearse a motor act to music or their own singing), great emphasis is placed on the child's own efforts to perform a given motor act, and high intensity. Children attend on a daily basis and the programme continues throughout the day and evening. Considerable claims have been made for the effectiveness of this approach in the popular press, although notably not by the Institute staff. Bairstow, Cochrane and Hur[11] reported a detailed evaluation of the conductive education approach as applied in a UK institute. The progress of children receiving conductive education was compared with the progress of children enrolled in the educational and therapy programmes in several special schools in Manchester, UK. The conductive education staff were trained and supported by staff from the Budapest Institute, who also selected all the children in the study. In this latter respect, the conductors concluded that a significant number of children with CP who were considered for the project would not benefit from conductive education, rejecting an estimated 65% of children with CP. A variety of techniques were employed in the initial and later assessments of the children in the study including a range of educational skills, language assessments, fine and gross motor measures, video analysis of specific tasks. The study group concluded that there were no grounds for believing that the children receiving conductive education made better progress than those receiving special education in the Manchester special schools. In particular, measures of hand skill progress, such as manipulation and object transfer, and gross motor function progress, showed no significant differences between the two groups, in spite of greater emphasis on physical skill development in the conductive education group. The study group concluded that while certain children responded well in the conductive education setting, there is insufficient evidence to recommend the widespread introduction of conductive education in the UK. In addition, it was recognised that there is a paucity of satisfactory data to support a number of the therapy practices undertaken in UK special educational provision.

Some further investigation of the effectiveness of different aspects of physical therapy is now available. Early intervention programmes remain popular, but supportive evidence in favour of such approaches remains elusive. In a randomised controlled trial of early physiotherapy in a group of 105 high risk infants, Weindling et al[12] were unable to demonstrate improved outcomes for those infants receiving therapy from birth compared to therapy commencing when abnormal neurological signs were recognised. Although it is difficult to demonstrate beneficial effects of early physiotherapy in these subjects, there may be significant positive effects in the families of the children. Evidence of the beneficial effects of strengthening exercise in CP has been shown in a number of studies. Carmick[13] used electrical stimulation to augment and strengthen gastrocnemius muscle in children with calf spasticity. Using electrical stimulation of the triceps surae during gait triggered by a remote switch, the study was able to show improved ankle motion in stance and swing, and this treatment had carry-over benefit for up to 5 months after the treatment programme had finished. This was a small observational study of 4 patients with no control data and details of the electrical stimulation component were not reported. Damiano and Abel[14] reported a prospective trial of strength training in 10 children (mean age 9.1 years) receiving a 6 week progressive resistance training programme. The disorders were either hemiplegia (4) or diplegia. Significant improvements in strength in both groups were recorded and there were improved gait parameters (velocity and cadence). Five children showed gains in gross motor function measures. Carry-over and duration were not reported. The effects of therapy directed to specific as opposed to general outcomes was examined by Bower et al.[15] This randomised controlled study of physiotherapy intervention contrasted the effects of intervention based upon general treatment aims (e.g. working towards sitting) with goal orientated therapy (e.g. sitting for a given period and function), in both 'intensive' and 'conventional' modes. 'Intensive' entailed daily therapy sessions 5 days per week. Treatment duration was 2 weeks in each group. This important study demonstrated that the only statistically significant difference was in favour of goal directed physiotherapy in the dimensions of the gross motor function measure scores,[16] where goals were set, compared to aim directed physiotherapy in the measures of the gross motor function measure scores where aims were set. There were indications of greater effectiveness of 'intensive' therapy compared to 'conventional' but these did not reach statistical significance. In the interpretation of these findings, it needs to be remembered that the trial treatment period was 2 weeks; nevertheless, these findings suggest that an effective treatment approach might include periods of intensive therapy aimed at specific goals as opposed to the conventional, regular, non intensive approach. Further studies of this question will undoubtedly be arduous but are essential such that definition of effective, timely and cost effective approaches can be achieved.

BOTULINUM TOXIN A

The role of botulinum toxin A in the management of CP has been the subject of considerable interest in recent years. The use of botulinum toxin A in children with CP was first described by Koman[17] in 1993 and several further studies have been reported since.[18–21]

Botulinum toxin A is the most studied of seven immunologically distinct toxins liberated by lysis of *Clostridium botulinum*. The toxins can be separated, crystallised and diluted with saline for clinical application by intramuscular injection. The use of botulinum toxin A has been reported in a variety of conditions including focal dystonias (blepharospasm, cervical dystonia), tremors, hemifacial spasm, tics, etc. More recently, attention has turned to the application of botulinum toxin A in CP. Botulinum toxin A cleaves synaptosomal associated protein, a cytoplasmic protein, which associates with the presynaptic membrane in the process of attachment of the synaptic vesicle to the membrane. When given by intramuscular injection, botulinum toxin A will diffuse into the muscle and, in some cases, may cross fascial planes, causing some local undesirable motor impairment, e.g. dysphagia following sternomastoid injections. Detectable effects following intramuscular injection of toxin occur after 2–13 days.[22] Multiple injections into a target muscle appear to be more effective and less likely to produce undesirable spread into adjacent areas. The duration of effect is usually 10–14 weeks, and measurable effects may persist for up to 26 weeks. In some children with CP, there appears to be a longer duration of action of up to 12 months, perhaps related to the effects initially of toxin on neuromuscular control and then, secondarily, on muscle growth.[23] It is important to appreciate that there are two preparations of botulinum toxin A, Botox (Allergan) and Dysport (Speywood), and that, although the measure of effectiveness relates to the LD_{50} for mice (mouse units), the 'potency' of the two preparations differs; the activity of 1 unit of Botox being approximately equivalent to 3 units of Dysport. The LD_{50} for monkeys by i.v. or i.m. injection is approximately 40 units/kg for Botox or 120 units/kg for Dysport and the dosing described for human usage is in the order of 2–8 units/kg body weight for Botox and 4–25 units/kg for Dysport.

Antibodies to botulinum toxin A develop in 3–10% of adult patients, in particular in those patients requiring frequent injections, or a high dose, or booster injections 2–3 weeks after previous injection treatment. Some authorities have reported even lower incidence of clinical antibody effects (2–3%)[24] and there is some evidence that children have fewer such complications.

In the upper limb, Corry et al[19] reported the effect of botulinum toxin A injection on elbow extension and hand function. Hand grasp score was improved, motor functional improvement was not demonstrated but patients reported significant beneficial cosmetic effects. In the lower limbs, Koman et al[17] conducted a double blind placebo controlled study in 12 CP patients age 4–11 years. Measures of effectiveness of treatment were by physician rating scale, observational gait analysis, physiotherapist examination, videotape recording of gait and Biodex isometric dynamometer. In 5/6 children treated with botulinum toxin A and in 2/6 control children, the physiotherapist assessment was rated as 'improved', the physician rating scale was improved, the parents' assessment was improved and the Biodex assessment was unsuccessful generally. Cosgrove et al[18] reported the results of botulinum toxin A treatment in a variety of spastic CP settings. Injection of the calf musculature was found to be effective in improving ankle motion in stance and swing phases of gait, the effect being better in the younger children (2–4 years) with some comparative reduction in effectiveness in the older children (6–8 years), particularly amongst those with hemiplegia. Of 23 treated patients, 17 showed a moderate or good response to the injection. Hamstring injection was almost universally effective and did not show the age decrement of below knee treatment. Mean improvements in knee extension of the order of 20° on passive testing were reported (21 groups in 14 patients, 1 non responder). Eames et al[21] measured gastrocnemius muscle length by gait analysis and showed peak effects following botulinum toxin A injection at 2 weeks to 3 months, with some residual effects on peak, but not mean, muscle length at 6 months post injection.[20]

Several further multicentre studies into the application of botulinum toxin A continue at the time of writing. The place of botulinum toxin A in the management of CP remains unclear. Its greatest value will probably lie in the postponement of surgical intervention until the child has achieved a mature gait pattern.[23] It can also be hoped that the extent of the eventual corrective surgery may be limited by careful application of the toxin in the growing child. Whether children will require less surgery and whether the timing of that surgery can be postponed remain important research questions. A useful review of the current status of botulinum toxin in the management of cerebral palsy has recently been published by Boyd and Kerr Graham.[23]

INTRATHECAL BACLOFEN

Baclofen is an analogue of gamma amino butyric acid and impedes excitatory neurotransmission at a spinal level. Oral baclofen has been in use in the management of spastic cerebral palsies for a number of years and in selected cases reduces tone by a factor in the order of 0.5–1.0 point on the Ashworth scale. More recently, the use of intrathecal baclofen by continuous infusion has been described.[24] This technique requires the placement of an intrathecal catheter and pump delivery system. The advantage of the technique lies in the much higher and continuous CSF baclofen level achieved (e.g. CSF level by oral administration 12–95 ng/ml, by intrathecal infusion 300–400 ng/ml).

In ambulatory patients, the most suitable for this technique are the 4–16 year-old children with spastic diplegia. Children who do less well with this technique are those who are slow, heavy or very weak. Poor motivation is also a contra-indication. In the non-ambulatory patients, those whose spasticity interferes with care are the most suitable. Treatment is preceded by a screening injection of 50 μg intrathecally by lumbar puncture and responses observed. If there is no response to this dose, 75 μg and then 100 μg may be tried. Patients who respond favourably may then be considered for an infusion system. The infusion pump requires replacement every 4–5 years. The infusion rate is usually in the order 0.1 ml/day, and percutaneous reloading of the system is required 2–4 monthly. Variable rate settings are possible, for example giving a higher dose during the early morning if required. Side effects include listlessness, apathy, urinary hesitancy, and weakness. Complications include a 5% incidence of pocket infection, catheter problems and accidental overdose caused by pump malfunction. Particular care should be taken in children who were born preterm and who may have some residual ventricular dilatation, as these children may develop CSF leak following catheter insertion. Pretreatment head CT scan is indicated in these children and blood patch at the time of catheter placement is recommended in those children who have residual ventricular dilatation. A blood patch is the injection of 2–3 ml of the patient's own blood into the CSF space down the catheter. This apparently forms a clot around the entry site of the catheter and prevents leakage. (Albright L, personal communication, 1997).

Outcome studies have shown 1–1.5 point reductions in spasticity on Ashworth scale, improved gross motor function measure scores and improved kinematics on gait analysis.[24]

SURGERY IN CEREBRAL PALSY

Selective posterior rhizotomy

There has been renewed interest over recent years in the procedure of selective posterior rhizotomy in patients with CP, especially in North America. Peacock[25] has popularised the approach. The procedure is conducted bilaterally under electromyographic control. Earlier approaches employed division of substantial numbers of the posterior rootlets but current practice has been refined to less extensive division, perhaps 40–50% of the rootlets. The procedure requires a period of postoperative intrathecal morphine analgesia followed by a period of phased rehabilitation over 6 weeks. Again two groups of patients are most suitable for this approach:

1. Where better ambulation is the expected outcome, These patients will need to have sufficient strength to be functional after their spasticity is reduced by the procedure. The best results are obtained amongst those children who are of good intelligence and well motivated.

2.   To improve care and relieve painful spasm. These patients are usually severely affected, non ambulant patients.

All treated patients will have increased weakness in the postoperative period. Complications include CSF leakage, dysaesthesia, sensory loss (rare), scoliosis, spine instability, hip dislocation, and valgus foot/midfoot break. Outcome studies have indicated significant reductions in spasticity, for example a change in Ashworth score of 1.1–1.5 versus 0–0.3 compared to intensive physiotherapy[26] and significant improvements in the Gross Motor Function Measure (5–11.3%) and dynamic joint ranges[27–29] following surgery. Stout et al[29] reported improved pelvic tilt and less need for subsequent psoas surgery when the rootlets treated included L1 to S1 as opposed to L2 to S1.

Orthopaedic surgical management of ambulant children with cerebral palsy

In children with cerebral palsy, abnormal muscle tone leads to abnormalities in function, contracture of affected muscles and secondary abnormalities of posture, such as bony torsions. While physiotherapy and medical treatment may prevent or delay the onset of significant contracture, some children will require surgical treatment to restore efficient musculoskeletal relationships. In these children, it has long been recognised that choice of surgical intervention in terms of timing, type and extent is difficult and is often unpredictable in its outcome, especially amongst ambulant children. As a consequence, surgeons have been cautious and have tended to treat only the most severely affected area at a particular time, and to treat areas sequentially. This serial approach to treatment (the 'birthday surgery syndrome' – Rang[30]) has been criticised in recent years as it has become clear that this approach frequently does not improve the long-term state of these patients.

The development and application of gait analysis to these patients has caused a radical change in the surgical approach. The development of computer and motion analysis systems over the past 20 years has facilitated the study of the principles underlying normal gait in adults and children. The systematic study of children's gait[31] has laid a foundation for the understanding of abnormal gait in children with cerebral palsy and other conditions. From this work, the principles underlying normal gait have been defined as well as the manner in which children with cerebral palsy deviate from the normal pattern. This has allowed the classification of certain types of movement disorder based upon gait analysis, for example, hemiplegic cerebral palsy (Fig. 8.1).[32] It can be seen that this classification is based upon the distal to proximal progression of involvement with increasing severity of cerebral palsy.

Two other points arise from consideration of this classification. Firstly, it can be seen that the predominant difficulties lie in the two joint muscles. This arises because these muscles are highly sophisticated in their action and timing. At different phases in normal gait contraction (either shortening, isometric or lengthening) of these bi-articular muscles subserve different functions. For example, in terminal stance and initial swing phase, the rectus femoris contracts concentrically as a hip flexor. In rapid walking the distal rectus femoris will also contract eccentrically to limit knee flexion. It is clear that precise timing of contraction is necessary in these muscles and this in turn

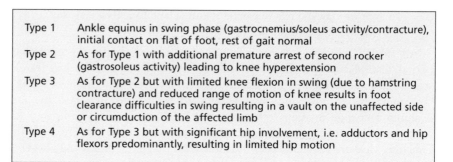

Type 1	Ankle equinus in swing phase (gastrocnemius/soleus activity/contracture), initial contact on flat of foot, rest of gait normal
Type 2	As for Type 1 with additional premature arrest of second rocker (gastrosoleus activity) leading to knee hyperextension
Type 3	As for Type 2 but with limited knee flexion in swing (due to hamstring contracture) and reduced range of motion of knee results in foot clearance difficulties in swing resulting in a vault on the unaffected side or circumduction of the affected limb
Type 4	As for Type 3 but with significant hip involvement, i.e. adductors and hip flexors predominantly, resulting in limited hip motion

Fig. 8.1 Classification of spastic hemiplegia (Gage).

requires an intact neurological mechanism to coordinate this activity. In cerebral palsy the timing of these muscles is impaired and the muscles are dysfunctional. In the case of rectus femoris, this commonly results in a constant-on firing pattern in swing phase, resulting in persistent knee extension and a stiff knee gait. The other major bi-articular muscles (gastrocnemius, hamstrings, psoas) are frequently of crucial importance in the gait pathology of children with CP.

Secondly, in mildly affected children the emphasis of the abnormality is in the peripheral bi-articular musculature. As a consequence peripheral control of the limb is more difficult and compensations for peripheral control difficulties occur in more proximal muscles/joints. An example of this principle would be the compensation of equinus in swing phase by excessive hip flexion to secure adequate ground clearance.

Gait analysis

The objective of gait analysis in the child with cerebral palsy is to provide a comprehensive picture of how the child is walking and to assess the relative contributions of secondary abnormalities (such as contracture and torsions) and compensatory mechanisms (such as vaulting, hip hiking, etc.). Separation of secondary abnormalities from compensatory mechanisms is essential and not always possible from traditional means of assessment (static examination, visual assessment). Visual assessment is particularly prone to error in the transverse and coronal planes and children with CP frequently have abnormalities of gait in all three planes. It is inevitable that reliance on visual assessment alone will lead to errors of interpretation of the abnormalities and incorrect surgical decision making. The importance of separating secondary abnormalities from compensatory mechanisms is vital as secondary abnormalities will require correction, whereas with correct treatment compensatory mechanisms will disappear spontaneously.

Gait analysis comprises evaluation of the patient by three-dimensional motion analysis using either an active or passive marker system attached to relevant bony landmarks. This information is computer analysed to recreate a model of the child's limbs and joints. From these data, continuous joint angle relationships in stance and swing phase are plotted. Kinetic data from floor-mounted force platforms are combined with these data to derive information about instantaneous joint moments and powers (Fig. 8.2).

> Static examination of the child
> Video tape recording in sagittal and coronal planes
> Three-dimensional motion analysis (Kinematics)
> Dynamic electromyography
> Force platform data (Kinetics)
> Energy cost assessment (O_2 consumption, PCI)

Fig. 8.2 Components of gait analysis.

When combined with electromyography of relevant muscle groups during walking, it is possible to build up a detailed picture of the contributions of different mechanisms occurring during the child's walking, for example the level of power generated at a particular joint or the phase of firing of a particular muscle group. The complexity of the gait abnormalities presented by children with CP are such that visual assessment of the child is inadequate to obtain a full understanding of the primary gait abnormalities and the compensatory mechanisms employed by the child. From the gait analysis information, the clinician has a deeper understanding of the patient's motion pattern and can make predictions about the probable outcome of surgical interventions, such as muscle lengthening procedures, derotations and tendon transfers. More recently models for absolute muscle length measures and prediction programmes for proposed interventions are being developed within the gait analysis computer software.[21]

The application of gait analysis techniques to children with CP has allowed the development of the simultaneous multilevel surgical approach.[32] Patients requiring correction of both soft tissue and bony problems are treated in a single treatment session. This approach has the obvious advantage of one set of operations compared to several, and one period of rehabilitation therapy. Gait analysis also allows proper objective review of the patient after surgery.

Recently published data concerning the relationship between gait analysis and surgical treatment have shown improved surgical results at 1 year postoperation in children with CP undergoing surgery after full gait analysis compared to those treated after clinical assessment alone.[33] Improved technical outcome has been shown following simultaneous event multi-level with an improved normality index (an index comprising 22 kinematic/kinetic variables) in more than 90% of patients, improved functional outcome as measured by oxygen consumption (overall reduction in O_2 consumption postoperatively of 35%) and significant postoperative gains as assessed by a functional questionnaire including strength, endurance and ability to keep up with peers (improvements in 63–70% in the latter three variables). Patient satisfaction was also excellent with 80% stating they would undergo procedures again.[34] Delp et al[35] have drawn attention to the misconceptions obtained from subjective assessment and which have been revealed by gait analysis. In this study of crouch gait spastic diplegia, only 3 of 14 subjects had hamstring shortening as defined by analysis, despite persistent knee flexion in stance phase. The importance of this observation is that one of the common operations in crouch gait diplegia, based upon visual analysis, is hamstring lengthening. De Luca et al[36] have recently shown that the surgical recommendations based upon static examination and visual assessment were altered in 52% of cases as a consequence of three-dimensional gait analysis. The most frequent changes in recommendations were with respect to rectus femoris transfer (17%), hamstring lengthening (12%), femoral derotation (12%) and tibial derotation (8%).

These data suggest that it is now advisable to postpone surgery in ambulant children until the gait pattern is mature (at least 6 years of age). Treatment by physiotherapy, splinting and the appropriate use of muscle relaxants (baclofen) or paralysis (botulinum toxin A) should be used to try to maintain joint ranges in the short-term. When the gait is mature, those children in whom surgery is considered necessary should undergo gait analysis and the surgical intervention planned as a single set of procedures.[37]

Key points for clinical practice

- Physical therapy remains the mainstay of therapy support for these children and early data suggest specific goal orientated intensive approaches are most effective.

- Dysphagia, reflux, aspiration and failure to thrive are common in cerebral palsy and major causes of morbidity in the more severely affected children. These problems require detailed assessment and treatment.

- Botulinum toxin A may offer the opportunity for postponing surgical therapy, but further evaluation is needed before the application of this agent can be recommended.

- Intrathecal baclofen may be helpful in some ambulant children and in some children with severe spasticity where care is an issue, but further research studies into its use are needed.

- Evidence is accumulating that surgical management of ambulant children is most suitably a simultaneous multilevel attempt to address the child's problems and this approach requires detailed pre-operative gait analysis.

References

1 Dahl M, Thommessen M, Rasmussen M, Selberg T. Feeding and nutritional characteristics in children with moderate or severe cerebral palsy. Acta Paediatr 1996; 85: 697–701

2 Wright R, Wright F, Carson C. Videofluoroscopic assessment in children with severe cerebral palsy presenting with dysphagia. Pediatr Radiol 1996; 26: 720–722

3 Mirrett P, Riski J, Glascott J, Johnson V. Videofluoroscopic assessment of dysphagia in children with severe spastic cerebral palsy. Dysphagia 1994; 9: 174–179

4 Evans P, Alberman E. Certified cause of death in children and young adults with cerebral palsy. Arch Dis Child 1990; 65: 325–329

5 Reyes A, Cash A, Green S, Booth I. Gastro-oesophageal reflux in children with cerebral palsy. Child Care Health Dev 1993; 19: 109–118

6 Borgstein E, Heij H, Beugelaar J, Ekkelkamp S, Vos A. Risks and benefits of anti reflux operations in neurologically impaired children. Eur J Paediatr 1994; 153: 248–251

7 Ramachandran V, Ashcroft K, Sharp R, Murphy P, Snyder C, Gittes G. Thalfundoplication in neurologically impaired children. J Pediatr Surg 1996; 31: 819–822

8 Herndon W, Troup P, Yngve M, Sullivan J. Effects of neurodevelopmental treatment on movement patterns in children with cerebral palsy. J Pediatr Orthoped 1987; 7: 395–400

9 Palmer F, Shapiro M, Wachtel M et al. The effects of physical therapy on cerebral palsy. N Engl J Med 1988; 318: 803–808

10 Tirosh E, Rabino S. Physiotherapy for children with cerebral palsy. Am J Dis Child 1989; 143: 552–555

11 Bairstow P, Cochrane R, Hur J. Evaluation of Conductive Education for Children with Cerebral Palsy. Final Report Part II. London: HMSO, 1993

12 Weindling AM, Hallam P, Gregg J, Klenka H, Rosenbloom L, Hutton JL. A randomised controlled trial of early physiotherapy for high risk infants. Acta Paediatr 1996; 85: 1107–1111

13 Carmick J. Managing equinus in children with cerebral palsy; electrical stimulation to strengthen the triceps surae muscle. Dev Med Child Neurol 1995; 37: 965–975

14 Damiano D, Abel M. Effectiveness of strength training in spastic cerebral palsy. Dev Med Child Neurol 1997; 39 (Suppl 75): 9–10

15 Bower E, McLellan D, Arney J, Campbell M. A randomised controlled trial of different intensities of physiotherapy an different goal setting procedures in 44 children with cerebral palsy. Dev Med Child Neurol 1996; 38: 226–237

16 Russell D, Rosenbaum P, Gowland C et al. Gross motor function measure manual. Hamilton, Ontario; Chedoke-McMaster Hospitals, 1990

17 Koman L, Mooney J, Smith B et al. Management of spasticity in cerebral palsy with botulinum A toxin: report of a preliminary, randomised, double blind trial. J Pediatr Orthoped 1994; 14: 299-303

18 Cosgrove A, Corry I, Graham HK. Botulinum toxin in the management of the lower limb in cerebral palsy. Dev Med Child Neurol 1994; 36: 386–396

19 Corry I, Cosgrove A, Walsh E et al. Botulinum toxin A in the hemiplegic upper limb: a double blind trial. Dev Med Child Neurol 1997; 39: 185–193

20 Eames N, Baker R, Cosgrove A et al. The effect of botulinum toxin A injection on gastrocnemius muscle growth in children with spastic cerebral palsy and predicting the likely response to injection. Gait Posture 1997; 5: 82

21 Eames N, Baker R, Cosgrove A. Defining gastrocnemius muscle length in ambulant children. Gait Posture 1997; 6: 9–17

22 Jankovic J. Botulinum toxin in movement disorders. Curr Opin Neurol 1994; 7: 4

23 Boyd R, Graham HK. Botulinum toxin A in the management of children with cerebral palsy: indications and outcome. Eur J Neurol 1997; 4 (Suppl 2): S15–S22

24 Albright A, Barron W, Fasick M et al. Continuous intrathecal baclofen infusion for spasticity of cerebral origin. JAMA 1993; 270: 2475–2477

25 Peacock W, Arens LJ, Berman B. Cerebral palsy spasticity. Selective dorsal rhizotomy. Pediatr Neurosci 1987; 13: 61–66

26 Steinbok P, Reiner A, Beauchamp R et al. A randomised clinical trial to compare selective posterior rhizotomy plus physiotherapy with physiotherapy alone in children with spastic diplegic cerebral palsy. Dev Med Child Neurol 1997; 39: 178–184

27 Boscarino L, Ounpuu S, Davis R et al. Effects of selective dorsal rhizotomy on gait in children with cerebral palsy. J Pediatr Orthoped 1993; 13: 174–179

28 Thomas S, Aiona M, Pierce R, Piatt J. Gait changes in children with spastic diplegia after selective dorsal rhizotomy. J Pediatr Orthoped 1996; 16: 747–752

29 Stout J, Dunn M, Gage J et al. The effects of L1 vs L2 selective dorsal rhizotomy on hip flexor spasticity in children with cerebral palsy. Abstracts American Academy for Cerebral Palsy and Developmental Medicine. Dev Med Child Neurol 1997; 38 (Suppl 74): 29

30 Rang M. Cerebral palsy. In: Morrissy RT. (ed) Pediatric Orthpaedics, 3rd edn. Philadelphia: Lippincott, 1990

31 Sutherland D, Olshen R, Cooper L, Woo S. The development of mature walking, J Bone Joint Surg 1980: 62A; 336–353

32 Gage JR. Gait Analysis in Cerebral Palsy. London: McKeith Press, 1991

33 Lee EH, Goh JC, Bose K. Value of gait analysis in the assessment of surgery in cerebral palsy. Arch Phys Med Rehabil 1996; 73: 642–646

34 Stout J, Selber P, Gage J. A comprehensive evaluation of treatment outcome in ambulatory cerebral palsy. Gait Posture 1997; 5: 80

35 Delp S, Arnold A, Speers R, Moore C. Hamstrings and psoas lengths during normal and crouch gait: implications for muscle tendon surgery. J Orthoped Res 1996; 14: 144–51

36 De Luca P, Davis RB, Oonpuu S, Rose S, Sirkin R. Alterations in surgical decision making in patients with cerebral palsy based on three dimensional gait analysis. J Pediatr Orthopaed 1997; 17: 608–614

37 Gage JR, DeLuca P, Renshaw TS. Gait analysis: principles and application. J Bone Joint Surg 1995; 77A: 1607–1623

M.Z. Mughal F.J. Hill

Effects of excessive consumption of soft drinks and declining intake of milk on children's teeth and bones

Recent dietary surveys of children and teenagers in the UK have shown a trend towards increasing consumption of sugary and acidic soft drinks. According to a recent UK food and drink marketing intelligence report,[1] the total sale of all soft drinks for all age groups, grew by almost 20% between 1991 and 1995. Much of this growth comes from an increase in the consumption of so-called diet and low sugar sector of the market. Cola drinks accounted for almost 50% of total sales by volume of all carbonated or fizzy drinks consumed in 1995. At the same time, there has been a steady decline in the consumption of milk in the UK since the 1970s.[2] Soft drinks are nutritionally very poor (Table 9.1). Their food energy comes solely from refined sugar. When they replace milk or other nutritious foods, their poor nutrient quality, high acidity and sugar content of non-diet drinks have the potential to lead to nutrient imbalance resulting in short, and long-term adverse effects on dental and bone health of growing children. This chapter reviews some of these dietary surveys and discusses possible adverse effects of excessive soft drink consumption and a falling consumption of milk on health of children.

COMPOSITION OF SOFT DRINKS

'Soft drinks' is a collective term to describe a wide variety of non-alcoholic beverages, which for the purpose of this review, will be used mainly to refer to flavoured or fruit juice containing drinks. They are available as concentrated squashes that require dilution before consumption or 'ready to drink' forms

M.Z. Mughal MBChB(Liverpool) FRCP(Lond) FRCPCH(UK) DCH(Eng), Consultant Paediatrician and Honorary Senior Lecturer in Child Health, Department of Paediatrics, Saint Mary's Hospital, Hathersage Road, Manchester M13 0JH, UK

F.J. Hill MDS FDSRCS(Eng) DOrth RCS(Eng) FDSRCPS(Glasgow), Consultant in Paediatric Dentistry, The University Dental Hospital of Manchester, Higher Cambridge Street, Manchester M15 6FH, UK

Table 9.1 Nutritional contribution of a glass of milk (150 ml) compared to a glass of non-diet cola

		Whole milk	Skimmed milk	Cola
Energy	(kcal)	102	72	59
Protein	(g)	5.0	5.1	trace
Fat	(g)	6.0	2.6	nil
Sodium	(mg)	85.5	85.5	12
Vitamin A	(µg)	87	36	nil
Thiamine	(mg)	0.06	0.06	nil
Riboflavin	(mg)	0.27	0.29	nil
Niacin	(mg)	1.30	1.35	nil
Vitamin B_6	(mg)	0.09	0.09	nil
Folic acid	(µg)	9	9	nil
Vitamin B_{12}	(µg)	0.6	0.6	nil
Pantothenic acid	(mg)	0.54	0.50	nil
Biotin	(µg)	3.0	3.2	nil
Vitamin C	(mg)	1.5	1.5	nil
Vitamin D	(µg)	0.05	0.02	nil
Vitamin E	(mg)	0.14	0.05	nil
Calcium	(mg)	179	183	6
Iron	(mg)	0.08	0.08	trace
Magnesium	(mg)	16.6	16.5	2
Phosphorous	(mg)	143	147	23
Potassium	(mg)	216	233	2
Selenium	(µg)	1.5	1.5	NA
Zinc	(mg)	0.6	0.6	trace
Iodine	(µg)	22.5	24	NA

NA = value not available. Adapted with permission from a figure in *Nutrition and Teenagers*,[64] by the National Dairy Council (copyright National Dairy Council)

contained in metal cans, cartons or bottles. The main ingredient in these drinks is water; carbonated (fizzy) drinks contain carbon dioxide (CO_2) gas (carbonic acid) under pressure. Most soft drinks get their sweet taste from either sugars such as sucrose, fructose and glucose, or artificial sweeteners such as aspartame, saccharin and acesulfame K in so-called 'diet' or 'light' drinks. Other ingredients depend on the brand type, but they may contain pure fruit juice, essences, various flavourings, preservatives, colouring agents and anti-oxidants. Most cola drinks also contain caffeine, which adds to their 'stimulant value'. As shown in Table 9.2, their pH values are usually below 4. Their acidity comes from natural fruit acids and acids (phosphoric, citric, malic, tartaric and carbonic acid) which are added to balance the sweetness, and to make them more 'refreshing'.[3]

SURVEYS OF SOFT DRINK AND MILK CONSUMPTION BY BRITISH CHILDREN

Infants and pre-school children

In a recent survey of infant feeding practices in Asian and Caucasian families

Table 9.2 The pH of each of the following drinks was measured using a Corning 150 pH/ion electrode, within 5 min of opening the can, carton or bottle. The pH value represents mean of three measurements made at room temperature

Beverage	pH
Carbonated canned soft drinks	
Coke (Coca-Cola)[1]	2.47
Diet Coke[1]	3.07
Pepsi (Pepsi-Cola)[2]	2.48
Diet-Pepsi[2]	2.91
Pepsi Max[2]	2.83
7-up[2]	2.89
Diet 7-up2	2.93
Tango-Orange[2]	2.82
Tango-Lemon[2]	2.67
R. Whites Lemonade[2]	2.70
Ribena Sparkling[3]	2.63
Lucozade Sport Orange[3]	3.28
Fruit juices (100%)	
Apple[4]	3.98
Pineapple[4]	3.94
Orange[4]	3.75
Water	
Manchester tap	7.15
Laboratory distilled	5.84
Still Mineral[4a]	7.39
Carbonated Mineral[4b]	4.71
Perrier Naturally Carbonated Mineral[1]	5.67

[1]Distributed by Coca-Cola and Schweppes Beverages Ltd, Uxbridge UB8 1EZ, UK
[2]Distributed by Britvic Soft Drinks Ltd, Chelmsford, UK
[3]Distributed by SmithKline Beecham, Brentford TW8 9BR, UK
[4]Sainsburys Pure Fruit Juices (made with concentrated fruit juices), Sainsburys Plc, Stamford Street, London SE1 9LL, UK
[4a]Sainsburys Caledonian Still Natural Mineral Water, Sainsburys Plc, Stamford Street, London SE1 9LL, UK
[4b]Sainsburys Caledonian Sparkling Natural Mineral Water, Sainsburys Plc, Stamford Street, London SE1 9LL, UK.

living in England,[4] mothers were asked about types of drinks, apart from milk given to their infants. When these infants were 9 months old, between a quarter to one-third of mothers in all ethnic groups gave pure or fresh fruit juice to their infants. Of Pakistani infants, 6% were being given fizzy drinks (white and Bangladeshi 1%, Indian 3%). By the age of 15 months, a quarter to one-half of infants in all ethnic groups were given sweetened fruit flavoured drinks: 14% of Pakistani, 8% of Indian and 6% of white and Bangladeshi infants drank fizzy drinks . Over a third of white infants never drank water by the time they were 15 months old.

The 1995 National Diet and Nutrition Survey[5] of 1658, 1.5–4.5 year old British children showed that 19% of the calorie requirements of children came from refined sugars. These types of sugars, which are usually associated with dental decay,[6] were mainly provided by non-diet soft drinks. Over two-thirds

Table 9.3 Median and ranges of total l/week of various drinks consumed by 11–16 year old Manchester boys and girls

Median l/week of drink	Males (n = 352)	Females (n = 372)	Significance (Mann-Whitney U test)
Cola beverages	1.99	1.32	$P < 0.001$
All fizzy drinks, including cola	5.14	3.57	$P < 0.005$
Milk	1.73	1.03	$P < 0.001$

of the children surveyed were regularly consuming diet and non-diet soft drinks, often several times a day. On average, the children surveyed consumed 1.5 l of non-diet, and 1 l of diet soft drinks per week; 17% of the children surveyed had active tooth decay.

In a survey of drinking habits of 105 infants and preschool children from Southampton, UK, Petter et al[7] reported that plain water consumption had largely been replaced by soft drinks; 50% of the infants and 73% of preschool children never drank plain water. They also found that 50% of the calorie requirements of infants and 15% of preschool children were provided by the sugar content of soft drinks. The authors speculated that these children had become conditioned to the sweet taste of drinks at an early age.

Older children and adolescents

The 1989 Department of Health report from the Sub-committee on Nutritional Surveillance survey of dietary habits of 10–11 and 14–15 year old British children revealed that the average consumption of cola beverages ranged between 0.54-0.70 l/week, for both gender groups.[8] In 10–11 year olds, the average weekly milk consumption was higher in boys (1.71 l) than in girls (1.3 l). A similar pattern was seen in the 14–15 year olds, but the girls in this age group were drinking even less milk than girls of the younger age group. In common with the national study, our own recent unpublished (1996) questionnaire survey of 724 11–16 year old (49% males, 51% females; 30% response rate) children attending secondary schools in Central Manchester showed a similar trend with respect to gender difference in self-reported consumption of milk (Table 9.3). However, as shown in Table 9.3, the average consumption of cola and all fizzy drinks was much higher than reported in the 1989 Department of Health survey.[8]

Boys in Manchester were drinking significantly more total fizzy drinks (including cola drinks) and milk than the girls. Consumption of all fizzy drinks was generally higher in the younger groups, especially among 12–14 year olds (Fig. 9.1). Total quantities of all fizzy drinks and milk consumed appeared to be vary among children of different ethnic groups. As shown Fig. 9.2, the Afro-Caribbeans were drinking almost twice the amount of fizzy beverages drunk by either the Asians (originating from India, Pakistan and Bangladesh) or the white Caucasians, while the Asians on average were consuming more cola drinks than Afro-Caribbean and white Caucasian children. Milk consumption was highest among the white Caucasians. Reasons for these observed

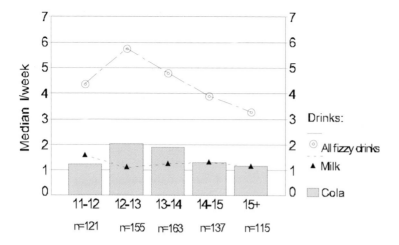

Fig. 9.1 Graph showing average weekly consumption of milk, cola and total fizzy beverages by Manchester children of different age groups.

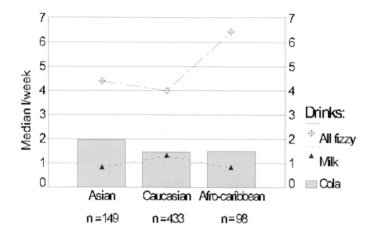

Fig. 9.2 Graph showing consumption of milk, cola and total fizzy beverages by white Caucasians, Asian and Afro-Caribbean 11–16 year old children from inner-city Manchester schools.

variations in consumption of fizzy drinks and milk among children from different ethnic origins are not apparent. However, a lower intake of milk among non-white children might be explained by a higher incidence of lactose intolerance in this group. For the whole group, we found that boys derived over 13%, and girls 11%, of their recommended daily calorie requirements from consumption of fizzy drinks.

In summary, dietary surveys suggest that children and adolescents appear to be consuming large quantities of soft drinks. Between 30–75% of infants and young children never drink tap water. While most children drink milk, its consumption was lower in pre-adolescent girls and decreased with increasing age.

DENTAL DECAY AND EROSION

The loss of dental tissue from consumption of soft drinks may occur from acids already in the drinks (dental erosion) or from those generated in the mouth, by fermentation of sugars that they contain (caries or decay).

Dental decay

Dental decay is characterised by decalcification of the tooth brought about by organic acids produced by fermentation of non-milk extrinsic sugars by acid forming bacteria (e.g. *Streptococcus mutans*) in the dental plaque. An individual's risk of developing dental caries depends on a number of biological and behavioural factors, including high consumption of fermentable sugars, high level of cariogenic bacteria in the mouth, exposure to fluoride, quality of oral hygiene, access to oral health services, socio-economic status and genetic factors.[9] However, animal[10] and human[11] studies have conclusively confirmed the causal relationship between excessive consumption of sugary foods and dental decay. The cariogenic potential of sugary food also depends on its stickiness and ability to stimulate saliva flow.[11,12]. In a trial which would now be considered to be unethical, Steinberg et al[13] randomised a group of 567 institutionalised mentally handicapped children and young adults aged 8–21 years to receive twice daily carbonated beverages, while the controls received water only. After 3 years, the experimental group had a non-significantly higher

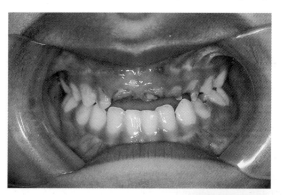

A

B

Fig. 9.3 Caries in the primary teeth of a 3 year old child associated with prolonged use of a sweetened feeding bottle. (A) Labial view. (B) Palatal view.

level of dental caries than the control subjects; however, the conclusions of this study are weakened by failure to control for consumption of other sugary foods during the study.

As part of the 1971–1974 US National Health and Nutritional survey, Ismail et al[14] looked at the relationship between consumption of soft drinks and dental cares scores in a sample of 3194 subjects aged 9–29 years. After controlling for confounding factors, such as age, gender, race, income, education and consumption of other sugary foods, they found significant associations between the amount and frequency of sugary soft drink consumption and high dental caries scores. The greatest risk in odds ratio was associated with the frequency of consumption of soft drinks between meals, rather than the actual amount consumed.

The National Diet and Nutrition Survey[6] included a dental health survey of 1658, 1.5–4.5 year old children from the UK: 17% had evidence of tooth decay, which in over 80% was untreated; 2% had filled teeth and a further 2% missing teeth due to decay. Consumption of sugary drinks at bedtime, children being left to brush their teeth themselves, and household expenditure on confectionery were all associated with caries prevalence. The subgroup with decay had higher than average intake of non-milk extrinsic sugars, which mainly came from sugary soft drinks and confectionery, than those without decay.

Infants and toddlers who are put to bed with feeding bottles containing milk or soft drinks, in order to soothe them and encourage them to sleep, are at risk of developing rampant dental decay (Fig. 9.3).[15] The decreased salivary flow and swallowing activity during sleep facilitate pooling of the ingested drink, and acids formed by their fermentation, against the teeth. Dental decay is less likely to occur at meal times when the saliva, and other foods and drinks consumed tend to dilute and neutralise the acid generated from fermentation of sugars.[16] Birkhed[17] measured pH changes in dental plaque after a group of teenagers rinsed their mouths with Coca-Cola® or dank the same volume of this drink from a glass, or through a drinking straw. The decrease in plaque pH was significantly lower when Coca-Cola® was consumed from a glass or through the straw, indicating the cariogenicity of soft drinks also depends on the mode of consumption. Herod[12] has reviewed the evidence from animal and human studies that cheese, but also milk, reduces the cariogenic potential of sugary foods. Chewing a piece of cheese stimulates saliva, reduces the levels of cariogenic bacteria and its high calcium and phosphate content appear to protect against demineralisation of the dental enamel.

Thus, based on present evidence, it is reasonable to conclude that the excessive consumption of sugary soft drinks is associated with an increased risk of dental decay. Further, the cariogenic potential of soft drinks is related to the amount consumed, the frequency of consumption especially in between meals, the time of the day (especially at night) and the way in which they are consumed. Milk or cheese, used as the 'final foods' at meal times may help to counteract the cariogenic effect of sugary soft drinks. Finally, it is well known that fluoridation of public water supplies in areas with low fluoride content (<1 ppm or 1 mg/l) has been shown to half the rate of dental caries in children.[18] However, the growing trend of children drinking soft drinks instead of less tap water[4,7] might undermine the benefits of public health fluoridation on children's dental health

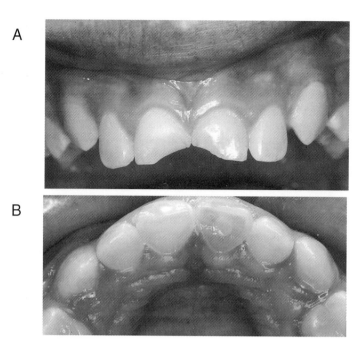

Fig. 9.4 Severe dental erosion of the upper permanent incisors in a 13 year old, associated with frequent consumption of acidic soft drinks. (A) Labial view. (B) Palatal view.

Dental erosion

Dental erosion is defined as chemical dissolution of the dental hard tissue by acids, which are not produced by intra-oral bacteria. It usually occurs on plaque-free sites. It may be caused by intrinsic or extrinsic acid sources. The intrinsic causes include regurgitation of acidic gastric contents into the mouth in patients suffering from gastro-oesophageal reflux and self-induced vomiting in disorders, such as anorexia nervosa.[19] The extrinsic causes include acidic foods, drinks, and medicines. Dental erosion is usually asymptomatic; however, an older child may present with disfigurement caused by loss of dental tissue (Fig. 9.4) or with painful sensitivity of the teeth.[20]

Acidic soft drinks

Recent clinical and prevalence studies suggest that dental erosion due to consumption of acidic soft drinks is becoming a common problem affecting both the deciduous and permanent teeth of British children. Millward et al[21] found evidence of tooth erosion in over 80% of 101 children aged 4–16 years, referred to their dental hospital. They also observed a significant ($P < 0.001$) positive correlation between the mean number of soft drinks and fruit juices consumed and the severity of dental erosion observed. Further, bedtime consumption of soft drinks was associated with more severe cases of erosion. Milosevic et al[22] found dental erosion in a third of over 1000 randomly selected 14 year old school children from Liverpool, UK. The National Child Dental Survey of 5–15 year old children in the UK[23] for the first time included assessment of dental erosion. Over half of 5–6 year olds showed evidence of erosion of their primary dentition and nearly a quarter of children had advanced erosion down to dentine. Almost a third of 15 year olds showed some erosion of the permanent dentition, which in 2% was severe with involvement of the dentine or pulp of the upper incisors. The National Diet and Nutrition Survey[6] showed that almost a fifth of 1.5–4.5 year old children had evidence of erosion affecting their deciduous teeth; 8% had severe erosion into dentine or dental pulp. Dental erosion was more common in those children with bedtime consumption of soft drinks. Thus, these studies suggest that dental erosion is a common problem among children in the UK, and that it is associated with consumption of large quantities of acidic soft drinks.

Dietary factors

Dietary factors responsible for dental erosion have recently been reviewed by Zero.[24] Most acidic drinks with pH of < 4.5 have the potential to cause dental erosion in the human mouth. Non-carbonated or still soft drinks contain acids from at least two sources: (i) fruit juices/extracts; and (ii) additives, that provide flavouring, for example, phosphoric acid and citric acid. The acidity and erosive potential of pure fruit juices vary according to the type of fruit from which the juice is prepared. Wynn and Haldi[25] studied the erosive action of various fruit juices on the lower molar teeth of rats. The juices were administered to the rats *ad libitum*. They found that grapefruit caused the most erosion, followed in descending order by grape, apple, pineapple, orange, prune and tomato juice.

In addition to containing fruit juice/extract and added acids, carbonated drinks also contain carbonic acid (CO_2 under pressure). As a rule, carbonation of drinks increases their acidity and the erosive potential. Mistry and Grenby[26] used a digital image analysis technique to study the erosion of rat molar teeth by carbonated and uncarbonated soft drinks. They found that rats administered carbonated orange drink (pH 2.61) had more dental erosion than those who drank uncarbonated or still orange drink (pH 3). The pH of some of the popular brands of diet and non-diet soft drinks is shown in Table 9.2. Unfortunately, the erosive dangers of 'diet' or 'low sugar' beverages appear to be less well appreciated both by children, parents and health professionals.

Other constituents of soft drinks may have a modifying effect on the degree and the rate of dental erosion. High calcium, phosphate and fluoride content appear to reduce the erosive capacity of soft drinks.[24,27] Evidence for this comes from elegant studies of Gadelia et al[28,29] in which they studied *in situ* the erosive effect of a popular brand of a cola drink on sections of tooth mounted in the human mouth, and the reparative effect of dairy products. They observed re-hardening of cola-softened enamel by a 5 min chewing period with cheddar cheese or a 1 hour exposure to cows' milk. These authors concluded that repair or remineralisation of cola-softened enamel occurred by the deposition of organic and mineral (calcium and phosphate) material contained in these dairy products. The consistency of cheese is such that its high concentration of minerals is kept in close proximity to the tooth surface. Fluoride is well known for its anti-cariogenic properties,[18] Its incorporation into the dental enamel makes the tooth more resistant to acid demineralisation. Using an in vitro model for studying dental erosion, Lussi et al[30] observed that soft drinks with the highest fluoride concentrations caused less dental erosion.

Drinking habits which increase the direct contact of acidic beverages with the teeth increase the risk of erosion. For example, Mackie and Hobson[31] described erosion of maxillary anterior teeth in 2 children caused by prolonged drinking of fruit-flavoured drink through a drinking straw placed directly against the affected teeth. In addition to causing dental decay (see above), the habit of drinking baby fruit juice from a drinking bottle, at bed-time, has been reported to have caused extensive dental erosion in a 2 year old girl.[32] Finally, saliva and its components protect the teeth against erosion by various mechanisms, which have been summarised by Meurman and ten Cate:[16] (i) increased salivary flow helps to dilute acids in the mouth, which also leads to their rapid removal through swallowing; (ii) salivary buffers partly neutralise acids in the mouth; (iii) calcium and phosphate ions in the saliva may allow repair or remineralisation of the acid etched areas of dental enamel; and (iv) salivary mucins protect against acid erosion.

OTHER EFFECTS OF EXCESSIVE CONSUMPTION OF SOFT DRINKS

Soft drinks as a disproportionate source of calories

Hourihane and Rolles[33] reported 8 children (mean age 20.8 ± 6 months, 4 boys and 4 girls) who presented with symptoms of anorexia, poor weight gain and loose stools, which they attributed to excessive intake of sugary soft drinks (fruit juice, squashes and fizzy drinks). The subjects were ingesting at least 30% of the recommended daily energy intake from fluids other than milk. Their symptoms, which could not be attributed to organic causes, resolved or improved when the subjects reduced the intake of soft drinks. In practice, this was achieved by increasing the intervals between drinks and/or by offering them more dilute drinks. The weight gain was more rapid in the 3 infants who were drinking more than 1.5 l of soft drinks/day. The authors named this the squash drinking syndrome which they felt was due to excessive intake of energy-rich drinks between meals, leading to poor appetite through disruption of the hunger-meal-satiety cycle, and thus failure to gain weight. The loose stools were attributed to the laxative effect of fruit juices. The authors speculated that some children who have been diagnosed as having toddler diarrhoea might actually be cases of the squash drinking syndrome. It is, however, important to emphasise that toddler diarrhoea is not usually characterised by failure to thrive.

Hypocalcaemia secondary to excessive consumption of phosphoric acid containing soft drinks

The potential of oral or parenteral phosphorus loads to cause hypocalcaemia has been recognised for over 20 years. Experimental studies on humans have shown that oral administration of phosphate salts to adult volunteers induces a drop in serum calcium concentration, and a rise in serum phosphorous and parathyroid hormone concentrations.[34] Mazariegos-Ramos et al[35] carried out a case-controlled study to assess whether the ingestion of soft drinks was a risk factor for the development of hypocalcaemia. They found a significant association between chronic ingestion of at least 1.5 l/week of phosphoric acid-containing soft drinks and low (< 2.2 mmol/l) plasma calcium concentration. In 17 of these children, the plasma calcium concentration rose from a mean value of 2.17 mmol/l to 2.35 mmol/l, one month after soft drink intake was discontinued. Although it is not mentioned by the authors, it is likely that the Mexican children with asymptomatic hypocalcaemia had low dietary intakes of calcium as they were recruited from an economically deprived population, the primary care facilities of a Mexican Institute of Social Security. The authors did, however, state that some mothers had substituted soft drinks for milk to feed their infants and that this may be due to low parental income levels and because soft drinks prices in Mexico are 3–5 times lower than in the USA.

Acidity of soft drinks and heartburn

Feldman and Bennett[36] reported that soft drinks had the lowest pH of many beverages and that the decreasing pH among soft drinks was correlated with reporting of symptoms of postprandial heartburn ($P < 0.001$)

Excessive caffeine consumption

Cola flavoured soft drinks usually contain caffeine, a stimulant drug that can cause insomnia, nervousness, irritability, anxiety and disturbances in the heart rate and rhythm.

Increased risk of kidney stones

Weiss et al[37] reported that drinking 3.4 l of a cola drink in a 48 hour period resulted in a decreased urinary excretion of magnesium and citrate (potential inhibitors of urinary stone formation) and an increased urinary excretion of oxalate, a known constituent of kidney stones. The authors concluded that these conditions could, in theory, enhance the formation of kidney stones.

Hazards of carbon dioxide content of fizzy drinks

Hadas-Halpren et al[38] described a case of emphysematous gastritis in a 16 year old boy secondary to ingestion of 1.5 l of a fizzy cola drink. Acute emphysematous gastritis is a life threatening disease in which gas-forming bacteria invade the gastric wall and cause its acute inflammation. Straub[41] described a double gastric rupture injury in a 19 year old patient after a motorbike accident. This injury was attributed, in part, to gastric dilatation caused by over-consumption of fizzy drinks, immediately prior to the accident.

DECLINING INTAKE OF MILK AND INCREASING CONSUMPTION OF COLA DRINKS

Childhood risk factors for development of osteoporosis during late adulthood

Osteoporosis is characterised by a decrease in the amount of normally mineralised bone leading to increased bone fragility and susceptibility to fracture. In the UK, it is recognised as a major public health problem as it affects 1 in 3 older women and 1 in 12 older men.[40] It leads to over 200 000 fractures per year, of which 85% occur in post-menopausal women.[41] In addition to causing pain, osteoporotic fractures can lead to deformity, permanent disability, loss of independence, and even death. As the population of elderly people increases, the prevalence of osteoporosis can be expected to increase, unless more preventative measures to delay its onset and diminish the severity are introduced.

Childhood origins of osteoporosis?

Childhood and adolescence are crucial times for skeletal development.[42–44] During this period, there is growth in size, strength and the amount of mineral (hydroxyapatite) in bone. The bone mass of a part of skeleton depends both on the volume and the amount of mineralised tissue contained within its periosteal envelope. The introduction of accurate, non-invasive and safe techniques for measurement of bone mass (the amount of hydroxyapatite) and density (the amount of hydroxyapatite in a given volume of bone tissue) has lead to an improved understanding of bone development during growth. The volumetric bone mineral density (g hydroxyapatite/cm^3) can be measured non-invasively in the vertebral body and long bones, using quantitative computer tomography (QCT). However, most paediatric studies of bone mass acquisition during growth and puberty have been carried out using dual energy x-ray absorptiometry (DXA) (Fig. 9.5), because of its greater precision and lower radiation dose than the QCT. DXA, however, provides measurement of areal bone mass (BMC) or mineral density (BMD) in g hydroxyapatite/cm^2, i.e. the amount of hydroxyapatite in a given area, rather than volume of skeleton. In other words, DXA measured bone mass and density is a two-dimensional projection of the three-dimensional bit of the bone, whose mass/density is being measured. Unlike QCT measured volumetric BMD, areal BMD tends to underestimate the BMD of small bones and exaggerate that of larger bones. Therefore, appropriate corrections have to be made to DXA measured BMC/BMD, to allow for changes in bone size accompanying skeletal growth.

The increase in bone mass parallels the tempo of linear growth. Theintz et al[45] used DXA to study longitudinally the increment in bone mass and BMD in the lumbar spine, femoral shaft and femoral neck, during puberty. In girls, the rate of increase in BMD was most rapid between 11–14 years of age, whereas in boys it was between 13–17 years of age. In girls, the rate of BMD increase declined rapidly after the age of 16 years, or 2 years after menarche. In women, 90–95% of the peak adult bone mass, defined as the amount of bone mass at the end of the skeletal maturation, is achieved by the second decade,[46] with bone growth during adolescence accounting for about half this figure.[47] Shortly after peak adult bone mass is attained, there is a progressive net loss of bone, which is more rapid in women after the menopause. Thus, two main factors that influence the occurrence of osteoporotic fracture are the amount of bone formed during growth and the rate at which it is subsequently lost. It follows that the factors affecting bone mass during growth may be important determinants of resistance to osteoporotic fracture, in latter life.

The magnitude of the peak adult bone mass is largely genetically determined,[48,49] however, 20–40% of the variability between individuals reflects adequate calcium intake, weight bearing physical activity and hormonal factors.[50,51] Thus, in an individual, the genetic potential for achieving peak adult bone mass is only realised when the modifiable factors that contribute to normal bone acquisition are favourable. Among the modifiable factors, adequate calcium intake during childhood and young adulthood is likely to be important for achieving peak adult bone mass. The only source of calcium available to the body is that contained in the diet. For most children, milk and other dairy products are the main source of calcium.[52,64]

Can the rate of bone mass acquisition be altered by calcium or milk supplementation?

A number of epidemiological and retrospective dietary recall studies have shown a positive association between life-long calcium intake and adult bone mass. In a study of two populations with different dietary calcium intakes in former Yugoslavia, Matkovic et al[53] showed that subjects consuming around 1000 mg/day of calcium had a higher metacarpal bone mass than subjects with a calcium intake of around 500 mg/day. A difference in bone mass and fracture rate in the two populations was already present by the age of 30 years, thus indicating that calcium intake during childhood and early adult life may be an important determinant of peak bone mass. However, genetic variation in the two populations could also account for part of the observed difference in bone mass. A retrospective study of postmenopausal women showed that those who reported drinking milk with every meal during childhood and adolescence had significantly higher areal bone density than those who reported drinking milk less frequently.[54] This suggests that differences in bone density due to calcium intake during childhood do persist into adulthood, although it could be due to a lifelong habit of high calcium/milk intake. However, results of this retrospective questionnaire study should be interpreted with caution because of inaccuracies in recall of childhood dietary information.

There are very few randomised intervention studies that have examined the effect of calcium or milk supplementation on bone growth or mineral density in children. The positive impact of milk consumption on longitudinal growth and, therefore, bone growth, has been known for several decades. A milk supplementation trial of 1425 school children aged 5–13 years from Scotland and Northern Ireland reported by Leighton and Clarke in 1929,[55] showed unequivocally that children who were randomised to a supplementary uptake of 0.75–1 pint of milk daily grew significantly faster, and put on more weight than the controls. Johnston et al[56] conducted a double-blind, placebo controlled calcium supplementation trial in North American monozygotic twins, thus controlling for the genetic factors affecting bone mass acquisition during pre- and postpubertal growth. In 23 pairs of prepubertal twins, calcium-supplemented twins, who received an additional 1000 mg of calcium citrate/malate per day for 3 years, had achieved small, but significantly higher, bone mineral density of radius and lumbar spine, compared with their placebo-controlled twin pairs. This positive effect of calcium supplementation on bone mass was not associated with any change in either bone area or height. The mean daily calcium intake of the twins given placebo was 908 mg, and that of the twins given calcium supplements was 1612 mg (894 mg from the diet and 718 mg from the supplement). There was no benefit of calcium supplementation on BMD in 23 pairs of twins who were postpubertal or who went through puberty during the trial. Unfortunately, the differences in bone mass did not persist after the supplement was discontinued.[57]

Recently, Cadogan et al[58] investigated the effect of milk supplementation on the gain in total body, areal bone mineral content (TBBMC; a two-dimensional projection of a three-dimensional true density, see above and Fig. 9.5) and density (TBBMD), measured by DXA in 12 year old white Caucasian girls from Sheffield, UK. The average baseline daily milk intake was 150 ml/day in both the intervention and control groups. The intervention group consumed, on average, an additional 300 ml/day throughout the 18 month trial period. The mean calcium intake of the group given milk was 1125 mg/day and that in the control group was 703 mg/day; the UK reference nutrient intake for girls of this age is 800 mg/day.[59] Compared with the control group, the intervention group had almost 1% and 3% greater increases of areal TBBMD ($P = 0.017$) and TBBMC ($P = 0.009$), respectively, at the end of trial. No differences were observed in the standing height of subjects in the two groups. Milk supplementation did not have a detectable effect on biochemical markers of bone formation and resorption. However, the serum concentration of insulin-like growth factor 1, which is known to have anabolic effects on the growing skeleton, was significantly higher in the milk supplemented group. The

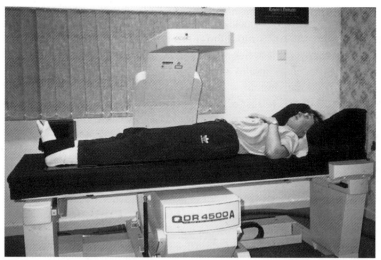

Fig. 9.5 The *Hologic QDR-4500 Acclaim* dual energy x-ray absorptiometer (DXA). Bone mineral measurements by DXA rely on the attenuation (absorption) of two different energy beams of x-ray photons across the whole body or a region of interest, e.g. the spine. Low energy photons penetrate the soft tissues whereas the high-energy photons penetrate both the soft tissues and the bone. A detector measures the exiting photons from the region of interest and the computer resolves attenuation into measurements of bone mineral, lean and fat soft tissue masses. DXA measured bone mineral content (BMC) is based on the two-dimensional projection of a three dimensional structure and therefore the values are dependent on the size, volume and mineral density of the bone being measured.

authors attributed the increase in serum concentration of insulin-like growth factor 1 to the higher intake of protein from milk. The authors speculated that if the observed 1–3% per year increase in bone mass resulting from a modest increase milk consumption was maintained, it could have a significant positive effect on peak adult bone mass.

In an elegantly designed and conducted double-blind, placebo controlled study, Bonjour et al[60] have recently examined the effects of a milk-derived calcium supplement on areal bone mineral density (BMD) in 149 prepubertal (mean age 7.9 years) Swiss girls. Calcium from a milk extract was used to fortify several food products (cakes, biscuits, fruit juices, powdered drinking chocolate, chocolate bars and yoghurts) which were eaten at breakfast or as snacks. The control (placebo) group was given similar products in terms of energy, protein, lipid and mineral content, but without added calcium. Subjects in the intervention group received an additional 850 mg calcium/day, increasing their average daily intake from 916 to 1723 mg of calcium/day. Among the girls who completed the 12 month intervention the DXA measured mean areal BMD gain at the radial and femoral sites, but not the lumbar spine were significantly greater in the calcium supplemented than the placebo group. The magnitude of the observed bone gain was greater in girls whose spontaneous calcium intake was below the median value of 880 mg/day. In this sub-group, described as 'spontaneously low-calcium consumers', calcium supplementation also led to a significant increase in the area of bones scanned by DXA and in standing height, which was still present 1 year after termination of the dietary intervention. From these data, the authors conclude that milk-derived calcium supplementation significantly increased bone mass acquisition in prepubertal girls, especially in those with lower spontaneous calcium intake. The authors suggested that milk derived-calcium, or other constituents of milk may increase bone mass by stimulating bone growth or modelling. They hypothesised that the contribution of the modelling effect on the skeleton would persist even after discontinuation of the calcium supplementation.

Taken together, the limited evidence from epidemiological and short-term calcium and milk supplementation studies suggest that adequate calcium intake during growth may positively influence skeletal growth and mineral density. These studies also suggest that a calcium intake below 900 mg/day may not be sufficient for optimal bone mass acquisition in prepubertal and adolescent girls. Thus, the current UK reference nutrient intake values for calcium,[59] for prepubertal girls of 550 mg/day and of 800 mg/day for adolescent girls may be insufficient for optimum skeletal development. Calcium derived from milk, or one or more of its other constituents, e.g. protein, appear to stimulate bone development. Pharmacological calcium supplements do not appear to stimulate bone modelling. Long-term prospective studies are needed to provide a definite answer to the question of whether or not increasing the intake of calcium during growth can reduce the burden of osteoporosis, through maximising achievement of the peak bone mass at skeletal maturity.

Ironically, eating behaviours of many teenagers such as dieting, skipping meals, living on snacks (including soft drinks) tends to occur at the time when they are rapidly accreting calcium and other minerals in their skeletons. Milk consumption among children and young adults in the UK has been declining since the 1970s,[2] and many children and adolescents are replacing milk with

Table 9.4 Average dietary phosphorous load calculated from the median l/week of cola beverage consumption by 11–16 year old Manchester school children

	Males	Females
Median consumption of Cola (l/week)	1.99	1.32
Daily phosphorous load from cola drinks (mg)	41.3	27.4
RDA for phosphorous for 11–18 year-olds (mg)	775	625
% RDA of phosphorous from cola drinks	5.3%	4.4%

nutrient-poor soft drinks. Thus, from a public health point of view, habitual low dietary calcium intake during childhood could result in a failure to achieve optimal peak bone mass which, in turn, might lead to a greater prevalence of symptomatic osteoporosis in later life. This might be particularly important for girls because of their proneness to osteoporosis after the menopause. As mentioned previously, recent dietary surveys show that adolescent girls have some of the lowest intakes of calcium rich milk and dairy products.

Increasing childhood consumption of cola drinks – a risk factor for development of osteoporosis?

Wyshak et al[61] reported a significant association between life-long carbonated beverage consumption and bone fractures occurring in a group of former female college athletes. The same group[62] using detailed food-frequency questionnaires and self-reported medical histories, reported a strong association between consumption of carbonated beverages and fractures in 8–16 year old girls, but not in boys. High dietary calcium intake had a protective effect against fracture risk. They postulated that high phosphorus content (from phosphoric acid) of cola drinks could cause an increase plasma phosphorous concentration and a lowering of plasma calcium concentration which, in turn, would lead to secondary hyperparathyroidism, skeletal demineralisation and an increased risk of fracture.

The amount of phosphorous derived from average volume of cola beverage consumed by 11–16 year old children attending secondary schools in Central Manchester appears to be small in comparison to the recommended dietary allowance (Table 9.4) for phosphorous, for this age group. Therefore, nutritive hyperparathyroidism due to excessive cola consumption probably only occurs when dietary intake of calcium is low. This notion is supported by the study of Calvo et al,[63] who showed that consumption of a diet high in phosphorus (1600 mg/day) and low in calcium (400 mg/day) by healthy volunteers resulted in reduced serum calcium and elevated serum parathyroid hormone concentrations, and increased urinary hydroxyproline excretion (indicating bone resorption).

Thus, it is proposed that the combination of high consumption of cola beverages and low calcium intake from the declining consumption of milk during childhood and adolescence could further compromise the achievement of the peak bone mass with increased risk of osteoporotic fracture in late adulthood.

CONCLUSION

Increasing consumption of soft drinks and falling consumption of milk is a source of concern for the health of children and adolescents. There is conclusive evidence that both diet and non-diet soft drinks lead to dental decay and/or erosion. There is circumstantial evidence that excessive consumption of sugary soft drinks by toddlers leads to blunting of the appetite, and secondary failure to thrive. Finally, it is proposed that the declining consumption of milk may adversely bone growth and mineral acquisition during childhood and adolescence, leading to inadequate achievement of the peak adult bone mass, with attendant risk of osteoporotic fracture in late adulthood. This is of particular importance to females because of their proneness to osteoporosis after the menopause. It is important that all health professionals are aware of the risk posed by such drinking behaviour to the short and long-term health of today's youngsters.

Key points for clinical practice

- Recent national nutritional surveys indicate that children and adolescents are consuming large quantities of soft drinks.

- Soft drinks are replacing the consumption of tap water.

- There is conclusive evidence that excessive consumption of soft drinks leads to dental decay and erosion.

- Based on current evidence, the following health education measures can be recommended for prevention of dental decay/erosion in children:
  1. Implementation of preventative dental health education measures, including fluoridation of drinking water, dietary advice, twice daily effective cleaning of the teeth with fluoride toothpaste and twice yearly dental examination.
  2. Avoidance of acidic soft drinks containing sugars between main meals. Ideally, discourage the consumption of these nutritionally poor drinks which are known to cause dental decay as well as erosion.
  3. If at all possible, sugary and acidic foods/drinks should be restricted to meal times, drunk quickly rather than sipped slowly.
  4. Fruit juices should be diluted.
  5. Consumption of less cariogenic and cariostatic snacks, e.g. chewing a piece of cheese as the final food after meals.
  6. Strongly discourage the habit of drinking milk/baby fruit juice from a drinking bottle, at bedtime.

- Milk consumption among children and young adults in the UK has been declining since the 1970s and many children and adolescents are replacing milk with nutrient-poor soft drinks.

- Girls who are particularly prone to osteoporosis after the menopause are consuming less milk than the boys, especially during the teen-years period when almost half of total body bone mass is laid down.

- Milk is an important source of calcium and other skeletal growth promoting nutrients. Increasing milk consumption or supplementation with milk derived calcium results in a significant bone gain in girls.

- Increased milk consumption during childhood may maximise the peak bone mass and reduce the risk of osteoporotic fracture in later life.

References

1 Mintel Marketing Intelligence. Food and Drink. Bristol: Mintel International, 1996

2 Slater JM. Fifty Years of National Food Survey. London: HMSO, 1991

3 Sorvari R, Rytomaa I. Drinks and dental health. Proc Finn Dent Soc 1991; 84: 621–631

4 Thompson M, Avery V. Infant Feeding in Asian Families. London: HMSO, 1997

5 Gregory JR, Collins DL, Davies PSW, Hughes JM, Clarke PC. National Diet and Nutritional Survey. Children aged 1.5–4.5 years. London: HMSO, 1995

6 Hindes K, Gregory JR. National Diet and Nutritional Survey. Children aged 1.5–4.5 years. Volume 2: Report of the Dental Survey. London: HMSO, 1995

7 Petter LP, Hourihane JO. Rolles D. Is water out of vogue? A survey of the drinking habits of 2–7 year olds. Arch Dis Child 1995; 72: 137–140

8 Department of Health. Diets of British Schoolchildren. Subcommittee on Nutritional Surveillance. Committee on Medical Aspects of Food Policy. Report on Health and Social Subjects. London: HMSO, 1989

9 Tinanoff N. Dental caries risk assessment and prevention. In: Johnson D, Tinanoff N. Dental health of the pre-school child. Dent Clin North Am 1995; 39: 709–719

10 Stephens RM. Effects of different types of human food on dental health of experimental animals. J Dent Res 1966; 45: 1551–1561

11 Gustafson G, Quensell CE, Lanke LS et al. The Vipeholm dental caries study: the effect of different levels of carbohydrate intake on dental caries activity in 436 individuals observed for 5 years. Acta Odontol Scand 1954; 11: 232–364

12 Herod EL. The effect of cheese on dental caries: a review of the literature. Aust Dent J 1991; 36: 120–125

13 Steinberg AD, Zimmerman OS, Barmer ML. The Lincoln dental caries study II. The effect of acidulated carbonated beverages on the incidence of dental caries. J Am Dent Assoc 1972; 85: 81–89

14 Ismail AI, Burt BA, Eklund SA. The cariogenicity of soft drinks in the United States. J Am Dent Assoc 1984; 109: 241–245

15 Blinkhorn AS, Mackie IC. Dietary counselling. In: Practical Treatment Planning for the paedodontic patient. London: Quintessence Publishing, 1992: 31–33

16 Meurman JH, ten Cate JM. Pathogenesis and modifying factors of dental erosion. Eur J Oral Sci 1996; 104: 199–206

17 Birkhed D. Sugar content, acidity, and effect on plaque pH of fruit juices, fruit drinks, carbonated beverages and sport drinks. Caries Res 1984; 18: 120–127

18 Murray JJ, Rugg-Gunn AJ, Jenkins GN. Fluoride in Dental Prevention, 3rd edn. Oxford: Butterworth-Heinemann, 1991

19 Bedi R. Dental management of a child with anorexia nervosa who presents with severe tooth erosion. Eur J Prosthodont Restor Dent 1992; 1: 13–17

20 Eccles JD, Jenkins WG. Dental erosion and diet. J Dent 1974; 2: 153–159

21 Millward A, Shaw L, Smith AJ, Rippin JW, Harrington E. The distribution and severity of tooth wear and the relationship between erosion and dietary constituents in a group of children. Int J Paediatr Dent 1994; 4: 151–157

22 Milosevic A, Young PJ, Lennon MA. The prevalence of tooth wear in 14-year-old school children in Liverpool. Community Dent Health 1994; 11: 83–86

23 O'Brien M. Children's dental health in the United Kingdom 1993. London: Office of Population Census and Surveys, 1994

24 Zero DT. Etiology of dental erosion – extrinsic factors. Eur J Oral Sci 1996; 104: 162–177

25 Wynn W, Haidi J. The erosive action of various fruit juices on the lower molar teeth of albino rat. J Nutr 1948; 35: 489–497

26 Mistry M, Grenby TH. Erosion by soft drinks of rat molar teeth assessed by digital image analysis. Caries Res 1993; 27: 21–25

27 Grenby TH. Lessening dental erosive potential by product modification. Eur J Oral Sci 1996; 104: 221–228

28 Gadelia I, Dakuar A, Shapira L, Lewinstein I, Goultschin J, Rahamim E. Enamel softening with Coca-Cola and rehardening with milk or saliva. Am J Dent 1991; 4: 120–122

29 Gedalia I, Ionat-Bendat D, Ben-Mosheh S, Shapira L. Tooth enamel softening with a cola type drink and rehardening with hard cheese or stimulated saliva in situ. J Oral Rehabil 1991; 18: 501–506

30 Lussi A, Jaeggi T, Jaeggi-Scharer S. Prediction of the erosive potential of some beverages. Caries Res 1995; 29: 349–354

31 Mackie IC, Hobson P. Case reports: dental erosion associated with unusual drinking habits in childhood. J Paediatr Dent 1986; 2: 89–94

32 Smith AJ, Shaw L. Baby fruit juice and tooth erosion. Br Dent J 1987; 162: 65–67

33 Hourihane JO, Rolles CJ. Morbidity from excessive intake of high energy fluids: the 'squash drinking syndrome'. Arch Dis Child 1995; 72: 141–143

34 Reiss E, Canterbury JM, Bercovitz MA, Kaplan EL .The role of phosphate in the secretion of parathyroid hormone in man. Clin Invest 1970; 49: 146–149

35 Mazariegos-Ramos E, Guerrero-Romero F, Rodriguez-Moran M, Lazcano-Burciaga G, Paniagua R, Amato D. Consumption of soft drinks with phosphoric acid as a risk factor for the development of hypocalcemia in children: a case-control study. J Pediatr 1995; 126: 940–942

36 Feldman M, Barnett C. Relationships between the acidity and osmolality of popular beverages and reported postprandial heartburn. Gastroenterology 1995; 108: 125–131

37 Weiss GH, Sluss PM, Linke CA. Changes in urinary magnesium, citrate, and oxalate levels due to cola consumption. Urology 1992; 39: 331–333

38 Hadas-Halpren I, Hiller N, Guberman D. Emphysematous gastritis secondary to ingestion of large amounts of Coca-Cola. Am J Gastroenterol 1993; 88; 127–129

39 Straub G. Double stomach rupture as isolated injury [in German]. Unfallchirurgie 1993; 19: 112–113

40 National Osteoporosis Society. News Letter. Bath, UK, 1997

41 Kanis JA, Pitt FA. Epidemiology of osteoporosis. Bone 1992; 13: S7–S15

42 Royer P. Growth and development of bone tissues. In: Davis JA, Dobbing J. (eds) Scientific Foundation of Paediatrics. London: William Heinemann Medical Books, 1974

43 Bonjour JP, Rizzoli R. Bone acquisition in adolescence. In: Marcus R, Feldman D, Kelsey J (eds) Osteoporosis. New York: Academic Press, 1996: 465–474

44 Parfitt AM. The two faces of growth: benefits and risks to bone integrity. Osteoporos Int 1994; 4: 382–398

45 Theintz G, Buchs B, Rizzoli R et al. Longitudinal monitoring of bone mass accumulation in healthy adolescents: evidence for a marked reduction after 16 years of age at the levels of lumbar spine and femoral neck in female subjects. J Clin Endocrinol Metab 1992; 75: 1060–1065

46 Matkovic V, Jelic T, Wadlaw GM et al. Timing of peak bone mass in Caucasian females and its implications for the prevention of osteoporosis. J Clin Invest 1994; 93: 700–808

47 Bonjour JP, Theintz G, Buchs B, Slosman D, Rizzoli R. Critical years and stages of puberty for spinal and femoral bone mass accumulation during adolescence. J Clin Endocrinol Metab 1991; 73: 555–563

48 Pocock NA, Eisman JA, Hopper JL, Yeates MG, Sambrook PN, Eberl S. Genetic determinants of bone mass in adults – a twin study. J Clin Invest 1987; 80: 706–710

49 Seeman E, Hopper JL, Bach LA et al. Reduced bone mass in daughters of women with osteoporosis. N Engl J Med 1989; 320: 554–558

50 Ott SM. Attainment of peak bone mass. J Clin Endocrinol Metab 1990; 71: 1082A–1082C

51 Matkovic V, Fontana D, Tominac C, Goel P, Chesnut III CH. Factors that influence peak bone mass formation: a study of calcium balance and the inheritance of bone mass in adolescent females. Am J Clin Nutr 1990; 52: 878–888

52 National Institutes of Health. Optimal Calcium Intake. Consensus Statement. Bethesda, MD: National Institutes of Health, 1994

53 Matkovic V, Kostial K, Simonovic I, Buzina R, Brodarec A, Nordin BEC. Bone status and fracture rates in two regions of Yugoslavia. Am J Clin Nutr 1979; 32: 540–549

54 Sandler RB, Slemenda CW, LaPorte RE et al. Postmenopausal bone density and milk consumption in childhood and adolescence. Am J Clin Nutr 1985; 42: 270–274

55 Leighton G, Clarke ML. Milk consumption and growth of school children. Lancet 1929; ii: 40–43

56 Johnston Jr CC, Miller JZ, Slemenda CW et al. Calcium supplementation and increases in bone mineral density in children. N Engl J Med 1992; 327: 82–87

57 Slemenda CW, Reister TK, Peacock M, Johnston Jr CC. Bone growth in children following cessation of calcium supplementation. J Bone Mineral Res 1993; 8: S154

58 Bonjour JP, Carrie AL, Ferrari S et al. Calcium-enriched foods and bone mass growth in prepubertal girls: a randomized, double-blind, placebo-controlled trial. J Clin Invest 1997; 99: 1287–1294

59 Cadogan J, Eastell R, Jones N, Barker ME. Milk intake and bone mineral acquisition in adolescent girls: randomised, controlled intervention trial. BMJ 1997; 315: 1255–1260

60 Department of Health. Dietary Reference Values for Energy and Nutrients for the United Kingdom. Report of the Panel of the Committee on Medical Aspects of Food Policy. London: HMSO, 1991

61 Wyshak G, Frisch RE, Albright TE, Albright NL, Schiff I, Witschi J. Non-alcoholic carbonated beverage consumption, among women former college athletes. J Orthop Res 1989; 7: 91–99

62 Wyshak G. Frisch RE. Carbonated beverages, dietary calcium, the dietary calcium/phosphorus ratio, and bone fractures in girls and boys. J Adolesc Health 1994; 15: 210–215

63 Calvo MS, Kumar R, Heath H. Elevated secretion and action of serum parathyroid hormone in young adults consuming high phosphorus, low calcium diets assembled from common foods. J Clin Endocrinol Metab 1988; 66: 823–829

64 National Dairy Council. Nutrition and Teenagers. Fact file number 5. London: National Dairy Council, 1995

J. Fernando del Rosario   Susan R. Orenstein

Gastrooesophageal reflux

Gastrooesophageal reflux disease (GERD) is the most common oesophageal disorder in children. It is distinguished from the physiological reflux that many healthy infants have by the presence of discomfort, or injury to the oesophagus and adjacent organs. This chapter will focus on current concepts pertaining to GERD.

EPIDEMIOLOGY

Up to 67% of healthy infants manifest more than one regurgitant gastro-oesophageal episode daily.[1] This is an underestimation of the frequency of reflux episodes in healthy infants since less than 20% of scintigraphically-detected or pH probe-detected reflux produce visible emesis.[2] The peak incidence of symptomatic infantile reflux, whether pathological (GERD) or not, is 4 months of age. This resolves in most infants by 1–2 years of age, unlike the pattern in children who develop reflux when they are older than 3 years, less than 50% of whom have spontaneous resolution of symptoms.[3] In many instances, regurgitation is looked upon by parents as an annoyance. Regurgitation only becomes a medical problem when vomiting is severe or when other symptoms, such as irritability or disinterest in eating, are present.[1] The latter two symptoms may indicate the development of oesophagitis, a common complication of GERD. GERD occurs when the frequency of reflux is increased, and overcomes the usual mucosal protective mechanisms

J. Fernando del Rosario MD, Assistant Professor of Medicine and Pediatrics, Director, Pediatric Gastroenterology, Allegheny Center for Digestive Health, Allegheny General Hospital, 320 E. North Ave, Pittsburgh, PA 15212–4772, USA

Susan R. Orenstein MD, Professor, Department of Pediatrics, Division of Pediatric Gastroenterology, University of Pittsburgh School of Medicine, Children's Hospital of Pittsburgh, 3705 Fifth Ave, Pittsburgh, PA 15213, USA

preventing injury to the oesophagus and adjacent organs, such as the hypopharynx, trachea, and lungs.

PATHOPHYSIOLOGY

There are three mechanisms for reflux: (i) transient lower oesophageal sphincter relaxation; (ii) transient increase in intra-abdominal pressure, which overcomes the resistance of the anti-reflux barrier; and (iii) spontaneous reflux through a permanently hypotonic sphincter.

Transient lower oesophageal sphincter relaxation, unassociated with swallowing, is the major mechanism allowing reflux to occur. Transient lower oesophageal sphincter relaxations are associated with the majority of reflux episodes in children.[4]

Contraction of the crural diaphragm around the gastrooesophageal junction helps prevent reflux during episodes of increased intra-abdominal pressure. This is not possible in the presence of a hiatus hernia; thus, the high incidence of GERD in people with hiatus hernias.

Low lower oesophageal sphincter tone is an uncommon primary cause of reflux disease. However, there are a number of hormones, neurotransmitters and medications that affect lower oesophageal sphincter tone (Table 10.1).[5] Caffeine has been thought to reduce lower oesophageal sphincter tone. However, a recent study, comparing the effects of caffeinated and decaffeinated coffee and tea on the frequency of reflux, suggests that other components of coffee may be responsible for the increase in reflux, rather than caffeine.[6] Alcoholic beverages,

Table 10.1 Pharmacological agents affecting lower oesophageal sphincter pressure

Agents	Lower oesophageal sphincter pressure	
	Increases	Decreases
Hormones and peptides	Angiotensin	Cholecystokinin
	Bombesin	Gastric inhibitory peptide
	Gastrin	Glucagon
	Motilin	Neurotensin
	Substance P	Progesterone
	Vasopressin	Secretin
	Pancreatic polypeptide	Vasoactive intestinal peptide
Neurotransmitters	α-adrenergic agonists	α-adrenergic antagonists
	Anticholinesterase	Anticholinergics
	β-adrenergic antagonists	β-adrenergic agonists
	Cholinergic agonists	Dopamine
Other	Cisapride	Calcium channel blockers
	Domperidone	Cyclic adenosine monophosphate
	Histamine (H_1)	Histamine (H_2)
	Indomethacin	Lidocaine
	Metoclopramide	Morphine
	Prostaglandin F_2-α	Prostaglandins E_1 and E_2
	Serotonin (neural receptor)	Serotonin (muscle receptor)
		Theophylline

From Clark[5] and reproduced with permission from WB Saunders.

such as wine and beer, have also been noted to provoke reflux, but the mechanism is unrelated to ethanol content.[7] These dietary constituents may provoke reflux in older children by lowering lower oesophageal sphincter tone.

Oesophageal and gastric motor function also influence the pathogenesis of reflux. Clearance of refluxate from the oesophagus is important in preventing reflux-related complications. Primary motor abnormalities of the upper gastro-intestinal tract may impair oesophageal clearance, and thus worsen reflux disease.[8] Peristaltic abnormalities, due to oesophagitis, can also delay oesophageal clearance, and make the oesophagitis worse.[4] Delayed gastric emptying contributes to GERD in children to a greater extent than in adults.[10]

CLINICAL PRESENTATIONS

Common clinical manifestations of reflux in infants and children include regurgitation, malnutrition, respiratory symptoms, and neurobehavioural symptoms. Oesophagitis occurs in up to 83% of infants with clinically significant reflux.[10] However, symptoms of oesophagitis, such as crying, complaints of heartburn or dysphagia, are less common manifestations of reflux in children than in adults with GERD.

Regurgitant reflux can vary from minimal and effortless drooling to a projectile form that is sometimes difficult to distinguish from a mechanical obstruction. Excessive regurgitation can give rise to choking and gagging episodes, as well as feeding refusal and failure to thrive.

Respiratory sequelae

Respiratory sequelae are among the most important manifestations of reflux in children, yet may be unassociated with typical reflux symptoms. Respiratory sequelae include chronic cough, wheezing, apnoea, hoarseness, stridor, and recurrent bronchitis or pneumonia caused by aspiration. Pulmonary disease and its consequent therapy can also exacerbate pre-existing reflux.[11] Thus, it is often difficult to determine whether reflux or pulmonary disease is the primary disorder.

Aspiration

The brain stem co-ordinates activities of the mouth, pharynx, larynx, oesophagus, and stomach to protect against aspiration and reflux-mediated respiratory disease. Respiratory disease occurs through various mechanisms when this elaborate system is disrupted and may occur even in the absence of aspiration, via oesophageal-respiratory neural reflexes (Fig. 10.1).[12] The upper oesophageal sphincter is the major barrier preventing material in the oesophagus from being regurgitated and aspirated. Even minute aspiration of oesophageal or gastric fluid (micro-aspiration) may be sufficient to stimulate airway neural elements or release of inflammatory mediators, resulting in laryngospasm.[12] Bronchospasm can result from alteration of the bronchi's baseline state of reactivity in response to reflux.[11]

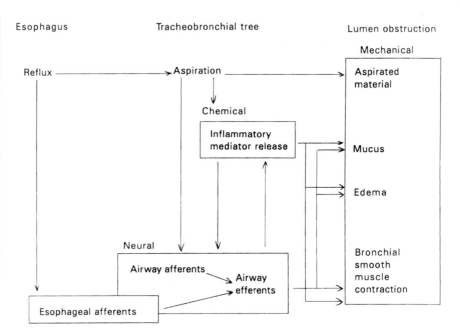

Esophagus   Tracheobronchial tree   Lumen obstruction

Fig. 10.1 Mechanisms for reflux-associated respiratory dysfunction. Reflux may produce respiratory disease directly, by mechanical occlusion of the lumen with aspirated material, or indirectly via neural or chemical induction of mucus secretion, oedema, or muscle contraction. Modified from Putnam et al[12] and reproduced with permission from William & Wilkins.

Asthma

The estimated prevalence of GERD among asthmatic patients is approximately 44%.[13] Reflux may be responsible for episodes of nocturnal cough in asthmatics. In some cases of severe, steroid-dependent asthma, medical or surgical anti-reflux therapy has resulted in improvement of their symptoms.[14]

The association between reflux and persistent wheezing in infants is not well established. However, one study of 12 infants with persistent wheezing refractory to bronchodilators and anti-inflammatory medications demonstrated clinical improvement in 50% of the infants after anti-reflux therapy, consisting of a prokinetic agent and a histamine antagonist, was instituted.[15]

Apnoea

Apnoea, triggered by reflux, is often an obstructive phenomenon, resulting from laryngospasm caused by laryngeal aspiration of gastric material or stimulation of vagal afferents.[16] Another proposed mechanism for reflux-induced apnoea is β-endorphin release triggered by oesophageal pain from reflux, resulting in a decrease in respiratory drive and modification of the chemolaryngeal reflex.[17]

Hoarse voice

Hoarseness may occur because of chronic reflux of gastric acid onto the vocal cords, resulting in inflammation and development of vocal cord nodules.

Laryngospasm secondary to aspiration of refluxate may result in stridor. Aspiration of gastric refluxate may also cause recurrent bronchitis or pneumonia. Children with neurologic impairment and inadequate protective mechanisms are particularly at risk for reflux-induced aspiration.

Other presentations

Sandifer's syndrome exemplifies neurobehavioural manifestations of reflux. Other behaviours include back-arching, feeding refusal, and rumination. Nonspecific irritability may be a manifestation of reflux-induced oesophagitis in nonverbal infants. This may take the form of extreme fussiness and sleep disturbance.

DIAGNOSIS

A variety of diagnostic modalities can be used in the evaluation of a child with suspected GERD. In many instances, a thorough history and physical examination may be sufficient to arrive at a diagnosis of GERD. The efficiency and completeness of the history is reliably and accurately enhanced in infants by utilizing an infant gastrooesophageal questionnaire.[18] Atypical reflux symptoms or the need to correlate GERD with another symptom warrants further testing. Figure 10.2A,B illustrates algorithms for the evaluation of reflux and reflux-related respiratory symptoms.[19]

Radiography

Fluoroscopic evaluation is most useful when an anatomical abnormality is a possible explanation of the symptoms, and should generally be performed prior to instituting prokinetic therapy for regurgitant reflux, to ensure the absence of a hiatus hernia, gastric outlet obstruction or malrotation, which would prompt consideration of alternative therapy. A modified barium swallow ('cookie swallow') is useful for documenting swallowing dysfunction or aspiration during swallowing.

Technetium scintigraphy ('milk scan') can demonstrate reflux following a physiologic non-acid meal (which the pH probe cannot detect), aspiration into the airway, and quantitative gastric emptying. The sensitivity for detection of reflux episodes is reported to be 59–93%,[20] and is markedly affected by technical issues, such as imaging frequency and duration. The main advantage of scintigraphy over fluoroscopy is a several-fold decrease in radiation exposure, facilitating longer imaging duration. In our institution, some infants with nocturnal symptoms suspected to be reflux-related undergo overnight scintigraphy, rather than oesophageal pH monitoring, to document reflux episodes, since scintigraphy is less invasive and cumbersome.

Endoscopy and biopsy

Endoscopy is useful to differentiate reflux from other gastrointestinal disease with similar symptoms. Suction oesophageal biopsy, which requires no

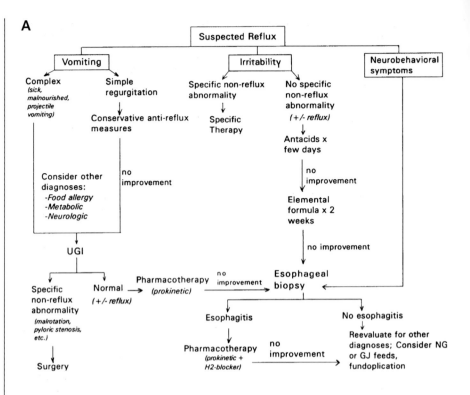

A

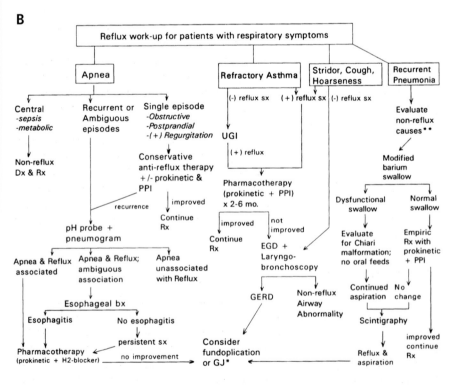

B

Fig. 10.2 (see next page for details)

Fig. 10.2 (see previous page) **(A)** Algorithm for the evaluation of infantile reflux. NG, nasogastric; GJ, gastrojejunostomy. **(B)** Algorithm for the evaluation of patients with chronic respiratory problems suspected to have reflux. Dotted lines, either approach is appropriate. NJ, nasojejunal; GJ, gastrojejunostomy.
*Oesophageal pH monitoring is helpful for patients with chronic respiratory disorders who have normal UGIs and no oesophagitis, and patients with oesophagitis who are symptomatic, despite maximal anti-reflux therapy. If there is excessive reflux, a fundoplication or GJ may be necessary.
**Non-reflux causes include cystic fibrosis, immunodeficiency, etc.
From del Rosario et al[19] and reproduced with permission from *The Gastroenterologist.*

sedation, provides an adequate specimen for evaluation of reflux oesophagopathy in infants with GERD,[21] and is less costly than a standard endoscopy.[22] Lower oesophageal sphincter location from the mouth is estimated using a published oesophageal length regression equation ($[0.226 \times$ height in cm$] +$ 6.7).[23] We then perform the biopsy at 87% or less of this calculated length.

Oesophageal pH monitoring

Twenty-four hour monitoring of distal oesophageal pH provides the clearest, longer-term documentation of frequency and duration of acid reflux episodes. This test is limited by its inability to detect reflux of non-acidic material. We circumvent this problem in infants by alternating formula feedings or breastfeeding, both of which can neutralize stomach contents, with apple juice feedings (pH 4) to increase detection of post-prandial reflux episodes. Another limiting factor is the need for meticulous documentation of symptoms (e.g. coughing, stridor, wheezing, apnoea) during oesophageal pH monitoring, to enable temporal correlation between symptoms and low distal oesophageal pH.

The optimum duration of oesophageal pH monitoring in infants and children has been a topic of debate. A recent study suggests that 1 and 4 hour pH studies (nap studies) underestimate GERD in infants,[24] and most evidence suggests the need for at least 18 hours of monitoring.

Simultaneous proximal and distal oesophageal pH monitoring has been suggested as a means to correlate respiratory symptoms with reflux.[25] In one study, proximal oesophageal pH monitoring documented pharyngeal reflux in 46% of patients with otherwise normal oesophageal acid exposure times by distal oesophageal pH monitoring.[26] Another group went as far as performing simultaneous tracheal and oesophageal pH measurements in asthmatic patients with GERD.[27]

Miscellaneous tests

Laryngoscopy can be performed to look for reflux-related changes (e.g. erythematous arytenoids, vocal cord nodules). Bronchoscopy with bronchoalveolar lavage can be done to sample tracheobronchial secretions for the presence of lipid-laden macrophages in order to document aspiration, keeping in mind that the presence of lipid-laden macrophages does not distinguish between aspiration of refluxate and aspiration during a swallow. The Bernstein test (intraluminal oesophageal acid perfusion) is effective in demonstrating causality between reflux and respiratory symptoms, and reflux and chest pain, but is infrequently performed in clinical practice. Oesophageal manometry is usually limited to those children with symptoms suggestive of oesophageal dysmotility, or in whom fundoplication is contemplated.[28]

THERAPY

Conservative

Conservative measures include positioning, dietary and environmental manipulation. The flat prone position when lying down and a completely vertical position when held are the most desirable positions for infants with reflux. The American Academy of Pediatrics exempts infants with reflux from the recommendation that the prone position be avoided to prevent SIDS, because the benefits of a prone position outweighs the risk of developing SIDS in infants with GERD. The right recumbent position has also been associated with fewer reflux episodes in adults,[29] but is challenging to maintain in infants.

Use of rice cereal to thicken formula is recommended for infants with regurgitant reflux, because of its increase of dietary caloric density and significant decrease of regurgitation frequency.[30] Fasting for several hours prior to bedtime, and avoidance of foods that have negative effects on lower oesophageal sphincter tone (peppermint, caffeinated beverages, fatty foods), gastric volume (carbonated beverages), or acidity (acidic beverages[31] or food) are helpful in older children.

Avoidance of cigarette smoke exposure is beneficial because passive inhalation has been associated with a reduction in lower oesophageal sphincter tone, delay in gastric emptying,[32] and development of oesophagitis in children.[33]

Pharmacotherapy

Treatment of GERD in children usually combines a prokinetic agent with either an H_2-receptor antagonist or a proton pump inhibitor. Anti-reflux therapy has also been successful in the treatment of reflux-associated respiratory disorders, as demonstrated by improved pulmonary function, and decreased nocturnal wheezing, stridor, hoarseness, and chronic cough.

In recent years, cisapride has supplanted metoclopramide as the prokinetic of choice. Cisapride has very few adverse effects, unlike metoclopramide, which has been associated with dystonic reactions and exacerbation of bronchospasm. However, one needs to be aware of the potential drug interactions between cisapride and certain antibiotics; specifically macrolides (erythromycin, clarithromycin, azithromycin), imidazoles (fluconazole, itraconazole, ketoconazole, miconazole), and troleandomycin.[34] These medications may interfere with the hepatic metabolism of cisapride, leading to high blood levels that may result in arrhythmias, which may be fatal. It is mandatory to avoid simultaneous use of these medications with cisapride.

H_2-receptor antagonists continue to be very effective acid inhibitors, but higher doses than previously believed may be required to provide efficacy in children.[35] Omeprazole has been reported to be safe and effective in the management of severe, refractory reflux oesophagitis in children, but is currently unavailable in a suspension. Various methods of circumventing this problem have been used in children, including mixing the granules in the omeprazole capsule with apple sauce, orange juice, cranberry juice, or yogurt to prevent premature dissolution of the granules after ingestion of the mixture.[36] Alternatively, the granules can be dissolved in 5 ml of sodium carbonate for children who receive tube feedings.[36] Lansoprazole has also been found to be efficacious in children,[37] but it is also unavailable in a suspension.

Surgery

Surgical fundoplication is an effective treatment for GERD and has good long-term results. In most cases of GERD, fundoplication is unnecessary.[38] Those who benefit most from surgery include children with reflux and aspiration, chronic lung disease, or neurological devastation; children with GERD refractory to aggressive pharmacotherapy; children who have developed reflux-induced oesophageal stricture or Barrett's oesophageal metaplasia.

Despite its high success rate, post-fundoplication complications in children are frequent.[39] They include herniation of the wrap through the hiatus, bowel obstruction due to adhesions, gas bloat, gastric dysmotility, and inability to belch or vomit when necessary. With the advent of laparoscopic fundoplication, surgical morbidity has decreased somewhat in the adult population, which may also occur in children.

An alternative to fundoplication is placement of a percutaneous gastro-jejunostomy tube under fluoroscopic or endoscopic guidance. This allows for enteral nutrition without exacerbation of reflux. This method is as effective as fundoplication in preventing reflux, but has lower morbidity.[40] However, acid-suppressing and prokinetic pharmacotherapy may still be necessary.

Key points for clinical practice

- Gastro-oesophageal reflux disease is the most common oesophageal disorder in children, and is frequently outgrown by 1–2 years of age. Most children who develop reflux older than 3 years will not have spontaneous resolution of symptoms.

- Transient lower oesophageal sphincter relaxation is the major mechanism allowing for reflux to occur. The presence of a hiatus hernia, or exposure to medications, food, and inhalants which decrease lower oesophageal sphincter tone, increases predisposition for reflux.

- Common manifestations of reflux in infants and children include regurgitation, non-specific irritability, and malnutrition. Gastro-oesophageal reflux disease should also be considered in patients with chronic respiratory symptoms (chronic cough, wheezing, apnoea, hoarseness, stridor, recurrent pneumonia) or asthma refractory to usual pharmacotherapy.

Key points for clinical practice (continued)

- Gastro-oesophageal reflux disease may be diagnosed by clinical history alone. However, a variety of diagnostic modalities are available to quantify reflux, correlate reflux symptoms, and assess for reflux-related complications.

- Prokinetic pharmacotherapy may have a greater role in children than in adults, because of the higher incidence of delayed gastric emptying in the former.

- Higher doses of H_2-receptor antagonists than previously believed may be necessary.

- Concurrent administration of cisapride with antibiotics and antifungals, which interfere with its hepatic metabolism (leading to high blood levels that may result in fatal arrhythmias) must be avoided.

- Laparoscopic fundoplication and percutaneous gastrojejunostomy may reduce morbidity in children with gastro-oesophageal reflux disease, who require surgical intervention.

References

1 Nelson SP, Chen EH, Syniar GM et al. Prevalence of symptoms of gastroesophageal reflux in infancy. A pediatric practice-based survey. Arch Pediatr Adolesc Med 1997; 151: 569–572

2 Orenstein SR, Deneault LG, Lutz JW et al. Regurgitant reflux, in contrast to nonregurgitant reflux, is associated with rectus abdominus contraction in infants. Gastroenterology 1991; 100: A135

3 Treem WR, Davis PM, Hyams JS. Gastroesophageal reflux in the older child: presentation, response to treatment and long-term follow-up. Clin Pediatr 1991; 30: 435–440

4 Cucchiara S, Staiano A, DiLorenzo C et al. Pathophysiology of gastroesophageal reflux and distal esophageal motility in children with gastroesophageal reflux disease. J Pediatr Gastroenterol Nutr 1988; 7: 830–836

5 Clark JH. Anatomy and physiology of the esophagus. In: Wyllie R, Hyams JS. (eds) Pediatric Gastrointestinal Disease, Pathophysiology, Diagnostic, Management. Philadelphia: WB Saunders, 1993; 316: 311–317

6 Wendl B, Pfeiffer A, Pehl C et al. Effect of decaffeination of coffee or tea on gastroesophageal reflux. Aliment Pharmacol Ther 1994; 8: 238–237

7 Pehl C, Wendl B, Pfeiffer A et al. Low-proof alcoholic beverages and gastroesophageal reflux. Dig Dis Sci 1993; 38: 93–96

8 Lundell L, Myers JC, Jamieson GG. Is motility impaired in the entire gastrointestinal tract in patients with gastroesophageal reflux disease? Scand J Gastroenterol 1996; 31: 131–135

9 Lin CH, Tolia V, Kuhns LR et al. Role of gastric emptying in infants with complicated gastroesophageal reflux. Pediatr Res 1989; 25: 118A

10 Black DD, Haggitt RC, Orenstein SR et al. Esophagitis in infants: morphometric histologic diagnosis and correlation with measures of gastroesophageal reflux. Gastroenterology 1990; 98: 1408–1414

11 Malfroot A, Dab I. Pathophysiology and mechanisms of gastroesophageal reflux in childhood asthma. Pediatr Pulmonol 1995; 11 (Suppl): 55–56

12 Putnam PE, Ricker DH, Orenstein SR. Gastroesophageal reflux. In: Beckerman R, Brouilette R, Hunt C. (eds). Respiratory Control Disorders in Infants and Children. Baltimore: William & Wilkins, 1991; 322–410

13 Gastal OL, Castell JA, Castell DO. Frequency and site of gastroesophageal reflux in patients with chest symptoms. Chest 1994; 106: 1793–1796

14 Irwin RS, Curley FJ, French CL. Difficult-to-control asthma: contributing factors and outcome of a systematic management protocol. Chest 1993; 103: 1662–1669

15 Eid NS, Shepherd RW, Thomson MA. Persistent wheezing and gastroesophageal reflux in infants. Pediatr Pulmonol 1994; 18: 39–44

16 Pransky SM, Kearns DB, Katz RM et al. Pediatric airway manifestations of gastroesophageal reflux. Ann Otol Rhinol Laryngol 1992; 101: 742–749

17 Beyaert C, Marchal F, Dousset B et al. Gastroesophageal reflux and acute-life-threatening episodes: role of a central respiratory depression. Biol Neonate 1995; 68: 87-90

18 Orenstein SR, Cohn JF, Shalaby TM et al. Reliability and validity of an infant gastroesophageal reflux questionnaire. Clin Pediatr 1993; 8: 472–484

19 del Rosario JF, Orenstein SR. Common pediatric esophageal disorders. Gastroenterologist 1998; 6(2): 104–121

20 Seibert JJ, Byrne WJ, Euler AR et al. Gastroesophageal reflux – the acid test: scintigraphy or pH probe? Am J Rhinol 1983; 140: 1087–1090

21 Putnam PE, Orenstein SR. Blind esophageal suction biopsy in children less than 2 years of age. Gastroenterology 1992; 102: A149

22 Orenstein SR. Gastroesophageal reflux. In: Feldman M. (ed) Gastroenterology and Hepatology: the Complete Visual Reference. (Pediatric GI problems; Vol.4, Hyman PE, vol. ed.). Philadelphia: Current Medicine, 1997; 24–27.

23 Strobel CT, Byrne WJ, Ament ME et al. Correlation of esophageal lengths in children with height: application of the Tuttle test without prior esophageal manometry. J Pediatr 1979; 103: 215–218

24 Graff MA, Kashian F, Carter M et al. Nap studies underestimate the incidence of gastroesophageal reflux. Pediatr Pulmonol 1994; 18: 258–260

25 Cucchiara S, Santamaria F, Minella R et al. Simultaneous prolonged recordings of proximal and distal intra-oesophageal pH in children with gastroesophageal reflux disease and respiratory symptoms. Am J Gastroenterol 1995; 90:1791–1796

26 Little JP, Matthews BL, Glock MS et al. Extraesophageal pediatric reflux: 24-hour double-probe pH monitoring of 222 children. Ann Otol Rhinol Laryngol Suppl 1997; 169: 1–16

27 Jack CI, Calverley PM, Donnelly RJ et al. Simultaneous tracheal and oesophageal pH measurements in asthmatic patients with gastroesophageal reflux. Thorax 1995; 50: 201–204

28 Slim K, Boulant J, Pezet D et al. Intraoperative manometry and fundoplications: prospective study. World J Surg 1996; 20: 55–58

29 Shay SS, Conwell DL, Mehindru V, Hertz B. The effect of posture on gastroesophageal reflux event frequency and composition during fasting. Am J Gastroenterol 1995; 91: 54–60

30 Orenstein SR, Magill HL, Brooks P. Thickening of infant feedings for therapy of gastroesophageal reflux. J Pediatr 1987; 110: 181–186

31 Feldman M, Barnett C. Relationships between the acidity and osmolality of popular beverages and reported postprandial heartburn. Gastroenterology 1995; 108: 125–131

32 Scott AM, Kellow JE, Shuter B et al. Effects of cigarette smoking on solid and liquid intragastric distribution and gastric emptying. Gastroenterology 1993; 104: 410–416

33 Shabib SM, Cutz E, Sherman PM. Passive smoking is a risk factor for esophagitis in children. J Pediatr 1995; 27: 435–437

34 Communication with Janssen Pharmaceutical Company

35 Lambert J, Mobassaleh M, Grand RJ. Efficacy of cimetidine for gastric acid suppression in pediatric patients. J Pediatr 1992; 120: 474–478

36 Gunasekaran TS, Hassall EG. Efficacy and safety of omeprazole for severe gastroesophageal reflux in children. J Pediatr 1993; 123: 148–154

37 Mikawa K, Nishina K, Maekawa N et al. Lansoprazole reduces preoperative gastric fluid acidity and volume in children. Can J Anaesth 1995; 42: 467–472

38 Wrap session: is the Nissen slipping? Can medical treatment replace surgery for severe gastroesophageal reflux disease in children? Am J Gastroenterol 1995; 90: 1212-1220

39 Samuk I, Afriat R, Klin B et al. Nissen fundoplication for gastroesophageal reflux in children. Harefuah 1994; 126: 311–315

40 Albanese CT, Towbin RB, Ulman I et al. Percutaneous gastrojejunostomy versus Nissen fundoplication for enteral feeding of the neurologically impaired child with gastroesophageal reflux. J Pediatr 1993; 123: 371–375

Robert J. Rothbaum

Gastrointestinal and hepatobiliary problems in cystic fibrosis

Cystic fibrosis (CF) is an autosomal recessive disorder of cAMP regulated chloride transport that results from a defect in the cystic fibrosis transmembrane regulator (CFTR). Described mutations may alter synthesis, intracellular transport, membrane insertion, or chloride channel function. The absence or dysfunction of CFTR results in diminished electrolyte and water secretion by duct epithelium. The concentration of macromolecules in the lumen of the affected duct increases significantly. Proteins precipitate into plugs, slow ductal flow, and produce duct obstruction. Pancreatic ductule obstruction leads to exocrine pancreatic insufficiency. At the air-fluid interface in the lung, secretions precipitate in small airways, initiating the cascade to chronic obstructive lung disease.

This chapter focuses on gastrointestinal issues such as gastrooesophageal reflux disease, biliary tract disease, intestinal obstruction syndrome, and colonic strictures. Current pathophysiology, manifestations, and management of exocrine pancreatic insufficiency and chronic lung disease form the subject of other reviews.[1]

GASTRO-OESOPHAGEAL REFLUX DISEASE

General symptoms

Some degree of gastrooesophageal reflux (GER) occurs in all individuals and can, therefore, be regarded as normal or physiological. In some instances, reflux of acidic gastric contents into the oesophagus leads to complications defined as gastrooesophageal reflux disease (GERD). GERD includes failure to

Robert J. Rothbaum MD, Associate Professor of Pediatrics, Division of Pediatric Gastroenterology and Nutrition, Department of Pediatrics, Washington University School of Medicine, St Louis Children's Hospital, One Children's Place, Box 8116, St Louis, MO 63110, USA

thrive, oesophagitis, oesophageal stricture, and pulmonary disease.[2] Oesophagitis may cause dysphagia, odynophagia (painful swallowing), or pyrosis (heartburn). Constant or periodic retrosternal discomfort or pain defines pyrosis. Infants with oesophagitis may have irritability and refusal to eat. Repeated vomiting may indicate GER, but not necessarily GERD. Failure to gain weight is uncommon in uncomplicated GER. Different mechanisms can produce a reduction in net energy intake: (i) dysphagia or dysmotility may interfere with ability to eat; (ii) feedings may be reduced or manipulated in an effort to decrease emesis; (iii) the volume of regurgitated material may be excessive. With GERD, children and adolescents may suffer epigastric or substernal pain after meals. These older patients report acid brash (reflux of acidic gastric contents into the pharynx) or water brash (a sudden increase in saliva production that accompanies acid reflux into the distal oesophagus). Dysphagia occurs with disordered oesophageal peristalsis or with oesophageal stricture.

Respiratory symptoms

Respiratory disease associated with GER presents as aspiration pneumonia, bronchospasm, hoarseness, or persistent cough.[3] Bronchospasm can follow direct acid irritation of the airway or may occur through a vagally mediated reflex following acid irritation of the distal oesophagus. Hoarseness and cough may result from laryngeal inflammation. A direct relationship between GER or GERD and pulmonary symptomatology is often difficult to prove. Continuous pulmonary symptoms do not allow for segregation of which symptoms are related to GER. Intermittent pulmonary symptoms often do not occur during the time of a particular study such as upper GI, radionucleotide milk scan, or prolonged pH study that documents reflux events. Lipid-laden macrophages identified in bronchoalveolar lavage fluid are not specific for aspiration of gastric contents. Such macrophages can be seen with inflammatory or obstructive lung disease alone. Often, the association of GER or GERD with pulmonary symptoms is only strongly suggested by improvement in the pulmonary symptoms following treatment of GER/GERD.

Reflux or chronic lung disease?

Because of concern that GER or GERD may exacerbate chronic obstructive lung disease in CF, clinical investigators examined this potential relationship several years ago. In the early 1980s, clinicians documented that complaints of regurgitation and heartburn were common in CF patients with significant respiratory disease. Feigelson et al evaluated 49 CF patients by oesophagoscopy performed in conjunction with bronchoscopy. All patients had 'marked' respiratory disease: 25 of the 49 had ulcerative oesophagitis. Only 16 of the 25 patients had any symptoms referable to the oesophagitis.[4] Thus, the influence of the oesophagitis on each patient's clinical condition was unclear.

pH studies

More recently, studies in larger groups of CF patients attempted to generalize these limited observations. Malfroot and Dab performed prolonged pH

Table 11.1 Factors preventing gastrooesophageal reflux disease

Defense mechanism	Function	CF-related problem
Lower oesophageal sphincter barriers Diaphragmatic crus Angle of His	Retention of acid contents in stomach	Medications decrease lower oesophageal sphincter tone Flattened diaphragm alters angle of His Frequent cough increases intra-abdominal pressure
Gravity	Keeps gastric contents in stomach when subject is upright or prone	Chest physiotherapy with head down
Primary peristalsis with swallowing Secondary peristalsis with reflux	Clear oesophagus of acidic material	Normal except with motility disorder of oesophagitis
Saliva	Dilutes and buffers acid reflux	Normal
Gastric emptying	Reduction of volume of gastric contents	Slowed by nocturnal or high density feeds
Oesophageal mucosal defense	Resistance of mucosa of oesophagus to acid injury	Not characterized

LES = Lower oesophageal sphincter

recording in the distal esophagus from 26 CF children younger than age 5 years. They found 81% of the children with abnormal pH studies shortly after the diagnosis of CF. With advancing age, general CF therapy, and cisapride, children with vomiting, poor weight gain, and recurrent wheezing improved over the course of one year. The anti-reflux therapy was, however, only a small component of their overall therapeutic regimen.[5] In other series of patients, increased time of acid exposure of the distal oesophagus has not been consistently related to oesophagitis or pulmonary disease.[6]

Defense mechanisms

Since all individuals have periodic acidic gastrooesophageal reflux but few develop GERD, several defense mechanisms protect against the development of oesophagitis or respiratory problems (Table 11.1). Alterations in any of these defense mechanisms may predispose to the development of acid-induced injury. The usual resting tone of the lower oesophageal sphincter limits spontaneous GER. In many patients with GERD, inappropriate relaxation of the lower oesophageal sphincter occurs, allowing for more frequent reflux of acid into the distal esophagus. Cucchiara documented such inappropriate lower oesophageal sphincter relaxation in 12 of 14 CF patients studied with prolonged pH and manometric studies.[7] Medications or foods that reduce lower oesophageal sphincter tone also increase oesophageal acid exposure. This increased acid exposure presumably produces mucosal damage and inflammation. Positioning can predispose to GER. Button et al showed that CF infants undergoing standard postural drainage, including head-down positions, had an increase in acid reflux episodes per hour in comparison to infants undergoing chest physiotherapy without their head down.[8] The duration of acid reflux episodes was not prolonged. Changes in the angle of His (the acute angle of entry of the oesophagus into the stomach) or in the angle of the oesophagus passing through the diaphragmatic crus may occur with pulmonary hyper-inflation or with scoliosis, decreasing the overall effectiveness of the lower oesophageal sphincter barrier. Swallowing disorders decrease the initiation of primary oesophageal peristalsis, reducing acid clearance from the distal oesophagus. With sleep, swallowing and saliva production are both reduced. Thus, acid reflux occurring during sleep may lead to prolonged exposure of the distal oesophagus to acid. Oesophagitis itself can produce a motility disorder that disrupts secondary peristalsis, leading to further retention of acid refluxate on already damaged mucosa. Defects in oesophageal mucosa that reduce resistance to acid-induced damage are hypothesized but not proven. Table 11.1 summarizes various conditions in CF that might diminish the effectiveness of usual defense mechanisms.

Investigations

In usual clinical practice, evaluation for GERD is performed in CF patients who have symptoms or signs directly referable to oesophagitis and on selected CF patients with respiratory tract disease refractory to usual therapy. Diagnostic tests for GERD include barium swallow, endoscopic visualization, oesophageal mucosal biopsy, and prolonged pH recordings from the distal oesophagus. Barium studies of the upper GI tract delineate anatomic abnormalities that predispose to gastric retention and subsequent acid reflux, such as gastric outlet obstruction, duodenal narrowing, or malrotation. Visualization of GER during an upper GI examination is common. Its presence does not predict underlying pathology. Its absence does not exclude GERD. The air contrast barium swallow is specific but not sensitive for the diagnosis of oesophagitis. If mucosal irregularity or 'ringed' oesophagus is present, then endoscopic or histologic oesophagitis will very likely be present. A normal barium swallow does not exclude oesophagitis. Oesophageal mucosal biopsy with or without upper gastrointestinal endoscopy is the 'gold standard' for the documentation of oesophagitis. Endoscopy may help define the extent and severity of the inflammation, allow identification of mucosal metaplasia (Barrett's oesophagus) and permit diagnosis of co-incident *Candida* or virus infection. A prolonged oesophageal pH study documents reflux of acid material into the distal oesophagus, but the findings do not correlate closely with the presence of oesophagitis.[6] A pH study may allow the correlation of specific symptoms (wheezing, apnoea, irritability, night awakening, etc.) with acid reflux.[3] Also, the pH study may permit documentation of medication effect, i.e. reduction of acid reflux following therapy. The Bernstein test (direct instillation of dilute acid into the distal oesophagus) is a provocation test that may elicit symptoms associated with GER. This test must be performed by personnel familiar with the technique and its interpretation.

No single test will directly connect pulmonary disease to GER. The most com-prehensive studies to link respiratory disease to GER have been performed in patients with posterior laryngitis and reactive airways disease. Posterior laryngitis presents as cough, throat clearing, throat burning and hoarseness. Refluxed gastric acid may cause the underlying intra-arytenoid oedema and erythema or ulceration. Reactive airways disease is familiar as cough or wheezing. Single probe pH studies, dual probe pH studies, upper gastrointestinal series x-rays, and radionuclide scans fail to predict, however, which patients will have improvement in respiratory complaints with anti-reflux therapy. Therapeutic trials of acid suppression with proton pump inhibitors over a period of 2–3 months provide the best evidence of a connection between GER and respiratory tract complaints. If the treated patient does not improve, then documentation of the effectiveness of acid suppression and inhibition of acidic GER with a gastric or oesophageal pH study may be necessary before admitting failure.

Management

GER usually requires no specific therapy. In infants, time and maturation lead to resolution in 95% of patients by age 18 months. Thickened feedings and positional changes may decrease emesis. Reduction in volume of feedings will not affect emesis but may limit overall energy intake and interfere with weight gain. Changes in lifestyle or medications represent initial therapy of GERD. Anatomy and gravity work to reduce the frequency of GER with the prone or right lateral position. GER occurs more often in the supine or left lateral decubitus positions. In infants, the presence of GERD might necessitate deviating from the recent American Academy of Pediatrics recommendation for supine position during infants' sleep. If large meals are avoided within 1–2 hours of retiring, then large volumes of acidic gastric contents will not be present in the stomach to reflux with the patient supine and sleeping. Avoidance of caffeine, chocolate, anti-cholinergics, theophylline, and, possibly, β-agonists, may reduce inappropriate relaxations of the lower oesophageal sphincter. Elevation of the head of the bed by 6 inches employs gravity as a force to keep acid contents in the stomach.

Medications that reduce gastric acid output are mainstays of therapy for oesophagitis since most oesophagitis is related to acid induced damage of the distal oesophageal mucosa. Proton pump inhibitors are more effective than histamine receptor antagonists for treatment of oesophagitis. These newer agents are also better documented as successful therapy for respiratory tract disorders thought to be related to GER. In treating oesophagitis, therapeutic benefit is usually assessed by diminished heartburn, dysphagia, or odynophagia. Treatment continues for 6–8 weeks, but many children and adults with oesophagitis have recurrent symptoms and require repeated courses of treatment. Resolution of oesophageal inflammation does not alter the previously noted factors that predispose to oesophagitis.

Fundoplication is not usually required for treatment of GERD. Oesophagitis refractory to medical therapy and recurrent symptomatic oesophageal stricture comprise the major indications for fundoplication. Occasional patients merit fundoplication because of excessive calorie loss from vomiting or a high index of suspicion of recurrent aspiration with associated chronic pulmonary disease. Fundoplication will reduce acid reflux and its associated problems, but postoperative problems are common. Up to 20% of postfundoplication patients report abdominal pain, bloating, or dysphagia after the surgery. About 15% of infants and children suffer persistent retching with feeding.[9,10] These symptoms usually improve during the first 6 postoperative months, but 10–20% of children will have recurrence of symptoms of GERD at a mean of 11 months after the original surgery. This period may, however, be long enough for oesophagitis to heal and for oesophageal clearance or defense mechanisms to improve.

HEPATIC DISORDERS

CFTR is present in biliary epithelium, but is not identifiable in hepatocytes. Possibly, abnormal electrolyte and water flux across biliary epithelium results in higher concentrations of macromolecules in CF bile. Biliary secretions may then inspissate in small ductules. Obstruction of bile flow may produce periportal inflammation followed by focal fibrosis. Histopathological findings consistent with this hypothesis are described in infants with CF. Almost one-third of CF infants examined by liver biopsy or autopsy had focal biliary fibrosis or mucous plugging of large intrahepatic bile ducts adjacent to the porta hepatis. Some infants had mucous obstruction of extrahepatic bile ducts. Table 11.2 outlines the full spectrum of hepatobiliary disorders that can develop over time.

Although defects in CFTR may potentiate the development of chronic liver disease, most CF individuals do not develop sufficient liver damage to alter their

Table 11.2 Hepatobiliary disorders in cystic fibrosis

Disorder	Clinical manifestation
Neonatal cholestasis	Transient neonatal direct hyperbilirubinemia ($\leq$ 2 months)
Hepatic steatosis	Enlarged liver
Focal biliary fibrosis	Hepatomegaly Elevated serum ALT, AST, or alkaline phosphatase

Multilobular biliary cirrhosis	Asymmetric firm hepatomegaly
	Splenomegaly with hypersplenism
	Complications of cirrhosis
	     Undernutrition, slow growth, and pubertal delay
	     Ascites
	     Variceal haemorrhage
	     Bacterial peritonitis
	     Portosystemic encephalopathy
	     Hypoxaemia
	     Liver synthetic failure

Microgallbladder	Asymptomatic
Cholelithiasis	Colicky right upper quadrant pain Elevated ALT, AST and/or alkaline phosphatase Gallstones evident on ultrasound
Bile duct strictures	Right upper quadrant pain Elevated ALT, AST or alkaline phosphatase Dilated extra- and/or intra-hepatic ducts on ultrasound or other imaging studies

clinical course. The most common clinical problems are asymptomatic elevation of serum transaminases (AST and ALT) and hepatomegaly. Up to 30% of CF patients may have elevated AST or ALT. Most of these patients have no other signs of liver dysfunction. Elevation of serum alkaline phosphatase may occur in 15–30% of patients.[11] Apparent hepatic enlargement (liver edge palpated 3 cm or more below the right costal margin) is often attributable to pulmonary overinflation. True hepatic enlargement (increase in liver span) is frequently due to hepatic steatosis. In untreated, undernourished patients, steatosis may be generalized and prominent. In treated patients, the fat accumulation is often focal but is not clearly zonal. There is no clear-cut relationship between hepatic steatosis and progressive liver disease.

Neonatal cholestasis

Neonatal cholestasis occurs in about 5% of CF infants. From one-quarter to one-half of these infants suffer meconium ileus in the newborn period, and many require surgery. Hypoxaemia, hypotension, bacterial or viral infection, and medications may accompany neonatal illness and surgery. In any newborn, transient cholestasis can follow these systemic problems. The CF infant with meconium ileus is more likely to experience problems that predispose to neonatal cholestasis and thus, is more likely to develop cholestasis than the CF infant without neonatal illness. Neonatal cholestasis can persist for as long as 2 months, but is not an indicator of potential long-term or chronic liver disease. Rarely, neonatal cholestasis in CF is associated with other disorders. Case reports describe coincident α_1-anti-trypsin deficiency, panhypopituitarism, and extrahepatic biliary atresia in CF infants with prolonged jaundice.

Cirrhosis

From 2–5% of CF patients develop macronodular, multilobular cirrhosis and portal hypertension.[12] No particular genotype is associated with an increased risk of cirrhosis. Almost all cirrhotic patients have pancreatic insufficiency. The male:female ratio is 2:1. About 35% of cirrhotic CF patients have a history of meconium ileus or distal intestinal obstruction syndrome versus about 12% in the general CF population.[13] Cirrhosis and portal hypertension develop silently and insidiously. A hard-edged, irregular liver and splenic enlargement are often first detected by careful physical examination between 4–14 years of age (mean 8.7 years) Superficial veins of the abdominal wall are dilated and prominent. Digital clubbing and oxygen desaturation occur with cirrhosis even without significant parenchymal pulmonary disease. For unclear reasons, hepatic cirrhosis can initiate precapillary shunting through the lung. The degree of elevation of serum transaminases or alkaline phosphatase or the duration of elevation do not clearly correspond with the risk of or presence of cirrhosis. Serum transaminases and alkaline phosphatase are mildly elevated or normal. In a recent report, 43 CF patients, aged 5 months to 35 years, underwent liver biopsy that identified steatosis or bridging fibrosis in 23% and 37%, respectively.[14] A clinical liver score grading the degree of hepato-splenomegaly and the extent of elevation of liver enzymes best predicted the severity of liver fibrosis. Liver synthetic and secretory function, evaluated with serum bilirubin, serum albumin, and prothrombin time, is initially normal. Increasing splenomegaly, shrinkage of the right hepatic lobe, and central prominence of the left lobe of the liver indicate progressive cirrhosis and portal hypertension, usually without overt symptoms.

Ursodeoxycholic acid

Ursodeoxycholic acid (UDCA) is a potent choleretic and hepatocyte protective agent. The increase in bile flow and cytoprotection resulting from the use of this agent could theoretically prevent bile ductular obstruction and hepatocyte damage in CF-related liver disease. In uncontrolled trials, administration of UDCA to CF patients with elevated transaminases or alkaline phosphatase produced a fall in these enzyme levels. In addition, hepatobiliary scintigraphy improved with UDCA therapy, potentially indicating improved bile flow.[15,16] In a small controlled trial, though, O'Brien et al substantiated the biochemical improvements but noted no change in scintigraphy in comparison to controls.[17] A Scandinavian study reported initial encouraging results with liver biopsy confirmation of less progression of liver fibrosis in UDCA-treated CF patients. Because the development of cirrhosis is uncommon and difficult to detect with non-invasive measures, definitive documentation that UDCA prevents progression to cirrhosis will be difficult to obtain. No other therapy is available, however, to ameliorate CF-related liver disease. In current clinical practice, therefore, many CF clinicians initiate UDCA therapy (10–30 mg/kg/day) in CF patients with elevated serum transaminases or alkaline phosphatase found in association with early evidence of fibrosis or cirrhosis on physical examination or imaging studies. Elevations of AST, ALT, and/or alkaline phosphatase improve or resolve to provide evidence of medication effect. Continuous UDCA therapy over years would be required to alter the long term progression of fibrosis.

Portal hypertension

The complications of portal hypertension rather than liver synthetic failure threaten the health of the CF patient.[12,18,19] Undernutrition, ascites, and gastro-intestinal haemorrhage constitute the most frequent clinical challenges. Porto-systemic encephalopathy is uncommon. Splenomegaly, sometimes painful, results in thrombocytopaenia and leukopaenia from hypersplenism, but these low counts do not usually contribute to clinical problems. Progressive jaundice is unusual. Prolongation of prothrombin time with normal partial thrombo-plastin time is often noted. Serum albumin is mildly depressed. Abdominal enlargement, respiratory muscle weakness, or CF-related chronic obstructive lung disease underlie decrements in pulmonary function.

Evaluation of nutritional status

Weight is an insufficient measure of nutritional status due to the increase in weight from hepatosplenomegaly, mesenteric oedema, and ascites. More detailed evaluation of lean body mass, such as triceps skin fold thickness or mid-arm circumference, indicates diminished muscle mass and fat stores.[20] Slow growth and delayed puberty are also frequent. These nutritional changes may be evident for months or years before more serious or acute complications occur. The exact aetiology of these decrements in nutritional status is unclear, but low nutrient intake is the most likely cause. Nutritional status may improve with aggressive provision of supplemental feedings via gastrostomy tube or parenteral nutrition.

Ascites

With progressive cirrhosis and portal hypertension, ascites may accumulate. Ascites often develops during or after gastrointestinal bleeding in cirrhotics. The patient/family should be advised of this common occurrence. Ascites requires treatment if the amount of fluid and abdominal distention are burdensome for the patient. The treatment of ascites in CF-related portal hypertension does not differ from that in other causes of portal hypertension and includes mild salt restriction and cautious use of diuretics. Spironolactone (2–3 mg/kg/day) is useful for initial therapy, but requires a few days to be effective. Thiazides and furosemide work faster but often produce hypokalaemia, hypochloraemia, and mild hyponatraemia.

Bacterial peritonitis

Spontaneous bacterial peritonitis is a serious complication of cirrhosis.[21] Fever, abdominal pain, increasing ascites, diarrhoea, and vomiting herald the onset of bacterial infection. Gastrointestinal haemorrhage can also be a presenting sign of bacterial peritonitis or bactaraemia. In peritonitis, diagnostic paracentesis demonstrates an absolute neutrophil count above 250 neutrophils/mm^3. An aliquot (10–30 ml) of ascitic fluid is sent for bacterial culture; the density of organisms may be quite low. Gram-negative bacteria, usually *Escherichia coli*, cause peritonitis in cirrhotics. CF patients may be at risk from *Pseudomonas* infection. Treatment with intravenous broad-spectrum antibiotics is promptly initiated. Intravenous antibiotic therapy continues for 5–7 days. Oral antibiotics that match bacterial susceptibility profiles extend therapy for another 7 days. Bacterial peritonitis often recurs, but prophylactic therapy with oral norfloxacin appears effective to prevent recurrent peritonitis in adults.

Gastrointestinal bleeding

Gastrointestinal haemorrhage is the most alarming complication of portal hypertension. The first episode of bleeding often occurs between 9–13 years of age. Avoidance of aspirin and non-steroidal anti-inflammatory agents may reduce the risk of bleeding. These medications produce oesophageal, gastric, or duodenal mucosal injury and impair platelet function. Haematemesis indicates bleeding from oesophageal or gastric varices. Melaena follows but may not appear for up to 24 hours. Haematochezia (fresh blood in stools) may indicate colonic variceal bleeding or rapid passage of blood from the upper gastrointestinal tract. Initial treatment focuses on maintenance of euvolaemia followed by transfusion of packed red blood cells. If prothrombin time and partial thromboplastin time are prolonged, 2–5 mg of parenteral vitamin K may correct the coagulopathy within several hours. More commonly, prothrombin time alone is prolonged, probably because of limited liver function to synthesize factor VII. Critically ill patients may require fresh frozen plasma and/or platelet transfusions. H_2-receptor antagonists are provided intravenously to reduce the deleterious effects of mucosal irritation from gastric acid and to prevent stress-related bleeding. In emergent situations, intravenous octreotide may slow oesophageal variceal bleeding without producing the confusing systemic vasoconstriction of intravenous vaso-pression. The timing and urgency of diagnostic or therapeutic endoscopic procedures vary among individual centres. Urgent endoscopic evaluation and attempted therapy during active bleeding is easily complicated by difficulty visualizing varices or ulcerations, potential regurgitation of blood, and problems with airway protection. Many upper gastrointestinal haemorrhages in children and adolescents are self-limited, providing a bleeding-free interval for stabilization and less problematic examination.

Recurrent oesophageal or gastric variceal haemorrhages often lead to thera-peutic intervention to ablate varices. Sclerotherapy requires 4–6 endoscopies and has multiple potential morbidities.[22,23] Oesophageal ulceration with self-limited rebleeding, oesophageal stricture, bacteraemia with metastatic foci of infection, mediastinal inflammation, and pulmonary congestion represent possible complications. Endoscopic band ligation necessitates fewer treatments and has a lower rate of rebleeding and complications.[24,25] Availability in paediatric centres may be limited, although banding devices of appropriate size for paediatric patients are now available. Additional bleeding during therapeutic procedures is not uncommon. Appropriate intravenous access, blood, and blood products must be readily available. The number and severity of bleeding episodes, the degree of pulmonary disease, the potential candidacy for liver transplantation, the experience of the treating physicians, and the wishes of the patient and family represent some of the considerations guiding the timing and intensity of therapeutic endoscopy.

Hepatocellular failure

Progressive hepatocellular failure and complications of portal hypertension may prompt consideration of liver transplantation. In the 1970s, various shunt procedures were recommended for recurrent gastrointestinal bleeding. Prophylactic shunts were considered in an effort to prevent bleeding episodes later in life when lung disease might be more severe. For selected patients with preserved liver synthetic function, portosystemic shunt procedures still may represent optimal treatment. However, the use of therapeutic endoscopic procedures, transjugular intrahepatic portosystemic shunting (TIPS), and liver transplantation have replaced operative shunts for many patients. TIPS may provide urgent decompression of the portal venous system and prevent further variceal haemorrhage. TIPS has been performed in CF patients. It provides only a transient solution for gastrointestinal haemorrhage or refractory ascites.[26] TIPS allows for stabilization of clinical status until liver transplantation can be performed.[26] Liver transplantation provides the dual benefits of replacing the diseased liver and decompressing the portal venous system. The risk of progressive liver disease with eventual failure of synthetic function and the risk of recurrent complications of portal hypertension can both be eliminated. Liver transplantation and the associated immuno-suppression do not lead to rapidly progressive pulmonary disease. Often, pulmonary function improves after liver transplantation.[18,20] Reduction in abdominal distention and improved muscle strength with better nutritional status probably underlie this improvement. Short-term survival (90%) for CF patients is similar to other patients undergoing liver transplantation. The decision to proceed with evaluation for transplantation or other therapeutic procedures requires the careful consideration and participation of the entire healthcare team. CF physicians, experienced hepatologists or gastroentero-logists, liver transplant surgeons, nurses, social workers, patient, and family join in consultation to decide which procedure is best-suited for managing the complications of cirrhosis and portal hypertension.

BILIARY TRACT DISORDERS

Gallstones

Cholelithiasis occurs in 5–15% of CF patients, the incidence increasing with age. In one review of 670 patients, 24 (3.6%) suffered symptomatic gallstone disease.[27] The youngest symptomatic patient was 4 years-old. CF-related gallstones contain calcium bilirubinate and proteins, but not a preponderance of cholesterol. The exact conditions that predispose to gallstone enucleation and enlargement in CF are not known. Since CF gallstones are not cholesterol stones, UDCA therapy is not effective in dissolving gallstones in CF patients.[28,29]

Symptoms from gallstones follow a characteristic pattern: pain is severe, colicky, and located in the right upper quadrant or epigastrium. Less commonly, pain will be referred to the right subscapular region. Pain lasts a few to several hours and then remits spontaneously. Presumably, pain occurs when a stone impacts in the cystic or common bile duct, producing obstruction and proximal distention of the duct or gallbladder. Stones residing in the gallbladder are often asymptomatic. Serum bilirubin elevation and transient mild elevation of serum alkaline phosphatase or serum transaminases may be present during or just after pain. Ultrasound reveals residual stones in the gallbladder or a stone within the cystic or common bile duct to confirm the diagnosis. In CF patients with characteristic pain and ultrasound findings, cholecystectomy is recommended because of the high risk of recurrent painful episodes and the potential for ascending cholangitis or cholecystitis. Laparoscopic cholecystectomy produces less morbidity than laparotomy and is the preferred procedure. Residual stones within the common bile duct can be detected and removed by laparoscopic techniques or by endoscopic retrograde cholangiopancreatography (ERCP). In some centres, the ERCP is performed immediately following the laparoscopic procedure, resulting in a single general anaesthetic.

Other biliary abnormalities

Particular anatomical abnormalities of the biliary tract occur with CF. Microgallbladder or very small thick-walled gall bladder is a common finding on ultrasound or at autopsy in CF patients. A microgallbladder may not fill or empty normally, but it does not appear to cause particular symptoms.[30] In 1988, Gaskin et al described a group of 61 patients with liver disease and CF, two-thirds of whom had abnormal biliary tracts identified by radionucleotide scanning. Transhepatic cholangiography demonstrated intrapancreatic compression of the distal common bile duct with proximal dilatation in 14 patients. Many of these latter patients underwent surgical diversion of the common bile duct. This paper is the only series to report such a high frequency of symptomatic bile duct abnormalities.[31] In subsequent studies, O'Brien found a far lower frequency of distal stricture of the common bile duct in CF patients with clinical liver disease. Intrahepatic duct irregularities were common, but only 1% of patients had documented distal abnormalities.[32] Potentially-affected CF patients have right upper quadrant pain with biochemical evidence of liver disease. If hepatobiliary ultrasound identifies dilatation of the extra- or intrahepatic biliary tract, then invasive studies, like endoscopic retrograde cholangiopancreatography or transhepatic cholangiography, delineate the exact biliary anatomy and site of presumed obstruction.

INTESTINAL DISORDERS

CFTR mRNA expression occurs throughout intestinal mucosal epithelium. CFTR is expressed at relatively high levels in duodenal mucosa with expression decreasing steadily down the length of the small bowel. In all areas with expression, CFTR concentration is highest in crypt cells and diminishes towards villous tips. Crypt cells secrete chloride in the normal intestine, establishing the electrochemical gradient for the movement of sodium and then water into the lumen. The presence of CFTR in crypt cells correlates with abnormalities in electrolyte flux in CF intestinal epithelia. A disturbance in chloride crypt secretion is, therefore, likely to reduce hydration of intestinal secretions and predispose to intestinal obstruction.

DISTAL INTESTINAL OBSTRUCTION SYNDROME

About 10–15% of CF newborns present with distal small bowel obstruction as neonatal meconium ileus. In the late 1960s, literature reports accumulated describing older CF patients who suffered distal small bowel obstruction due to inspissated intestinal contents in the terminal ileum. Originally, this clinical problem was labelled meconium ileus equivalent, but it is now called distal intestinal obstruction syndrome (DIOS). In the initial descriptions of DIOS, clinicians proposed that the condition occurred when CF patients failed to take adequate enzyme supplementation. Subsequent experience suggests that most patients with DIOS are actually taking their enzymes in appropriate dosages. CF patients with DIOS may have more severe residual steatorrhoea, even with pancreatic enzyme treatment. Persistent steatorrhoea may slow intestinal transit as neurotensin, a GI hormone delaying motility, is secreted from the distal ileum when unabsorbed fat reaches that location. Inherently slow intestinal motility, narcotics, anti-cholingergics, postoperative ileus, or abnormal intraluminal secretions may also potentiate DIOS.

Symptoms

DIOS may present with acute or chronic symptoms. The cardinal features include: crampy abdominal pain, often in the right lower quadrant or lower abdomen, a palpable mass in the right lower quadrant, and decreased frequency of defaecation. Abdominal distention and bilious vomiting, signs of actual or impending small bowel obstruction, can predominate. Approximately 10% of CF patients will suffer this form of DIOS.[33] Signs of dehydration and intravascular volume depletion occur with fluid losses from vomiting or reduced intake and with fluid and electrolyte secretion into the lumen of obstructed small bowel. Abdominal plain films (flat plate and upright films) show bubbly faecal material in the right lower quadrant or throughout the colon. With acute obstruction, air-fluid levels appear in dilated proximal small bowel loops. Affected CF patients are almost always older than age 5 years and often average above age 15 years. In the chronic form of DIOS, the colicky abdominal pain may be provoked by meals, resulting in anorexia as a method of avoiding pain. The attacks of pain may remit for weeks or months, but return associated with right lower quadrant mass and relative constipation. Physical examination reveals a mass or fullness in the right lower quadrant. The rectal examination may be normal or may reveal accumulated faeces. If these 'classic' physical and radiological findings are not present, then alternative aetiologies of abdominal pain and/or obstruction must be considered. Often, DIOS is incorrectly implicated as a cause of abdominal pain in a CF patient.[34,35] This error delays the diagnosis of appendicitis, intussusception, small bowel obstruction due to adhesions, or fibrosing colonopathy and may lead to inappropriate therapy.

Management

The treatment of DIOS is directed at non-operative relief of the small bowel or colonic obstruction. The two most common approaches are enema with a radiopaque hypertonic solution (Gastrografin® or Hypaque®) and voluminous intestinal perfusion of a balanced electrolyte solution. Table 11.3 details the advantages, disadvantages, and cautions relevant to each procedure. Gastrografin® enema confirms the diagnosis and may dislodge inspissated material from the distal ileum or colon. In DIOS, the enema shows a non-dilated colon and filling defects outlined in the distal ileum. Contrast material should reflux into the more proximal dilated small bowel. The hypertonic solution draws fluid into the small bowel lumen allowing for washout of the thick faecal material into the colon. If the course of DIOS is chronic or if there is not evidence of complete small bowel obstruction, intestinal lavage treatment provides an alternative therapy to mobilize inspissated intestinal contents. Lavage treatment provides a large volume of isotonic fluid flowing from the stomach to the distal small bowel to dilute the impacted material. Older CF patients may take sufficient lavage solution by mouth; younger patients often require an infusion through a nasogastric tube.[36]

Table 11.3 Advantages, disadvantages, and cautions about distal intestinal obstruction syndrome treatment

Advantages of hypertonic enema	Advantages of lavage
Exact diagnosis established	Less discomfort with procedure
Post-evacuation films document resolution	Less x-ray exposure
	Therapy at home
Disadvantages	Disadvantages
Intravascular volume depletion	Exact diagnosis not delineated
Patient discomfort	Vomiting
X-ray exposure	Contra-indicated in total obstruction
Examination may fail to relieve obstruction	Nasogastric tube may be needed
Repeat examination may be required	Intraluminal fluid shifts may occur
Cautions	Cautions
Intravenous line needed	Large volume of solution required
Experienced radiologist and clinician required during procedure	Abdominal distention may occur
Patient discomfort may be considerable	

Recurrences of DIOS are common. Increased fluid intake or bulk or lubricant laxatives have been offered as prophylactic therapies, but are not proven unequivocally effective. CF patients treated with a continual course of cisapride had fewer recurrences of DIOS that required intestinal lavage treatment than CF patients treated with placebo.[37] Cisapride treatment did not, however, abolish all recurrences of DIOS. An alternative therapy with anecdotal support is periodic intake of intestinal lavage solution in amounts less than that used in aggressive lavage treatments. Patients ingest lavage solution in amounts similar to that used as preparation for colonoscopy whenever they begin to have crampy abdominal pain or on a regularly defined schedule. No controlled study of this therapy is available.

INTUSSUSCEPTION

Ileo-colic intussusception occurs in CF patients, reportedly at increased frequency and at an older age than in the general population. Idiopathic (non-CF) intussusception generally afflicts children ages 9 months to 2 years. In CF, the patient may be in the second decade.[38] The symptoms and signs can mimic the findings in DIOS. Early in the course, intussusception causes severe colicky pain, but without radiological signs of obstruction. Obstructive signs appear after the accumulation of bowel wall oedema with ischaemia. Abdominal ultrasound may be useful to identify intussusception, demonstrating the 'target sign' at the lead point of intussusception. Gastrografin® enema can be diagnostic and may prove therapeutic for the intussusception. Hydrostatic reduction is often accomplished during a diagnostic contrast enema. If the intussusception is not reducible by this manoeuvre, then surgical exploration is required.

APPENDICITIS

Acute appendicitis can mimic the presenting signs of the acute form of DIOS. Fever and leukocytosis may be present. The appendix is often perforated by the time the diagnosis is established, but the perforation is contained by surrounding structures.[39,40] The frequent use of broad spectrum antibiotics in CF patients may prevent severe complications of appendiceal perforation, blunting the clinical presentation. Contrast enema often shows deformity of the caecum with mass effect and not the findings expected in DIOS. Abdominal CT scan readily defines intra-abdominal abscess or fluid collection near the caecum. In normal individuals, non-filling of the appendix during contrast enema may indicate appendicitis. In a retrospective review of contrast enemas in series of CF patients, non-filling of the appendix was not a reliable sign for the presence of appendicitis. Histological studies showed that non-filling may be due to mucous plugging of the appendiceal lumen.[41] This appendiceal distention has been implicated as a cause of recurrent right lower quadrant pain or repeated intussusception.[42] With laparoscopic appendectomy and percutaneous drainage of appendiceal abscess, the morbidity of laparotomy may be avoided in many CF patients with appendiceal disease.

FIBROSING COLONOPATHY

Several CF centres recently reported the occurrence of segmental colon fibrosis and stricture in CF patients who had been treated with very high dose pancreatic enzyme supplements.[43-45] Most of the patients were between ages 2–8 years. A recent case control study of US CF patients documented a mean daily dose of 50 000 units lipase/kg/day in fibrosing colonopathy patients versus a mean dose of 19 000 units/kg/day in age-matched controls.[46] Also, affected children were more often taking H_2-receptor antagonists, corticosteroids, and aerosolized dornase alfa. Presenting symptoms included crampy abdominal pain and 3 or more loose stools per day with visible or microscopic blood. Some patients suffered colicky pain, decreased stools, and vomiting, suggesting partial distal bowel obstruction. Patients were often treated initially for possible DIOS. Contrast enemas revealed, however, narrowing and lack of distensibility of segments of the colon. The caecum and right colon were damaged most severely. Colonoscopic biopsies showed non-specific chronic inflammation, focal acute inflammation with crypt abscesses, and a prominence of mucosal eosinophils.[47] Characteristic pathological changes in resected specimens clearly differentiated the disorder from inflammatory bowel disease or infectious colitis: submucosal fibrosis, scarring and thickening of the muscularis propria, and fibrosis of the lamina propria affected both strictured and non-strictured areas. In some patients, short segments of resected terminal ileum contained linear ulcerations with transmural inflammation.

In reported patients, symptoms did not respond well to anti-inflammatory medications or to reduction of supplemental pancreatic enzymes. Most patients required resection of affected colon, but at least two improved with provision of parenteral nutrition, discontinuation of enzymes, and a specialized low fat oral diet. After 3–4 months, their colonopathy symptoms and radiological changes

Table 11.4 Abdominal pain problems in CF

Location	Character	Associated findings	Aetiology
Substernal	Burning	Haematemesis	Oesophagitis
Epigastric	Meal-related		Gastritis
RUQ, epigastric	Colicky	Elevated LFTs*	Cholelithiasis
RUQ	Periodic	Elevated LFTs	Bile duct stricture
RLQ, diffuse	Periodic	RLQ mass	DIOS
RLQ, diffuse	Colicky	Right-sided mass	Intussusception
RLQ, focal	Constant	Fever, leukocytosis	Appendicitis
Diffuse	Colicky	Distention, bilious vomiting	Small bowel obstruction
Diffuse	Periodic	Diarrhoea, rectal bleeding	Fibrosing colonopathy
Diffuse	Periodic	Faecal impaction	Constipation

*LFTs = serum ALT, AST or alkaline phosphatase.
RUQ = right upper quadrant.
RLQ = right lower quadrant.

remitted. A usual oral diet and pancreatic enzymes had not been re-introduced at the time of the published report.[43] In the 1997 summary report, 30 of 31 affected US patients had undergone subtotal colectomy. One patient required total colectomy.[46]

Aetiology and pathogenesis

The exact aetiology of fibrosing colonopathy is unknown. The association with intake of high doses of pancreatic enzymes was strong enough, however, to initiate the removal of high potency pancreatic enzyme supplements from the commercial market in the US. In the 1997 US study, although all patients took delayed release enzymes formulations, no specific enzyme product demonstrated an increased risk for development of colonopathy. Investigators hypothesized that actual enzyme content, enzyme coating, or additional medications may contribute to the colon damage.

Characteristic fibrosing colonopathy afflicted relatively few CF patients, but bowel wall thickening, a possible precursor of more severe disease, has recently been detected in a much larger segment of the CF population. Cross-sectional surveys demonstrate that mean ileal and colon wall thickness in CF children and adults exceeds that in normal individuals when measured by ultrasound. Considerable overlap exists, however, between values in CF and controls.[48,49] For example, in CF patients, caecal wall measures a mean of 2.7 mm (range 1.0–5.0 mm) versus controls with a mean of 1.4 mm (range 0.7–1.9 mm).[48] Thickening is most notable in the submucosa of the colon. Mean bowel wall thickness does not correlate with lipase dosage, previous abdominal surgery, or type of enzyme preparation. The studied individuals are asymptomatic, obviating any correlation with symptoms suggesting bowel dysfunction. Bowel wall thickness increases with age in both CF and control individuals. Two studies relate high dose enzyme strength to maximum colon wall thickness, but could not correlate total daily enzyme dosage with the ultrasound findings.[45,49] In one study, maximal colonic wall thickness did not progress over 1 year. A second study showed reduction in wall thickness with decrease in enzyme dosage in selected patients. The significance and time course of these observed differences in small bowel and colonic wall thickness require additional clarification with longitudinal studies in CF and normal populations.

Abdominal pain

Cystic fibrosis patients are vulnerable to several serious intra-abdominal conditions that present with abdominal pain. Table 11.4 provides a succinct outline of these potential problems. Abnormal biliary tract and intestinal secretions, resulting from the basic CFTR defect, may represent the initial factor behind these complications. The CF patient with acute abdominal pain requires careful evaluation for multiple diagnoses ranging from cholelithiasis to small bowel obstruction. The CF patient with chronic recurrent pain may harbour a CF-related problem or a more benign diagnosis. Chronic DIOS, constipation, recurrent abdominal pain, and irritable bowel syndrome become considerations in individuals with less severe illness. Because of the potential for serious illness, however, CF patients often require more extensive evaluation and investigation than the patient without underlying disease.

Key points for clinical practice

- Gastro-oesophageal reflux is not in itself a disease; some degree of reflux occurs in normal individuals. Complications of gastro-oesophageal reflux include failure to thrive, oesophagitis, and respiratory tract disease.

- No single test identifies gastro-oesophageal reflux as a contributing factor in respiratory tract disease. Improvement in respiratory tract symptoms or signs with medical or surgical therapy of gastro-oesophageal reflux provides the strongest evidence of a connection.

- Neonatal cholestasis, steatosis, or elevation of serum transaminases are not predictors of chronic liver disease in cystic fibrosis patients.

- Careful physical examination is the first clue to cirrhosis. The usual physical findings include prominence of superficial abdominal veins, palpable hard-edged liver, and progressive splenomegaly.

- Complications of portal hypertension, not liver synthetic failure, threaten the health of cirrhotic cystic fibrosis patients.

- Liver transplantation cures cirrhosis and portal hypertension. Pulmonary function and nutritional status also improve. Immunosuppression does not potentiate progressive lung disease.

- Cholelithiasis is often asymptomatic, not requiring intervention. Laparoscopic cholecystectomy is preferred for surgical management of symptomatic gallstone disease.

Key points for clinical practice (continued)

- Distal intestinal obstruction syndrome afflicts about 10% of cystic fibrosis patients. Crampy abdominal pain, right lower quadrant fullness, and diminished defaecation are diagnostic hallmarks.

- Appendicitis, intussusception, small bowel obstruction from adhesions, and fibrosing colonopathy can mimic distal intestinal obstruction syndrome. The diagnosis of distal intestinal obstruction syndrome requires characteristic symptoms, signs, and x-ray findings.

- Therapy of distal intestinal obstruction syndrome includes gastro-intestinal lavage or hypertonic enema with a radiopaque solution. Lavage produces less discomfort, but contrast enema provides exact diagnosis and can detect different or additional diagnoses.

- Fibrosing colonopathy presents with abdominal pain and diarrhoea, often with haematochezia (fresh blood in stools). Patients taking high doses of supplemental pancreatic enzymes are at risk. Once colonopathy produces symptoms, resection of damaged colon is usually necessary to ameliorate clinical problems

- Thickening of intestinal and colonic wall is sometimes evident from detailed abdominal ultrasound. The relationship of this thickening to abdominal symptoms is unclear.

References

1 Orenstein D, Stern R. (eds) Treatment of the Hospitalized Cystic Fibrosis Patient. New York: Marcel Dekker, 1998

2 Katz P. Pathogenesis and management of gastroesophageal reflux disease. J Clin Gastroenterol 1991; 13 (suppl 2): S6–S15

3 Orenstein S, Orenstein D. Gastroesophageal reflux and respiratory disease in children. J Pediatr 1988; 112: 847–858

4 Feigelson J, Girault F, Pecan Y. Gastro-oesophageal reflux and oesophagitis in cystic fibrosis. Acta Paediatr Scand 1987; 76: 989–990

5 Malfroot A, Dab I. New insights on gastro-oesophageal reflux in cystic fibrosis by longitudinal follow up. Arch Dis Child 1991; 66: 1339–1345

6 Ferreira C, Lohous MJ, Bensoussan A, Yazbeck S, Brochu P, Roy CC. Prolonged pH monitoring is of limited usefulness for gastroesophageal reflux. Am J Dis Child 1993; 147: 662–664

7 Cucchiara S, Santamaria F, Andreotti MR et al. Mechanisms of gastro-oesophageal reflux in cystic fibrosis. Arch Dis Child 1991; 66: 617–622

8 Button BM, Heine RG, Catto-Smith AG, Phelan PD, Olinsky A. Postural drainage and gastro-oesophageal reflux in infants with cystic fibrosis. Arch Dis Child 1997; 76: 148–150

9 Low D, Mercer C, James E, Hill L, Post nissen syndrome. Surg Gynecol Obstet 1988; 167: 1–5

10 Negre J. Post-fundoplication symptoms. Ann Surg 1983; 198: 697–700

11 Roy C, Weber A, Morin C et al. Hepatobiliary disease in cystic fibrosis: a survey of current issues and concepts. J Pediatr Gastroenterol Nutr 1982; 1: 469–478

12 Psacharopoulous HT, Howard ER, Portmann B, Mowat AP, Williams R. Hepatic complications of cystic fibrosis. Lancet 1981; ii: 78–80

13 Colombo C, Apostolo MG, Ferrari M et al. Analysis of risk factors for the development of liver disease associated with cystic fibrosis. J Pediatr 1994; 24: 393–399

14 Potter CJ, Fishbein M, Hammond S, McCoy K, Qualman S. Can the histologic changes of cystic fibrosis-associated hepatobiliary disease be predicted by clinical criteria? J Pediatr Gastroenterol Nutr 1997; 25: 32–36

15 Colombo C, Castellani MR, Balistreri WF, Seregni E, Assaisso ML, Giunta A. Scintigraphic documentation of an improvement in hepatobiliary excretory function after treatment with ursodeoxycholic acid in patients with cystic fibrosis and associated liver disease. Hepatology 1992; 15: 677–684

16 Galabert C, Montet JC, Lengrand D et al. Effects of ursodeoxycholic acid on liver function in patients with cystic fibrosis and chronic cholestasis. J Pediatr 1992; 121: 138–141

17 O'Brien S, Fitzgerald MX, Hegarty JE. A controlled trial of ursodeoxycholic acid treatment in cystic fibrosis-related liver disease. Eur J Gastroenterol Hepatol 1992; 4: 857–863

18 Mack DR, Traystman MD, Colombo JL et al. Clinical denouement and mutation analysis of patients with cystic fibrosis undergoing liver transplantation for biliary cirrhosis. J Pediatr 1995; 127: 881–887

19 Stern R, Stevens D, Boat T, Doershuk C, Izant R, Symptomatic hepatic disease in cystic fibrosis: incidence, course, and outcome of portal systemic shunting. Gastroenterology 1976; 70: 645–649

20 Noble-Jamieson G, Barnes N, Jamieson N, Friend P, Calne R. Liver transplantation for hepatic cirrhosis in cystic fibrosis. J R Soc Med 1996; 89 (Suppl. 27): 31–37

21 Runyon B. Spontaneous bacterial peritonitis: an explosion of information. Hepatology 1988; 8: 171–175

22 Paquet K, Lazar A. Current therapeutic strategy in bleeding esophageal varices in babies and children and long-term results of endoscopic paravariceal sclerotherapy over twenty years. Eur J Pediatr Surg 1994; 4: 165–172

23 Goenka A, Dasilva M, Cleghorn G, Patrick M, Shepherd R. Therapeutic upper gastrointestinal endoscopy in children: an audit of 443 procedures and literature review. J Gastroenterol 1991; 8: 44–51

24 Fox V, Carr-Locke D, Connors P, Leichtner A. Endoscopic ligation of esophageal varices in children. J. Pediatr Gastroenterol Nutr 1995; 20: 202–208

25 Laine L, Cook D. Endoscopic ligation compared with sclerotherapy for treatment of esophageal variceal bleeding. Ann Intern Med 1995; 123: 280–287

26 Kerns S, Hawkins I. Transjugular intrahepatic portosystemic shunt in a child with cystic fibrosis. Am J Respir 1992; 159: 1277–1278

27 Stern RC, Rothstein FC, Doershuk CF. Treatment and prognosis of symptomatic gallbladder disease in patients with cystic fibrosis. J Pediatr Gastroenterol Nutr 1986; 5: 35–40

28 Angelico M, Gandin C, Canuzzi P et al. Gallstones in cystic fibrosis: a critical reappraisal. Hepatology 1991; 14: 768–775

29 Colombo C, Bertolini E, Assaisso ML, Bettinardi N, Giunta A, Podda M. Failure of ursodeoxycholic acid to dissolve radiolucent gallstones in patients with cystic fibrosis. Acta Paediatr 1993; 82: 562–565

30 Quillin SP, Siegel MJ, Rothbaum R. Hepatobiliary sonography in cystic fibrosis. Pediatr Radiol 1993; 23: 1–3

31 Gaskin KJ, Waters DLM, Howman-Giles R et al. Liver disease and common-bile-duct stenosis in cystic fibrosis. N Engl J Med 1988; 318: 340–346

32 O'Brien S, Keogan M, Casey M et al. Biliary complications of cystic fibrosis. Gut 1992; 33: 387–391

33 Matseshe JW, Go VLW, DiMagno EP. Meconium ileus equivalent complicating cystic fibrosis in postneonatal children and young adults. Gastroenterology 1977; 72: 732–736

34 Dik H, Nicolai JJ, Schipper J, Heijerman HGM, Bakker W. Erroneous diagnosis of distal intestinal obstruction syndrome in cystic fibrosis: clinical impact of abdominal ultrasonography. Eur J Gastroenterol Hepatol 1995; 7: 279–281

35 Dalzell AM, Heaf DP, Carty H. Pathology mimicking distal intestinal obstruction syndrome in cystic fibrosis. Arch Dis Child 1990; 65: 540–541

36 Koletzko S, Stringer DA, Cleghorn GJ, Durie PR. Lavage treatment of distal intestinal obstruction syndrome in children with cystic fibrosis. Pediatrics 1989; 83: 727–733

37 Koletzko S, Corey M, Ellis L, Spino M, Stringer DA, Durie PR. Effects of cisapride in patients with cystic fibrosis and distal intestinal obstruction syndrome. J Pediatr 1990; 117: 815–822

38 Holmes M, Murphy V, Taylor M, Denham B. Intussusception in cystic fibrosis. Arch Dis Child 1991; 66: 726–727

39 Shields MD, Levison H, Reisman JJ, Durie PR, Canny GJ. Appendicitis in cystic fibrosis. Arch Dis Child 1990; 65: 307–310

40 Allen ED, Pfaff JK, Taussig LM, McCoy KS. The clinical spectrum of chronic appendiceal abscess in cystic fibrosis. Am J Dis Child 1992; 146: 1190–1193

41 Fletcher BD, Abramowsky CR. Contrast enemas in cystic fibrosis: implications of appendiceal nonfilling. Am J Respir 1981; 137: 323–326

42 Coughlin JP, Gauderer MWL, Stern RC, Doershuk CF, Izant Jr RJ, Zollinger Jr RM. The spectrum of appendiceal disease in cystic fibrosis. J Pediatr Surg 1990; 25: 835–839

43 Schwarzenberg SJ, Wielinski Cl, Shamieh I et al. Cystic fibrosis associated colitis and fibrosing colonopathy. J Pediatr 1995; 127: 565–570

44 Freiman JP, FitzSimmons SC. Colonic strictures in patients with cystic fibrosis: results of a survey of 114 cystic fibrosis care centres in the United States. J Pediatr Gastroenterol Nutr 1996; 22: 153–156

45 Sweeney EJM, Oades PJ, Buchdahl R, Rosenthal M, Busch A. Relation of thickening of colon wall to pancreatic-enzyme treatment in cystic fibrosis. Lancet 1995; 345: 752–756

46 FitzSimmons SC, Burkhart GA, Borowitz D et al. High-dose pancreatic-enzyme supplements and fibrosing colonopathy in children with cystic fibrosis. N Engl J Med 1997; 336: 1283–1289

47 Pawel BR, De Chadarvian J-P, Franco ME. The pathology of fibrosing colonopathy of cystic fibrosis: a study 12 cases and review of the literature. Hum Pathol 1997; 28: 395–399

48 Haber HP, Benda N, Fitzke G et al. Colonic wall thickness measured by ultrasound: striking differences in patients with cystic fibrosis versus healthy controls. Gut 1997; 40: 406–411

49 Pohl M, Krackhardt B, Posselt HG, Lembcke B. Ultrasound studies of the intestinal wall in patients with cystic fibrosis. J Pediatr Gastroenterol Nutr 1997; 25: 317–320

David C. Morley

Low-technology approaches to child care in the third world

Just as long as the health interventions we are involved with, remain in the formal clinic or hospital environment, there will be barriers which separate the mother and child from 'owning' or 'participating' in their health care. The responsibility and control of health changes must become part of everyday behaviour from hygiene and sanitation to sexual behaviour, child nutrition and development. Only when this 'owning' and 'participation' takes place will the interventions become successful and sustainable. Health workers need to think in simple terms and always observe and question the way that families live and behave. For example:

> *On arrival from the UK to undertake research in an African village, the author was surprised to find that well babies rarely cried. In their early months they were in constant skin contact with their mother or some other member of the family. Small babies had their heads covered with brightly coloured woolly hats. They did not have nappies as within a week of birth the mother from the movement on her back recognised when her infant was about to urinate or defaecate.*

It was only over years that the significance of these observations and their importance to infants became apparent.

LOW TECHNOLOGY APPROACHES APPROPRIATE TO EACH AGE GROUP

Preconceptual care

There is strong evidence that much low birthweight and congenital disabilities which cause great suffering and can take up so much of paediatric care, can be

Prof. David Morley CBE MD(Cantab) FRCP, 51 Eastmoor Park, Harpenden, Herts AL5 1BN, UK

prevented in the weeks prior to conception.[1,2] Paediatricians and other health workers seldom have opportunities to influence future parents in this period for their first baby. However, they may have for subsequent births. After examining each new-born and congratulating the mother on a healthy child, the health worker can advise the parents on an adequate birth interval and their lifestyle and health in the preconceptual period for any future births. As the child health care worker sees young children in the under five's clinics, they should know the 'vulnerable' month on the child's growth chart.[3] This is identified from a study of birth intervals as the month when 5% of mothers conceive. Before this month, the mother and father should be advised on the advantages of a long birth interval and appropriate preconceptual care. This will involve avoiding tobacco, alcohol, slimming diets, and conceiving in the period following a flu-like illness. Recent research suggests also that, in developing countries, pregnancy during a period of food shortage may increase the mortality by as much as 10-fold,[4] when the child is grown up, in the age group 20–25 years. This is a finding of potential considerable significance and suggests that the development of the immune system may be affected during the pregnancy.

The neonate

Thanks to activities by national governments supported by WHO, and particularly UNICEF, the under five mortality in children has dramatically

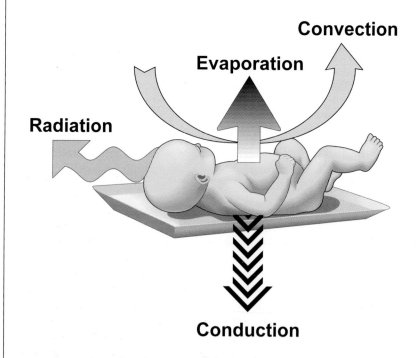

Fig. 12.1 Those caring for the newborn and young infants need to know how the infant loses heat and the steps to take to keep the infant warm.

fallen in most countries. Unfortunately the decline in mortality has been less significant in the neonatal period. Much of the mortality in this period arises from failures in temperature control, preventing infections and establishing adequate breastfeeding.

Warmth

The WHO advises that where the birthweight is between 1.5–2 kg a room temperature of 32–34°C is required, for babies between 2–2.5 kg a range of 30–32°C, while infants greater than 2.5 kg require a temperature of 28–30°C. Even this rather lower temperature may be considered hot for adults, even in tropical countries. Health workers need to know the several ways in which small babies can lose heat (Fig. 12.1). All those caring for the new-born must know the following:

* Immediately after birth, wrap baby in a warm dry cloth while any necessary resuscitation, is being given.
* The heads of small babies should always be covered with a warm cap or blanket.
* Any surface on which a baby is placed must be covered with a warm cloth.
* Draughts from windows or doors will cool a baby.
* **Never use hot water bottles, heated stones, etc.**

'Kangaroo mother care'

The simplest of all low technology developments has been the acceptance of the value of close contact between the mother and the baby. In societies where this is acceptable, the contact should be skin-to-skin between the breasts as probably occurred in prehistoric times. There is now a group of doctors and nurses who have developed this concept which has been aptly called 'Kangaroo care'.[5]

Infection

The dying umbilical cord is a wonderful culture medium. At one time in parts of the world 60 out of every 1000 neonates died from neonatal tetanus from infection of the umbilical stump at or soon after birth. Neonatal tetanus is now uncommon, and any case seen requires a drive to cover all mothers with tetanus toxoid in pregnancy. Perhaps almost as important, but less well recognised, are the antibiotic resistant organisms that the umbilicus can collect from the hospital environment, such as the multiple antibiotic resistant *Staphylococcus aureus*. This dangerous infection is less likely if the stay in hospital in minimal and, wherever possible, all the handling and toilet of the baby is undertaken by the mother. Whether at home or in hospital the proud new mother must be aware of the need to protect her new-born from handling or being kissed by relatives, particularly those with respiratory infections. For this she will need the support of health workers in societies where by custom the newborn infant is passed around from relative to relative.

Breastfeeding

For most babies born in developing countries, successful nutrition depends almost entirely on establishing and maintaining adequate breast feeding for around 2 years. For a proportion of mothers in all societies, establishing breastfeeding is not easy. In the past, health professionals have frequently not had the knowledge or commitment of time and patience to help the mother achieve appropriate breastfeeding. Senior staff must have the time to spend demonstrating to junior staff the great patience needed to help a mother to achieve her baby latching on to the breast (Fig. 12.2). It is now more widely appreciated that by allowing a baby to suck from a feeding bottle the baby develops 'nipple confusion'. Fortunately there are now many hospitals in the developing world where feeding bottles are excluded. Feeding is achieved from a cup using expressed breast milk except for a few small or ill infants who require tube feeding.

'Not enough milk'

Almost every woman can produce enough milk for her baby: (i) if she wants to; (ii) if the baby suckles in a good position; and (iii) if the baby suckles frequently.

Much emphasis is fortunately now placed on establishing breastfeeding. Unfortunately due to failures in growth monitoring, which will be discussed later, the success of the mothers breastfeeding over the ensuing months is not carefully monitored in terms of adequate weight gain.

The mother needs encouragement from the health worker and support from her family, who must provide her with the time to breastfeed and release her from many of her chores. With this support, a high proportion of mothers can provide large quantities of breast milk through the first 8 months of life. They must understand that the volume of milk depends on stimulation of the nipple by frequent sucking and the mother limiting her physical exertion.

Figure 12.3 shows the simplified growth records of two infants using the easily remembered figures 8, 4 and 2. We start the baby with a reasonable birth weight of 3.2 kg (8 × 4 = 3.2). If, over the next 8 months, the infant averages a gain of 800 g/month his/her weight at 9 months will be just over the 50th centile (the upper line). If the infant now gains at an average of 200 g/month he/she will remain around the 50th centile.

If another baby averages 400 g in the first 8 months, he/she will arrive on the 3rd centile (lower line) at 9 months. If this infant now also gains at 200 g/month he/she will remain around the 3rd centile. Health workers, with experience in

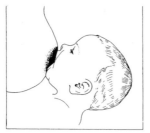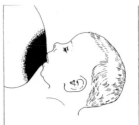

Fig. 12.2 Suckling in a good position. This baby is close to the breast with the mouth wide open and not as in the second figure.

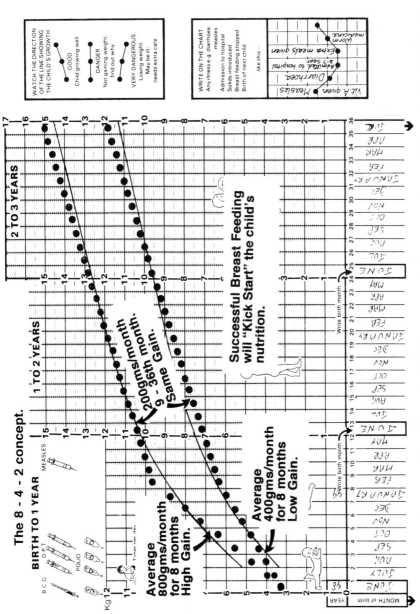

Fig. 12.3 A simplified growth record involves the numbers 8, 4, and 2. This demonstrates the importance of successful breast feeding in the first 8 months of life.

developing countries, know well that if a child is on the 50th centile at 9 months of age, that child has a good chance of overcoming the common infections and maintaining a satisfactory nutritional state during the important first 3 years of life. In general, the child who is only on the 3rd centile or below this by the age of 9 months is much less likely to achieve satisfactory nutrition and overcome infections in the next 2 years. If mothers are encouraged in their breastfeeding and receive family support, many more infants can be around the 50th centile by 9 months.

THE INFANT AND PRE-SCHOOL CHILD

Immunisation

Due to a sustained effort by governments supported by international agencies, around 80% of the world's children were fully immunised in 1990 and a high proportion of their mothers had received tetanus toxoid. Since then immunisation coverage has been further extended in many countries. There is a real possibility that poliomyelitis will be eradicated within the first decade of the next century. In terms of lives saved, this has been the most successful public health measure in any decade.

Unfortunately 'severe measles' still occurs far too often. This is due to the failure of so many health workers to ensure that at every contact after 9 months children who have escaped immunisation are immunised as quickly as possible. The advent of measles vaccine has stimulated epidemiological research into the severity of diseases, such as measles, which has wider significance.

Size of infecting dose

One of the errors the author of this chapter made in a previous book[6] was to suggest that severe measles was due to the poor nutrition of children catching measles. Aaby,[7] in his important studies in Guinea Bissau, showed that the mortality of measles did not correlate with nutritional state as assessed by a variety of anthropometric measurements. Instead, he showed there was a 4-fold increase in mortality between secondary and index infections presumably due to the size of infecting dose. Many studies, including those from historical records of measles in Europe, have now demonstrated that the severity of measles and its mortality in households was far greater in secondary cases rather than the index case.

There are reasons to believe that the findings on measles relate to other droplet borne infectious diseases and health workers need to take this into account when talking with mothers. We need to explain that respiratory and other infections are likely to spread through a family, but that if younger members can sleep in separate beds and are not handled more than necessary by members with an infection, then they are less likely to have a severe illness. The size of the infecting dose is likely to be a major reason why those living in poverty and overcrowded conditions have more severe illness.[8]

Diarrhoea, vomiting, coughs and colds

These are universal. Fortunately WHO and other organisations have now worked out schemes for their appropriate treatment.

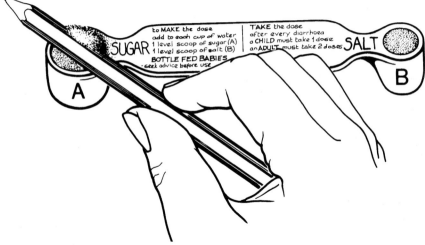

Fig. 12.4 A two-ended spoon to make up sugar and salt solutions for oral rehydration. This solution can be mixed with a cereal gruel to halve the size of the diarrhoeal stools.

Diarrhoea

In developing countries, every child is likely to have on average 10 significant bouts of diarrhoea before the age of 5 years. At least one of these led to dehydration; before oral rehydration was understood around one in every 10 dehydrated child would die.

Fortunately, knowledge of oral rehydration has spread through many communities. Much emphasis is still placed on providing pre-packaged salts for dilution in a litre of water. However, to provide and distribute adequate packages to treat all cases of diarrhoea may involve half of the Ministry of Health's budget. For this reason, there is a place for the home-made oral rehydration solution. Various measures such as spoons or bottle tops have been used. A two-ended plastic spoon (Fig. 12.4) is particularly appropriate. These solutions need to be made up with a cereal or used alongside the local cereal 'pap' or porridge.[9] The value of the cereal is not only that it helps in the nutrition of the child but, more importantly, research shows that by using cereal the volume of the diarrhoeal stool is reduced to a half. It is stopping or reducing the diarrhoea which is so important to the grandmother and other decision makers in the family. Perhaps more time needs to be spent on explaining the physiology of gut peristalsis as part of health education. Most adults realise they pass a stool after a meal, due to reflex movement of the whole gut. For this reason, the child is more likely to have a diarrhoeal stool after any feed. This, however, does NOT mean that the food caused the diarrhoea, as is so commonly assumed, and led to the universal belief in not feeding children with diarrhoea. It is now well researched that food is well absorbed even in acute episodes of diarrhoea.

Vomiting

The majority of diarrhoeal illnesses are associated with vomiting which worries parents trying to follow instructions to feed fluids. The parents need

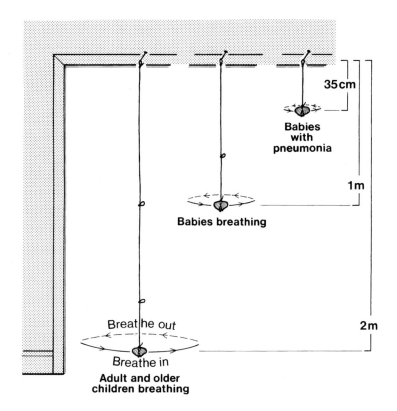

35 cm

Babies
with
pneumonia

1 m

Babies breathing

Breathe out

2 m

Breathe in
**Adult and older
children breathing**

Fig. 12.5 A simple method of demonstrating rapid breathing.

to be fore-warned and have a utensil ready to catch the vomit. They should be reassured when they see the volume of vomit is less than a quarter of the fluid the child has drunk.

Coughs and colds

The unsatisfactory management of upper respiratory infections and the failure to understand that so many coughs are due to a postnasal drip, leads to a major waste of limited resources in health care. WHO has emphasised the importance of rapid breathing to distinguish infections which involve the lower respiratory tract. To teach recognition of rapid respiration to mothers or children in schools, a pendulum created with a stone and a piece of string allows for a simple demonstration (Fig. 12.5). This is particularly effective if the mothers or children are encouraged to breathe in time with the stone as it swings. In this way, they are likely to appreciate and remember the importance of recognising rapid breathing in small children and bring them for antibiotic treatment.

Feeding in convalescence

Repeated infections, particularly diarrhoea and vomiting, can devastate the child's nutrition. The health workers need to know and advise on locally affordable foods which are 'energy dense' and usually contain a high quantity of locally produced cooking oil. All children, particularly those undernourished, require frequent feeding, at least 5 times a day. If the parent can afford any processed food, they may be encouraged to buy skimmed or full cream milk. This is rubbed into local cooking oil to produce a high energy food. The oil disappears and when cold water is added, the oil remains in suspension while it is fed to the child.

Stimulating environment

Educational psychologists have now presented overwhelming evidence on the importance of development of speech and play in a child's later success in schooling, broader education and career. In most countries, government departments of education are stretched even to provide primary schooling from the age of 6 or 7 years. Except perhaps in the capital city, there will be few opportunities for nursery and pre-school education. Health workers have a responsibility to encourage a stimulating environment as they are the only workers regularly in contact with the mother and her pre-school children. They need to impress on the mother the need to 'bathe' her child in words from an early age. Toys appropriate for the age are needed and there is now experience of making these using cardboard boxes, bottle tops and other waste material to be found in almost all communities worldwide.[10] A number of successful programmes have involved school children in construction of these toys and then encouraging them to use these toys to play with their younger siblings (see Child-to-Child below).

THE HEALTH WORKER'S PLACE IN COMMUNITY DEVELOPMENT

Throughout this chapter, there is an underlying concern for developing a greater knowledge of health within the community. In the past, health workers have accepted their responsibility in community development to involve maintaining the health of the community they serve. However, the health worker has the potential to be a major player in community development. There are many examples of this around the world, perhaps the most outstanding is that of the Doctors Arole in India.[11] After a long and wide in-depth health training, they settled in this remote and poverty stricken area centred on the small town of Jamkhed in Maharashtra. They worked through local farmers' clubs side-stepping the caste ridden, corrupt power structures in the villages. In a population of around 200 000, the infant mortality rate was brought down to a figure of 30 or 40 and, at the same time, the agriculture of the area was improved so that there was no longer need for the men to migrate for part of the year to the cities with all the problems that this created. On a visit, Dr Arole made a significant remark:

The farmers' clubs trust my advice on agricultural matters because they believe my concern is for their welfare. They realise how the community health volunteers have created a safer motherhood and their children no longer die. They so often consider that the agricultural extension officers give advice in response to government directions.

Health workers have the opportunity to create trust in the population and offer guidance in so many aspects of their life. The Aroles improved the local economy through better agriculture and income generating programmes, so that the poor could escape the bondage of indebtedness. They appreciated that such a methodology cannot be taught appropriately in a medical school or university setting, and now run training courses for different levels of workers from India and beyond, in their village environment of Jamkhed.

Child-to-Child

The Child-to-Child approach was initiated jointly between the Institutes of Child Health and Education in London University for the International Year of the Child in 1979. Child-to-Child identified that it is the small children who are at greatest risk in most communities, and are cared for by older children for more than half the day. By teaching older children, who are also the future parents, simple health activities, they are able to care for small children more effectively. All sixty countries[12] involved have their own 'programme' and way of developing Child-to-Child. Across the world there has been a movement away from the original Child-to-Child concept which involved older children caring for younger children; now children in Child-to-Child programmes communicate also to peer groups, to their parents and to their communities. Child-to-Child crosses the disciplines of health and education and has become one of the more effective methods of health education. The activities take children out of the classroom and into the home and community. This is a challenge to teachers who may feel less secure outside the classroom. They need the support of those in health who should be more accustomed to involvement with the community.

Child-to-Child has built on the excellent UNICEF/WHO/UNESCO publication *Facts for Life*[13] by taking the important messages set out there into the classroom through a book *Children for Health*.[14] These ideas have been developed further by the concept of involving the school as a driving force for improving health and nutrition in the communities they serve through another book *Health Promotion in our Schools*.[15] When children learn to take decisions about health in school they lead healthier lives and spread health messages to their families. Any school, however modest its means, can become health promoting and improve the health of the children in the community it serves.

Measuring adequate growth

Health workers concerned with the health of children know the importance of measurement. The science of nutrition in childhood depends on anthropometric measurements as a measure of its success. For research workers the body mass index (weight in kg/height m^2) has proved satisfactory and removes the need to discover the age of the child, which in many situations is still difficult. For rapid assessment by communities themselves, the arm circumference remains one of the most satisfactory methods and in its simplest form can consist of no more that a coloured strip. However, neither of these methods are appropriate for the ongoing measurement of a child which can be understood by the parents, the family and the community health worker. For this, regular weighing and plotting of the weight of a child is essential.

Growth monitoring

The concept of growth monitoring arose out of a paediatrician's experience using a simple weight-for-age growth chart in the West African village of Imesi-Ile.[16] As well as simplicity, this chart introduced two new concepts. The first was a monthly calendar system starting with the child's month of birth (Fig. 12.3) to record passage of time and thus removing the need to calculate the child's age. This is a concept still to be adopted in industrial countries. The second concept was that the charts became the first widely used home-based health record and were provided with a strong polythene envelope suitable for safe keeping by the family. Their use was accepted by WHO, UNICEF and many non-governmental organisations and weight-for-age charts were introduced in most developing countries in the 1970s.

In the 1980s several assessments of the value of various aspects of national primary health care were made, and, unlike oral rehydration and immunisation, the cost of the equipment and time taken in growth monitoring could not be justified on a cost/benefit basis. There was evidence that it worked well in many church related and other non-governmental organisation programmes, but failed when attempts were made to introduce it as a national programme.[17] The reasons for this discrepancy became apparent from colleagues in Child-to-Child concerned with primary education. The latter pointed out the complexity of a line graph. Jean Piaget (1896–1980), the Swiss psychologist, noted for his studies of thought processes especially in children, suggested that the comprehension of the line graph was one of the more complex concepts in education. The graphic representation of information has not been taught in the majority of primary schools in developing countries, nor is graph paper usually available. The weight-for-age line graph was the first attempt to use graphic information of this type at family level and was attempted in countries where education was limited, particularly among women. Perhaps it is not too surprising that the majority of locally trained health workers, and even some doctors, had difficulty in completing a weight-for-age curve and, even more, in making decisions based on it.[18]

Growth monitoring is described here in detail to illustrate a possible important trend in healthcare in which the individual, mother and family, become involved in decision making as a result of measurements which they make themselves.

A new technology and a new concept

Most weighing scales indicate a weight with a pointer on a dial, or give a digital reading. The Direct Recording Scale (Fig. 12.6) introduces a new method of weighing which removes several steps in the growth monitoring process. The scale is low cost, unbreakable and kept in the community. The mother in, or close to, her home, places her child in trousers suspended by loops of cloth below the scale. She sees a large spring, which stretches 1 cm/kg, move up her child's chart which has been so positioned in the scale that it reflects the infant's age in months. She inserts a ball pen through a hole in the pointer at the top of the scale and makes that month's entry onto her child's chart. She observes that the stretching of the spring is related to her child's

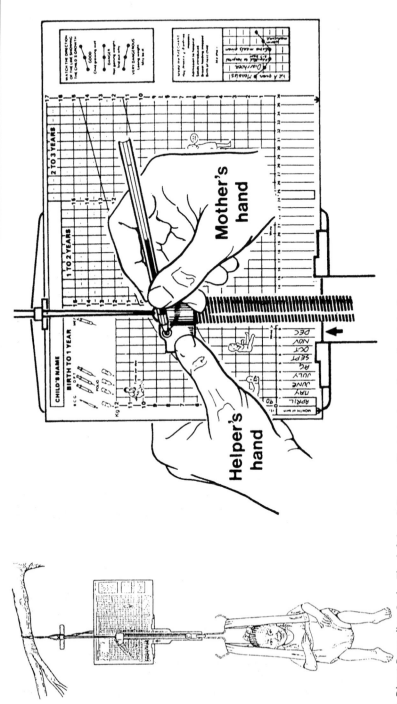

Fig. 12.6 Direct Recording Scale. The left hand diagram illustrates how the scale can be hung from a branch, a beam, or a nail in the lintel of a door. As the weighing is done in or near the home the child should not be frightened when placed in the trousers. By lowering the scale so the infants feet are on the ground it can be used as a 'baby bouncer' without harming the spring. Thus the child will come to enjoy weighing. The right hand diagram shows how the mother uses a ball pen to insert the next point on the chart's growth curve.

weight and she can compare the dot she has made this month with the previous month. The weight-for-age curve is directly recorded without reading from a scale or any use of the 'number'. The majority of illiterate mothers come to understand what they are doing and the meaning of the growth curve within 9 months.[19]

Teaching the use of the scale

A simple method to assist mothers and junior health workers within hours to understand the growth curve better was considered essential and has been developed.[20] This involves a bucket hung below the scale and a plastic bottle cut in such a way that it will hold 200 ml at one end and 400 ml the other. The mothers under guidance empty volumes of water into the bucket and create for themselves, on a chart, adequate and inadequate growth curves. In this way, they learn the meaning of a growth curve in a matter of hours. Use of the scales amongst the Maasai[21] has now been extended and currently there are 359 scales in the Maasai community, an average of 12.5 children (range 4–17 months) are weighed each month on each scale.

In a more recent study, the understanding of the growth curve by the rest of the family was investigated. After 2 years, not only the mother, their daughters and significantly, grandmothers, but also half the older boys and fathers comprehended the meaning of the growth curve. In the families where the mothers weighed their infant using the Direct Recording Scale, a smaller proportion were found to be suffering from periods of growth failure compared with families where the infant was weighed by community health workers with a dial scale.

There are obvious gains to be achieved by trying to shift technologies out of the clinic situation into and involving the family and the community. The weighing and charting of their children's weights by the mother may be a further step in the fight to overcome undernutrition in developing countries.

PROVISION OF APPROPRIATE TRAINING MATERIAL FOR DEVELOPING COUNTRIES

Teaching Aids at Low Cost (TALC), a small non-governmental organisation was developed in the 1960s. The original concept was to improve teaching in health training institutions by providing low cost transparencies. Thirty years later TALC has distributed 7 million transparencies in sets of 24 each with a detailed script. A special effort was made to provide material to understand, prevent, and manage HIV/AIDS. For this, over 200 000 slides and 250 000 books have been distributed by TALC. Since the middle of the 1980s, the number of slides being distributed has diminished, partly due to lack of finance, but also to fewer slide projectors being available due to difficulties in maintenance and lack of finance for purchase. Recent information suggests that the major producers of slide projectors are giving up production as, in the industrialised world, digitalisation of images will allow other methods of projection. Although there is great emphasis on the future of such electronic

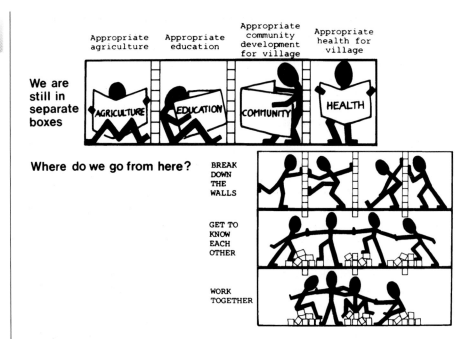

Fig. 12.7 The disciplines that need to work together for health.

communication in industrialised countries, for the majority of health workers in the third world, the book will remain the appropriate technology for the promotion of health, prevention of disease and clinical care for many years to come.

TALC has now become a major distributor of books to developing countries and has sent out over a million. The books must be low cost, as the average book on healthcare in Europe costs more than a month's salary for many health workers in countries of the south. English is a second language for the vast majority of workers. For books to be useful, they have to be written in appropriate simple English and, if possible, be well illustrated. TALC has now a range of such books, but it is not enough just to make these books available. As the following experience suggests.

> *When visiting one of the best community health workers in a south American country, the worker was asked to use his copy of Where there is no Doctor to find out how he would manage an outbreak of poliomyelitis in a local village. He thumbed through the book, and then threw it down and said he would refer the patient to a hospital in spite of the fact that many of the villages in this area are cut off during the wet season. This health worker like so many community health workers had never been taught to use the index of a book.*

This not uncommon experience suggests that where health workers are literate they should always be taught around a book, and given exercises which involve using the index. A similar problem exists with students taking more advanced courses as health workers. They were described in a letter from the director of a training programme with many years of experience, who wrote as follows:

We tried to create a 'reading' culture amongst our students, particularly as we got more into problem-based learning. However, we discovered that students who had been in schools following the 'parrot-fashion' style of teaching had no inclination and little ability to read. We, therefore, brought our 'book-list' down to 5 key books, and included the price of them in school fees. Students were given the books, and all problems were confined to the texts within these books, apart from problems in the community. Other sessions were given to specified reading. Without such discipline, books were carried around to protect papers carried inside them – or to look important.

As books are so expensive, the concept of library packs of 15–20 books has been developed. These would form the basis of small libraries limited to no more than 30–50 books for health centres and hospitals. Unfortunately, there is little experience of running such libraries democratically in health units. Unless such methods are developed, many of the books will either disappear or be kept locked in a cupboard and unused. There is a great need to create a situation where all health workers take a pride in furthering their own training and, as a result, preventive and curative child care will be improved.

This chapter attempts to show that 'Low Technology' to be effective must be available and understood by the mothers and families and the community health workers. It must embrace the needs the people express, many of which are not related to health, but health workers still need to respond to them. Health care will be more effective when it breaks down the walls that so easily imprison health and other disciplines (Fig 12.7).

Key points for clinical practice

- The wise health worker observes, listens and learns from the mother and grandmother.

- Resources applied to preconceptual care may achieve more than those applied to antenatal care.

- Newborns at all times must be kept as close to their mothers as possible.

- The nutrition of infants depends on successful breast feeding throughout at least the first year.

- Successful immunisation surpasses all other health measures in effectiveness.

- The size of infecting dose and severity of the related illness demand greater attention.

- Because of their ability to cut the maternal and child mortality, doctors have an unequalled opportunity to gain the trust of individuals and the community, and a responsibility to use this trust to assist in community development.

- Opportunities exist and must be grasped by health workers to co-operate with other disciplines to accelerate community development.

Key points for clinical practice (continued)

- Health workers have a duty to encourage a stimulating environment for the small child.

- Involvement by paediatricians in primary school education through a programme such as Child-to-Child can be an effective use of their time.

- Family measurement of child growth can be a stimulus to numeracy.

- Success in growth monitoring can be achieved when the complexity of a weight for age line graph is understood, and the family involved in weighing.

- Training courses need to be around a text book. Involvement by the trainee in the use of the index to the contents of the book is essential.

References

1 Wynn A, Wynn M. The problem of low birthweight; the cost and possible prevention. Nutr Health 1997; 11: 159–184

2 Wynn A, Wynn M. No nation can arise above the level of its women: new thoughts on maternal nutrition. J Nutr Environ Med 1995; 5: 163–185

3 Morley D, Woodland M. See How They Grow. Basingstoke: Macmillan, 1979; 135

4 Moore S, Cole T, Poskitt EM et al. Season of birth predicts mortality in rural Gambia. Nature 1997; 388: 434

5 Cattaneo A, Tamburlini G. The international network on 'kangaroo care' gives addresses of interested groups. Int Child Health 1979; 8: 105

6 Morley D. Paediatric Priorities in the Developing World. London: Butterworths, 1973

7 Aaby P, Bukh J, Lisse IM, Smiths AJ. Spacing, crowding and child mortality in Guinea Bissau. Lancet 1983; ii: 161

8 Feuerstein M-T. Poverty and Health. Basingstoke: Macmillan, 1979

9 Molla AM, Molla A, Rohde J, Greenhough WB. Turning off diarrhoea: the role of food and ORS. J Pediatr Gastroenterol Nutr1989; 8: 81–84

10 Carlile J. Toys for Fun: A book of toys for pre-school children. Basingstoke: Macmillan, 1988

11 Arole M, Arole R. Jamkhed: A Comprehensive Rural Health Project. Basingstoke: Macmillan 1994

12 Child-to-Child Trust. Directory of Child-to-Child Activities World Wide. London: Child-to-Child Trust, 1966 [Available from: Child-to-Child Trust, Institute of Education, 20 Bedford Way, London WC1H 0AL, UK]

13 UNICEF/WHO/UNESCO/UNFPA. Facts for Life. St Albans: TALC, 1993 [Available from TALC, PO Box 49, St Albans AL1 5TX, UK]

14 Hawes H, Scotchmer C. Children for Health. St Albans: TALC, 1993 [Available from TALC, PO Box 49, St Albans AL1 5TX, UK]

15 Hawes H. Health Promotion in Our Schools. St Albans: TALC 1997. [Available from TALC, PO Box 49, St Albans AL1 5TX, UK]

16 King Maurice (Ed) Chapter 26.5, Medical Care in Developing Countries. Nairobi: Oxford University Press, 1966

17 Nabarro D, Chinnock P. Growth monitoring: inappropriate promotion of an appropriate technology. Soc Sci Med 1994; 26: 941–948

18 Morley D. Will growth monitoring continue to be part of primary health care? S Afr Med J 1994; 84(Suppl): 15–16

19 Meegan M, Morley D, Brown R. Child weighing by the unschooled: a report of a controlled study of growth monitoring over 12 months of Maasai children using the direct recording scale. Trans R Soc Trop Med Hygiene 1994; 88: 635–637

20 Hardip S, Wilkinson D, Morley D. Growth-monitoring teaching aid to improve mothers' understanding. Lancet 1997; 350: 562

21 Meegan M, Morley D. Growth monitoring: family participation: effective community development. Tropical Medicine 1998; In press

22 Savage-King F, Burgess A. Nutrition for Developing Countries. Oxford: Oxford University Press, 1993

Third world: appropriate technologies

Nicholas Banatvala   Bruce Laurence   Timothy Healing

Paediatric care in disaster and refugee settings

THE DISASTER SETTING

The United Nations Children's Fund defines an emergency as *a situation of hardship and human suffering arising from events which cause physical loss or damage, social and/or economic disruption with which the country or community concerned is unable to fully cope alone.*[1] For the health care professional, an emergency can be viewed as a dramatic deterioration in a population's health. This is often most impressively and easily reflected by mortality rates which are frequently used as a health indicator in emergencies.[2] Crude mortality rates of greater than 1/10 000/day define a very serious situation in a relief programme, while more than 5/10 000/day define a major catastrophe.[3] In both refugee and famine situations, excess mortality occurs in all age groups, but particularly among children.[2,3]

Disasters can be of several types, both natural (e.g. earthquakes, floods and drought) and man-made (e.g. wars, chemical incidents).[4,5] Some may be a combination of both (e.g. a famine may result from a combination of war and drought). Disasters may strike suddenly (earthquakes) or insidiously (drought). Regardless of the type, they frequently lead to mass population movements in which people may become internally displaced within their home country, or refugees (fleeing across an internationally recognised boundary).[4,5]

In rapid onset natural disasters, much of the immediate care is provided by local personnel – international relief simply cannot be organised fast enough. For example, in most earthquakes, 95% of those recovered are discovered and

Dr **Nicholas Banatvala**, Medical Adviser, MERLIN (Medical Emergency Relief International), 14 David Mews, Porter Street, London, W1M 1HW, UK

Dr **Bruce Laurence**, Medical Director, MERLIN (Medical Emergency Relief International), 14 David Mews, Porter Street, London, W1M 1HW, UK

Dr **Timothy Healing**, Epidemiologist, MERLIN (Medical Emergency Relief International), 14 David Mews, Porter Street, London, W1M 1HW, UK

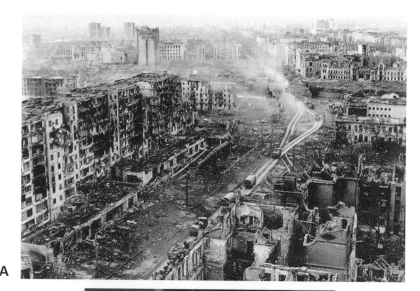

A

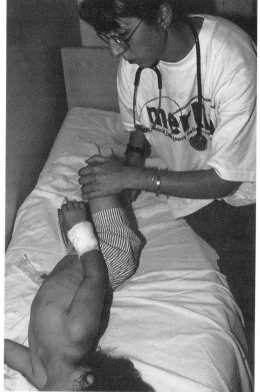

B

Fig. 13.1 (A) Devastation following aerial bombardment to Grozny City, Chechnya. **(B)** The health care infrastructure was destroyed and resulted in an epidemic of polio.

treated in the first 24 hours. International aid is of greatest value in re-supply and reconstruction during the emergency, and in capacity building in the immediate aftermath. In longer term (chronic) disasters, such as wars, international agencies have a greater role to play, although the greatest source of personnel should still be the affected communities themselves – many of whom, as in any society, have experience in child healthcare.

Medical staff working for agencies undertaking health care in disasters face two particular challenges. First, health is part of a much wider picture (e.g. political and environmental). Secondly, a population approach to health care delivery is required (the public health perspective) which is often unfamiliar to practising clinicians.[6] In the early days of medical relief, emergency medicine was primarily about managing trauma injuries directly caused by natural or man-made disaster. First-aid, resuscitation and surgery, with provision of basic curative health services for common diseases were priorities. In time, agencies and governments understood that major disasters, especially in poor countries, and in displaced populations, needed a response much more grounded in public health measures. The term 'Emergency Public Health' is now commonly used by agencies such as MERLIN and Médecins sans Frontières to describe the theory behind what they practice. More recently, interest has focused on telemedicine, geographic information, and early warning systems to either minimise or prevent the adverse health consequences of disasters.[7]

The relief environment is not straightforward. Affected populations, host population governments, local health services, local and international government and non governmental organisations and those providing funds for relief or implementing programmes – all have their own complex agendas.[8] Again, such an environment is alien to most doctors.

The logistic difficulties of working in emergencies are immense and those providing health care will need to work within such constraints. For example, the geographic remoteness, atrocious weather conditions and civil war led to logistic difficulties in mounting a rapid and effective response to the 1998 Afghanistan earthquakes.

This chapter focuses primarily on emergencies caused by conflict, which inevitably lead to population displacement. Activities associated with these so-called complex emergencies is what the majority of relief agencies have focused most of their attention on in the last decade. General principles of emergency health care are well illustrated with the study of such emergencies. This is because not only do risks to health increase, but, at the same time, the ability of a society to cope with those risks is diminished by conflict or displacement. This is through destruction of the infrastructure, damage to services in all sectors and the disruption of the social framework. It should also be added that most conflicts leading to displacement now occur in the poor countries of the world, which are already least able to provide for their basic needs. The description here is also slanted towards the viewpoint of a medical relief agency. This is partly because it is that of the authors, and partly because most western paediatricians encountering this sort of situation will do so through this type of channel (Figs 13.1 & 13.2).

THE CHILD

In any population, children are a vulnerable group, who are dependent on others and developing physically and emotionally. In any disaster, children are in an even more precarious status.[9] They are more susceptible to malnutrition

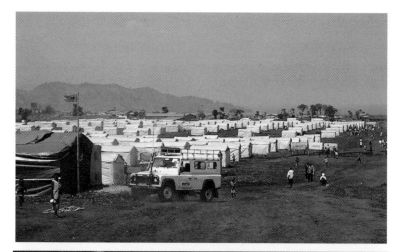

A

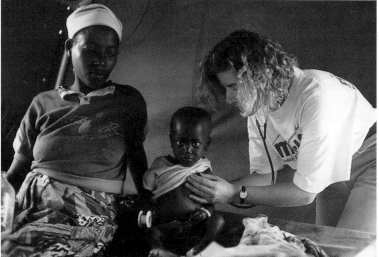

B

Fig. 13.2 (**A**) The traditional densely populated refugee camp with (**B**) organised and efficient health care delivery. This is often considerably easier to organise than in urban jungles, such as Chechnya.

and disease, and less able to fend for themselves. Children suffer not only physically, but also psychologically. They see their lives disrupted, education may cease, and far too often in modern war they are targeted for atrocities, or made into fighters, with devastating consequences for their future development. Furthermore, children may become separated from their families, and sub-camps of unaccompanied children are a common feature of the modern refugee camp.

It is easy to forget in a modern advanced society, where so much is taken for granted, that the major determinants of health are outside the 'health sector'. In any country, clean water, adequate food, sanitation and shelter will have a more significant impact on morbidity and mortality than do the health services. It may be argued that this is not the business of a paediatrician. However, it is often the task of medical relief agencies to plan, co-ordinate, or implement work in a

---

Rapid initial assessment

What has happened, to whom, where, when and with what consequences for the communities and individual households?

Do problems exist – or might they develop with regards
    shelter and clothing?
    water for drinking and hygiene?
    health – immediate problems or threats?
    children in need of special care (unaccompanied, traumatised)?
    logistic means to maintain service and deliver assistance?

To what extent and in what ways can the government and communities themselves cope?

What further needs must be met immediately to assure survival – how should this be targeted?

On what sectors and geographic areas should ongoing assessment focus?

What additional manpower and expertise is needed to make a thorough assessment?

Source: *Assisting in emergencies - a resource handbook for UNICEF field staff.*[1]

variety of sectors, and any doctor or nurse working for such an agency will often have a very wide range of responsibilities, including planning and management, far beyond what they would have in a normal health service role.

Care of children in emergencies is, therefore, based on an understanding of their place in the emergency context; of the different influences on children's health in these circumstances, and of practical and structured ways in which to put this understanding into practice. No agency can undertake such work alone. Their role is rather to support the local community and secure its participation in the recovery process. For children, priorities must include preservation of a stable family environment and meeting the goals of child survival and development. Assistance should form a coherent, integrated package designed to meet specifically identified needs, i.e. a programme with clear objectives, rather than disjointed *ad hoc* actions. These principles are presented more fully elsewhere.[1]

The Convention on the Rights of the Child, which received near-universal ratification in 1994, sets comprehensive standards to virtually every aspect of a child's life. The convention is based around a triangle of 'rights' for children: non-discrimination, participation and best interests, and conservation of ethnic, religious and linguistic culture are recognised as human rights. These basic principles act as the cornerstones for humanitarian relief.[10]

GUIDING PRINCIPLES IN HUMANITARIAN RELIEF

Rapid initial assessment

Almost all agencies will assess the impact of a disaster before mobilising resources. Even a brief 24 hour reconnaissance can prevent importation of inappropriate materials and omission of essential items. Table 13.1 outlines the key issues that should be assessed during an on-site visit. If camps are being developed for displaced populations, the siting of tents, water supply and latrines in relation to one another is critical. As many camps develop around water sources, washing facilities should be downstream from drinking water supply, and latrines even further downstream.[11]

Effective disaster programming

Proposed action requires defining priorities and objectives in collaboration with other agencies and community leaders. Practical strategies for implementing the

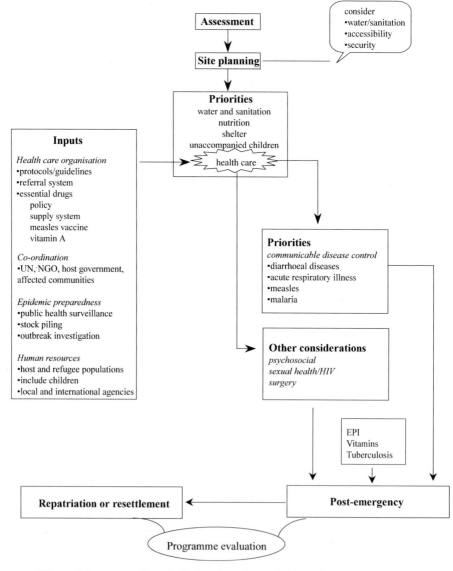

EPI, expanded programme of immunisation; HIV, human immunodeficiency virus; NGO, non-governmental organsiations; UN, United Nations agencies.

Fig. 13.3 A scheme outlining key strategies and activities in a disaster.

Table 13.2 Principles in health care delivery in an emergency

Principle	Issues
Equity	Provision of health care to all members of an afflicted population according to need
	Identification and assistance to groups which are especially vulnerable through age, gender, disability, ethnicity or geography
Multi-sectoralism	Recognition that health is determined by much more than health care services
	Co-ordination of different sectors to achieve maximum benefits with maximum efficiency
Participation	Active involvement of the beneficiary population in the relief effort – especially if relief is long term
	Movement of children from passive recipients of relief, to active participants in the relief programme with the advantages in health promotion of Child-to-Child teaching
Health promotion and disease prevention	The disaster environment is especially favourable to disease outbreaks and it is essential to be aggressive in preventing disease occurring and spreading before it overwhelms any available curative services
Sustainability and appropriate technology	Sustainability depends on running programmes with staff from the beneficiary populations with appropriate technology
	In extreme and early stages, may be necessary to use some high-technology approaches to meet needs

programme, gaining agreements with host governments, and ensuring rapid deployment of funding are all essential to the success of a disaster programme. The remainder of the chapter focuses on key issues that affect children's health in the emergency setting. Throughout, an attempt is made to discuss health issues not only in relation to their relative importance but in terms of preventive care available (health promotion, hygiene promotion though water and sanitation, vaccination), opportunities for surveillance, and appropriate curative responses. A schema of essential concepts surrounding paediatric health care in disasters with principle activities is illustrated in Figure 13.3.

Primary health care

The basic principles of primary health care are highly relevant to the maintenance of child health in an emergency, and some of those principles are listed in Table 13.2.

HEALTH CARE PRIORITIES

Purely 'relief' inputs should be kept to the minimum, and specifically targeted at the most vulnerable. Once survival is assured, efforts should be focused on the restoration and improvement of community and family life, household protection, the rehabilitation and development of services for children and their parents, and reducing their vulnerability to future disasters. There is widespread agreement on priorities in child health during emergencies. These are to prevent and respond to measles, diarrhoeal diseases (including cholera and dysentery), acute respiratory infection, malaria, and malnutrition.[12] Displaced populations are at risk of measles epidemics, which can have a very high mortality, and measles vaccination is, therefore, a priority.[12] Throughout, host and migrant community skills and local health structures should be used, and except in the most dire emergency, careful consideration given before parallel health structures are set up as they are difficult to sustain. Health care should be available for both the indigenous population as well as the displaced. If funds are only available to those of refugee or displaced status, this can cause resentment and prevent community integration.

Nutrition

Malnutrition in childhood inhibits physical and mental development and increases vulnerability to infection. Poor nutrition is one of the most important factors predisposing refugee children and those affected by disasters to a high mortality.[13] Protein energy malnutrition is often found when droughts or disruptions associated with conflict have been developing for some time and adequate action has not been taken early enough. Food is a powerful political weapon, lack of which can result from inadequate supplies, but also poor purchasing power. Maldistribution of available supplies within the community or household is also important, but the situation can be compounded by high rates of disease and ignorance or taboos with regard to dietary habits.[3]

The prevalence of acute malnutrition in children under 5 years of age is generally used as an indicator for the entire population, since this group is especially sensitive to a reduction in available food and international reference values are readily available.[3,14] Nutritional status is best measured by assessing the child's weight (W) and height (H) and the presence of bilateral ankle oedema, but the mid upper arm circumference (MUAC) is also widely used.[3,14] Surveys provide rapid assessment of a population's nutritional status and results are presented by prevalence of severe (percent of children with W/H under minus 3 Z scores) and moderate (percent of children with W/H between under minus 2 but less than minus 3 Z scores) malnutrition (Z scores are the number of standard deviations above or below the median value of the international accepted reference population[3]). Taken together, they provide a global malnutrition rate. The results of such assessments along with security, availability of resources, and concurrent epidemic disease (e.g. measles or dysentery) or very high crude mortality rates may require one or a combination of the following emergency food interventions:

(i) general food distribution (ensures adequate food rations for all);

(ii) supplementary feeding (provides food and medical follow-up for moderately malnourished and vulnerable groups, e.g. pregnant women); and

(iii) therapeutic feeding (special, intensive feeding provided under close medical supervision for severely malnourished children).

Supplementary feeding programmes should never be a substitute for a proper ration in the general feeding programme. Therapeutic feeding is expensive and one of the most technically specialist areas of emergency paediatric health care. Technical details, guidelines and algorithms are provided elsewhere,[14] but these are no substitute for ensuring a response that is logistically, financially and culturally appropriate. Contrary to popular belief, starving children will not always eat culturally alien food.

Breast feeding reduces the risk of infant infection and in a disaster the benefits are even greater. Health promotion should encourage breast feeding, and mothers should receive supplementary feeding if necessary as malnourished mothers may not be able to feed their infants. If a mother cannot breast feed or has died, efforts should be made to find a wet nurse.

The importance of micronutrient deficiency is also well recognised.[15] Vitamin C (scurvy), niacin (pellagra), thiamine (beri-beri), iron (anaemia) and iodine (goitre and cretinism) deficiencies have all caused problems in different disasters. Pregnant and lactating women should be given iron and folate supplements and educated in the importance of compliance. There remains debate regarding the role of iron in the moderately malnourished child, but the severely malnourished should not receive supplements initially because of the increased risk of infection. Mass supplementation or fortifying food is a method of reaching large numbers of persons. Ferrous sulphate (supplemented with vitamin C to enhance absorption) is used to treat anaemia.

The lack of vitamin A is one of the most serious nutritional deficiency diseases in young children in developing countries and is a common cause of blindness and children up to 15 years of age should receive vitamin A prophylaxis every 4–6 months.[14] The clinical manifestations of vitamin A deficiency include night blindness, ocular lesions such as Bitot's spots, and xeropthalmia. Most refugee's rations contain less than the daily recommended allowance of 2500 IU of vitamin A and the distribution of this vitamin to children is one of the most effective interventions leading to reduced morbidity and mortality in refugee populations.[16,17] Vitamin A supplements should also be given to children over 6 months old with measles (especially if they are malnourished) as it greatly decreases the frequency of complications such as diarrhoea and pneumonia.[16]

Communicable disease

In most disasters, even wars, many more people die from illness than from trauma.[3] Malnutrition, crowding and stress increase susceptibility to illness and the breakdown of infrastructures means that the risk of exposure to disease is increased and opportunities for preventive health care (e.g. vaccination) are reduced.[2] Excess mortality occurs in all age groups, but particularly in children under 14 years of age. Orphaned and separated children and pregnant women are especially vulnerable.

The illnesses that cause problems after a disaster are generally those which were always common in the area; rare or exotic diseases do not usually emerge, although migrants may introduce novel infections into a host community. Lack of resistance to infection, immaturity of the immune system in the very young, together with immunosuppression associated with malnutrition, renders children especially vulnerable.

Acute respiratory infection, diarrhoeal diseases, measles and malaria consistently account for 60–95% of all deaths in refugees and displaced populations. Typhoid, meningitis and tuberculosis can also be associated with widespread mortality and morbidity in a disaster. The triad of prevention, early recognition and effective and appropriate response are often best considered in the disaster setting through an integrated health service delivery that is co-ordinated by one agency and ensures community participation.

Acute respiratory illness

Malnutrition, vitamin A deficiency, chilling associated with poor shelter, over-crowding and pollution (inadequate ventilation in shelters) make the refugee child particularly susceptible to acute respiratory infection, and since acute respiratory infection accounts for at least 25% of deaths in those under 5 years in developing countries, it is hardly surprising that acute respiratory infection (90% of which is pneumonia) causes widespread mortality in disasters. Both viral and bacterial pneumonias occur, the common causes of the later being *Streptococcus pneumoniae* and *Haemophilus influenzae*. Accessible health care, trained health care staff, and use of recognised protocols will ensure early diagnosis and effective case management, and reduce mortality.

Immunisation against measles (in the immediate phase) and diphtheria and pertussis (once the population is stabilised) is the most effective preventive measure available and along with a reduction in the risk factors above, will reduce acute respiratory infection-associated deaths in the relief setting. Diagnosis of acute respiratory infection is clinical and differentiation between upper and lower respiratory tract infection is often difficult. Case definitions are useful for surveillance purposes. Where antibiotics are indicated, national policies of the host country will guide the prescriber. Co-trimoxazole is usually the oral treatment of choice, ampicillin or chloramphenicol for intravenous therapy. Children with associated malnutrition should be given nutritional support.

Diarrhoea

Disasters, with inadequate water supply (both quantity and quality), over-crowding, poor sanitation and malnutrition, provide the ideal setting for outbreaks of diarrhoeal disease and children can die rapidly and in massive numbers.[3] Young children in particular may be highly susceptible to such infections. In 1994, one million Rwandan refugees in Goma were exposed to cholera and dysentery, death rates of up to 800 per 10 000 were recorded among some groups of children.[18]

Diarrhoeal diseases are broadly divided into bloody and non-bloody diarrhoea by the case definitions used in aid programmes.[12] Many organisms may be involved. Dysentery is caused by the highly infectious *Shigella* species, especially *Shigella dysenteriae* but a number of other organisms can give very similar symptoms, including *Campylobacter* species, some strains of *Escherichia coli*. *Vibrio cholerae* (O:1 and O:139) and many viruses are responsible for epidemics of non-bloody diarrhoea.[19] Cholera is a particularly emotive disease and governments may be reluctant to admit outbreaks in their spheres of influence. Communities may try to blame minority groups or refugee groups for an outbreak, which can hamper control measures.

Prevention of diarrhoeal diseases consists of ensuring adequate (calculated at 15–20 l/person/day) clean water.[3] It is better to supply large amounts of reasonably clean water rather than small amounts which are very pure. Organisations with specific knowledge of water and sanitation systems (e.g. Oxfam) are often well placed to take a lead role. Malnutrition increases the severity and duration of diarrhoeal diseases, and diarrhoeal illness, in turn, leads to malnutrition promoting a vicious cycle. Health education with provision of sufficient latrines (ideally one latrine per family or else a minimum of 1/20 persons) or defaecation field, supplies of soap, and proper washing facilities (clean water and waste water disposal) together with the promotion of breast feeding is of supreme importance: community participation, an important tool in implementing such measures, is often under-utilised. Effective surveillance makes it possible to detect epidemics in the early stages and to take appropriate action: a single death from diarrhoea in a person over five years of age, or a person presenting with bloody diarrhoea should trigger an investigation for cholera or dysentery respectively.

The frequency and rapidity with which outbreaks of diarrhoeal illness can occur mean that outbreak preparedness is essential.[20] This should include the rapid establishment of a surveillance system and plans for outbreak investigation and epidemic control. Diarrhoeal illness is best treated by the use of oral re-hydration salts and stocks of oral re-hydration salts and of equipment for re-hydration (disposable cups, water carriers, water purifying tablets, etc.) should be obtained as soon as possible after an aid programme commences.[20] Training of health care workers in the use of oral re-hydration salts should also be started immediately. Many of the deaths in the Goma outbreak could have been prevented by more rapid re-hydration, better use of oral re-hydration therapy, use of more appropriate intravenous fluids, and proper training of health workers in the management of severe cholera.[21] Although intravenous fluid will be required in the severely dehydrated child, where ever possible oral fluids should be given and treatment of both sporadic or epidemic diarrhoea should not be primarily a clinic activity, rather decentralised re-hydration points should be scattered around refugee camps or in way stations along routes that refugees are using. The large scale of many oral re-hydration salts' programmes demands well co-ordinated logistic support and adequate supplies of safe water. These may affect the location of re-hydration points. Scepticism about the effectiveness of oral re-hydration salts among local health care workers and carers may need to be overcome if treatment campaigns are to work.

Rapid laboratory confirmation of the organisms responsible for outbreaks is essential, as is the determination of antimicrobial sensitivity patterns although treatment with antibiotics is secondary to the use of oral re-hydration salts and should be reserved for extreme cases. Multiple drug resistance is becoming common amongst enteric pathogens. Traditional standbys such as co-trimoxazole, ampicillin and nalidixic acid are now ineffective in many instances reducing treatment options to the use of expensive drugs such as ciprofloxacin. Unfortunately the indiscriminate use of antibiotics in many countries has meant that a number of micro-organisms (e.g. some strains of *S. dysenteriae*) are now developing resistance to this agent as well. Cholera in children should generally be treated by re-hydration but if an antibiotic is required then co-trimoxazole is the treatment of choice. Tetracycline is equally effective, but is not licensed for paediatric use in many countries. Vaccination campaigns in a cholera epidemic are not recommended. This is because the currently available vaccine: (i) frequently lacks the required potency; (ii) even when potent, the vaccine is not very effective (not all those vaccinated are protected); (iii) any protection that does occur lasts only for 3–6 months; and (iv) vaccination does not reduce the incidence of asyptomatic infections or prevent the spread of disease.[38]

Typhoid fever

Typhoid fever has also been reported among populations affected by disasters.[22,23] Spread by the same routes as other gastro-intestinal pathogens and programmes to supply clean water and safe food will greatly reduce the threat of typhoid outbreaks. Untreated typhoid has a mortality which can approach 20%. Unlike the treatment of most enteric infections, antibiotics are used for the treatment of typhoid (chloramphenicol, amoxycillin and co-trimoxazole are the agents of choice) but an increasing problem is the spread of multiple resistant *Salmonella typhi* in disaster affected countries.[23] The development of such strains has further stimulated interest in the use of vaccines in the disaster setting.

Measles

Measles was first recognised as an important cause of refugee deaths during the 1980s when outbreaks were reported from refugee camps in Africa and Asia.[3] Case fatality rates can be as high as 32% (as was documented in Sudan in 1985 when 2000 deaths occurred over 4 months).[3] Measles immunisation has been recognised as the first health priority in a displaced population and this has greatly reduced the problem. Children between 6 months and 15 years should be targeted in the immunisation campaign and, at the same time, given vitamin A (the host population should also be included where there is contact with the displaced community).[24] Newly arriving children should be offered measles vaccination as a matter of urgency and a second dose given to all those who received a primary dose at less than 9 months of age.

Mortality is usually caused by the complications of measles and a reduction in case fatality rates can be achieved through the vigorous management of pneumonia, malnutrition and gastro-enteritis and encouraging breast feeding. Topical antibiotics should be given to all children to prevent conjunctivitis.

Malaria and other vector borne diseases

Disasters with their frequent population movements can lead to outbreaks of malaria as non-immune individuals are exposed to malaria parasites for the first time, or infected individuals move into areas previously free of the disease.[3,25] The priority is for rapid treatment especially where *Plasmodium falciparum* is endemic as this can kill in 48 hours. Information campaigns to ensure that those with fever come forward for treatment are essential. Impregnated bed nets have shown great promise in reducing the incidence of malaria. Such programmes will be more effective if social factors are also considered, for example in some cultures adults may protect themselves with the nets rather than use them for children or males may be protected before females. Other vectors which can cause problems include flies, lice and fleas (often a problem in newly established camps) together with bugs, ticks and rodents (which become an increasing problem in camps operating for some time).

Vector control in refugee camps is not simple. The disease burden, level of knowledge, finance and technical skill will determine the relative roles of health promotion, sanitation, environmental health and biological control methods.[26] Education programmes need to accompany any vector control activities since control may involve the use of toxic compounds (insecticides, rodenticides). Children, who are naturally curious, are especially at risk of accidental poisoning.

Other diseases

Other epidemics in emergency settings include meningitis, typhus (louse borne, murine typhus, scrub typhus), other rodent borne diseases such as relapsing fever, plague, Lassa fever, and arthropod borne diseases such as yellow fever and dengue.[19] An awareness of the endemic and epidemic diseases in an area where an aid programme is being undertaken will permit proper outbreak preparedness. Good surveillance will ensure that cases are detected early and that outbreaks can be prevented or minimised.

Large outbreaks of meningitis are caused by *Neisseria meningitidis* and over-crowding, poor hygiene and population movements are risk factors.[27] Routine vaccination of displaced persons or refugees during non-epidemic periods is not cost-effective, however a vaccine campaign should be considered if there is evidence of an impending outbreak.[28]

Sexual health

Rape and other forms of sexual violence are not uncommon in refugee/internally displaced people situations and every effort should be made to protect children from these, and to ensure that victims receive remedial assistance for their recovery.[10] Prevention of the sexual abuse of children and the identification of those who have been affected is far from easy. The maintenance of order in refugee camps, and the prevention of prostitution and child abuse, requires the active involvement of the whole community.

The breakdown of the social order may see an increase in the incidence of sexually transmitted diseases. Children who have been abused or raped should be assessed for sexually transmitted disease infections and, where possible, counselled. Children breast fed by HIV positive mothers are at risk of HIV infection but at a population level, breast feeding is to be encouraged as the benefit from a reduction in non-HIV related disease is so great.[29]

A more detailed appraisal on how best to improve sexual health is usually left to the early stages of the postemergency phase, although provision of condoms along with basic sexual health education at a community level, should be undertaken in the emergency phase of a disaster.

Mental health and psycho-social needs

Children suffer severe trauma in wars and other disasters and many will require psychological assessment and assistance. In addition to many of the horrors witnessed, the artificial environment of a refugee centre makes normal childhood activities impossible, leading to poor emotional development. Direct support to the child, helping the child through support to the family, and assisting both child and family through services to the community are all methods of protecting children.[10] A daily routine should be aimed at wherever possible and children should be given accurate information concerning their current situation, their rights and responsibilities and the possibilities of durable solutions. Direct assistance to the child includes play, education, counselling and support groups.[30] Child-to-Child care is particularly effective in generating community participation and as a tool for health and hygiene promotion.[31] Such activities provide opportunities for identifying particular hazards, such as land mines.

Children may become unaccompanied before, during and after an emergency. The unaccompanied child falls into a number of groups; those that are alone with parental consent (abandoned, entrusted, or those living independently) or those alone against the parents wishes (lost, abducted, runaway or orphaned). Children from each category will require specific help. Children may also be conscripted, both with and without their consent. Rapid and strenuous efforts to trace the family of unaccompanied children should be made. Social service information offices should be set up to receive reports and register unaccompanied children and the parents of such children. Care and supervision should be provided while tracing is being undertaken and, where necessary, temporary or permanent fostering instituted. At the same time, action should be directed at preventing further family separations, and developing policies and provisions to remove administrative, political or military barriers to family reunion. Principles underlying the care of unaccompanied children have been reported in detail elsewhere.[32]

The Universal Declaration of Human Rights, the Declaration of the Rights of the Child and the Geneva Convention all support this principle.[33] Experience has shown that, even in situations of armed conflict, children can continue to receive formal education and when schooling is disrupted or non-existent, alternative educational services can be provided.[34]

MOVING TO THE POSTEMERGENCY PHASE

Conflict often leads to a chronic disaster. The political and economic climate may lead to the population being displaced for months or years. The term 'complex emergency' is often used to describe situations such as Afghanistan, Sierra Leone, Jaffna in Sri Lanka and Chechnya. Over the last decade, the proportion of internally displaced people has risen and the number of refugees reduced. That international law is less effective for the internally displaced does not assist in finding a solution to the problems faced by such individuals.

Once the excess mortality associated with the emergency is controlled (often defined as mortality rates falling to less than 1 per 10 000 per day) and food, water, sanitation and shelter are available, relief enters the postemergency phase. This phase only ends when a permanent solution is found, such as repatriation of the displaced or integration of these individuals into the host community. Health programmes in the postemergency phase will need to consolidate earlier activities and address wider needs, ideally through the existing health care system. Throughout, there should be sufficient capacity to handle new emergencies such as population movement, disease outbreaks, or trauma from an upsurge in fighting.

Rehabilitation will encroach upon health sector reform, and is necessary for the health service to meet the new needs within the new finances available to the health sector. The introduction of agencies with experience in health sector rehabilitation into the situation and the proper integration of their work with that of the providers of emergency aid that are already working in the area, will improve the chances of introducing sustainable reforms. This in turn will ultimately reduce the needs for external assistance. HIV, sexual transmitted diseases, and tuberculosis programmes and enhanced psychosocial and mental health care will need to be developed. The expanded programme of immunisation, (DTP, polio, BCG in addition to measles) should be integrated into existing health programmes and basic curative care be made available to diagnose and treat common childhood conditions, such as anaemia and skin infections, in addition to those described in more detail earlier. The resources associated with the expanded programme of immunisation mean that a programme should only be implemented if the population is expected to remain stable for several months, that adequate resources are available to enable the programme to be completed, and that the programme can be incorporated in to the host country's national immunisation programme.

Liaison with national AIDS programmes is essential in designing appropriate approaches to the control of HIV in the postemergency phase.[35] This will include health promotion, provision of condoms, and training in the management of sexually transmitted diseases. The development of a tuberculosis programme needs to be considered very carefully.[36] More harm than good can come from treating patients who complete only part of their treatment, either because they migrate elsewhere, drug supply runs out or compliance precludes full treatment. Such patients are at risk of developing resistant disease. A poor security situation is a contra-indication to commencing a tuberculosis programme.

CHALLENGES FOR THE FUTURE

While the practice of paediatric care in the disaster setting has developed rapidly over the last 15 years, there remain major challenges for the future.[37] Effective and appropriate research and development are essential to ensure that evidence is available to improve the care of the refugee and other children caught in disasters. In caring for such children, the practitioner must respond to the supreme challenge of acting with the highest levels of ethics; indeed it can be argued that the ethical imperative is at its greatest for this, the most vulnerable group of individuals imaginable in our society.

Key points for clinical practice

- In a disaster, children are a vulnerable group, who are dependent on others and are developing physically and emotionally. A holistic approach to care is essential.

- In most disasters, even wars, many more people die from illness than from trauma: clean water, adequate food, sanitation and shelter will have a greater impact on morbidity and mortality than health services.

- Priorities in child health during emergencies are prevention and control of measles, diarrhoeal diseases, acute respiratory infection, malaria, and malnutrition.

- Culturally appropriate psycho-social care is integral to child health in a disaster and includes family tracing, family support, Child-to-Child care, counselling, and attempting to create routine and provide education.

- Planning and co-ordination are essential to the success of any child health care disaster programme.

References

1 United Nations Children Fund. Assisting in Emergencies, a resource handbook for United Nations Children Fund field staff. New York: United Nations Children Fund, 1986

2 Toole MJ, Waldman RJ. Prevention of excess mortality in refugees and displaced populations in developing countries. JAMA 1990; 263: 3296–3302

3 Centers for Disease Control and Prevention. Famine-affected, refugee, and displaced populations: recommendations for public health issues. MMWR Morb Mortal Wkly Rep 1992; 41 (RR-13)

4 Levy BS, Sidel VW. (eds) War and Public Health. Oxford: Oxford University Press, 1997

5 Noji EK. (ed) The Public Health Consequences of Disasters. Oxford: Oxford University Press, 1997

6 Slim H. The continuing metamorphosis of the humanitarian practitioner: some new colours for an endangered chameleon. Disasters 1995; 19: 110–126

7 Llewellyn CH. The role of telemedicine in disaster medicine. J Med Syst 1995; 19: 29–34

8 International Federation of Red Cross and Red Crescent. World disaster report. Oxford: Oxford University Press, 1996

9 Toole MJ, Waldman RJ. Refugees and displaced persons. War, hunger, and public health. JAMA 1993; 270: 600–605

10 United Nations High Commission for Refugees. Refugee children – guidelines on protection and care. Geneva: United Nations High Commission for Refugees, 1994

11 United Nations High Commission for Refugees. Water manual for refugee situations. Geneva: United Nations Children Fund, 1992

12 Médécins sans Frontières. Refugee health – an approach to emergency situations. London: Macmillan, 1997

13 Toole MJ, Nieburg P, Waldman RJ. The association between inadequate rations, undernutrition prevalence, and mortality in refugee camps: case studies of refugee populations in Eastern Thailand, 1979–1980 and Eastern Sudan, 1984–1985. J Trop Pediatr 1988; 24: 218–223

14 Médécins sans Frontières. Nutrition guidelines. Paris: Médécins sans Frontières, 1995

15 Toole MJ. Micronutrient deficiencies in refugees. Lancet 1992; 339: 1214–1216

16 Beaton G, Martorell R. Effectiveness of vitamin A supplementation in the control of young child morbidity and mortality in developing countries. ACC/SNN. Nutrition Policy Discussion Paper No. 13. 1993

17 Semba RD. Vitamin A, immunity and infection. Clin Infect Dis 1994; 19: 489–499

18 Goma Epidemiolgy Group. Public health impact of Rwandese refugee crisis: what happened in Goma, Zaire in July 1994? Lancet 1995; 345: 339–345

19 Benenson AS. (ed) Control of communicable diseases manual. Washington DC: American Public Health Association, 1995

20 LaMont-Gregory E, Henry CJ, Ryan TJ. Evidence-based humanitarian relief interventions. Lancet 1995; 346: 312–313

21 Siddique AK, Salam A, Islam MS et al. Why treatment centres failed to prevent cholera deaths among Rwandan refugees in Goma, Zaire. Lancet 1995; 345: 359–361

22 Reisinger EC, Grasmug E, Krejs GJ. Antibody response after vaccination against typhoid fever in Kurdish refugee camp. Lancet 1994; 343: 918–919

23 Murdoch DM, Banatvala N, Bone A, Shoismatulloev BI, Ward LR, Threlfall EJ. Epidemic ciprofloxacin-resistant *Salmonella typhi* in Tajikistan. Lancet 1998; 351: 339

24 Toole MJ, Steketee RW, Waldman RJ, Nieburg P. Measles prevention and control in emergency settings. Bull World Health Organ 1989; 67: 381–388

25 Seleman M. Malaria in Afghan refugees in Pakistan. Trans R Soc Trop Med Hyg 1988; 82: 44–47

26 United Nations High Commission for Refugees. Vector and pest control in refugee situations. Geneva: United Nations High Commission for Refugees, 1997

27 Moore PS, Toole MJ, Nieburg P, Waldman RJ, Broome CV. Surveillance and control of meningococcal meningitis epidemics in refugee populations. WHO Bull 1990; 58: 587–596

28 World Health Organization. Control of epidemic meningococcal disease. Lyons: Marcel Merieux, 1995

29 United Nations High Commission for Refugees. Reproductive health in refugee situations, an inter-agency field manual. Geneva: United Nations High Commission for Refugees, 1995

30 Bonnerjea L. Disasters, family tracing and children's rights: some questions about the best interests of separated children. Disasters 1994; 18: 277–283

31 Hanbury C. (ed) Child-to-Child and Living in Camps. London: CTC Trust, 1993

32 Williamson J, Moser A. Unaccompanied children in emergencies – a field guide for their care and protection. Geneva: International Social Services, 1988

33 Ressler EM, Tortorici JM, Marcelino A. Children in war, a guide to the provision of services. New York: United Nations Children Fund, 1993

34 Dodge CP, Mohammed A, Kuch PJ. Profile of the displaced in Khartoum. Disasters 1987; 11: 243–250

35 United Nations High Commission for Refugees, World Health Organization, UNAIDS. Guidelines for HIV interventions in emergency settings. Geneva: UNAIDS, 1996

36 World Health Organization. Tuberculosis control in refugee situations, an inter-agency field manual. Geneva: World Health Organization, 1997

37 Howarth JP, Healing TJ, Banatvala N. Health care in disaster and refugee settings. Lancet 1997; 349: 14–17

38 World Health Organization. Guidelines for cholera control. Geneva: World Health Organization, 1993

T.J. David

Paediatric literature review – 1997

ALLERGY AND IMMUNOLOGY

Allergy

Romano A, Quaratino D, Papa G et al. Aminopenicillin allergy. Arch Dis Child 1997; 76: 513–517. *The label of penicillin allergy was incorrect in most cases.*

Immunology

Filipovich AH. Hemophagocytic lymphohistiocytosis: a lethal disorder of immune regulation. J Pediatr 1997; 130: 337–338. *Review. See also pp 352–365.*

Morgan G. What, if any, is the effect of malnutrition on immunological competence? Lancet 1997; 349: 1693–1695. *Review.*

Rosen FS. Severe combined immunodeficiency: a pediatric emergency. J Pediatr 1997; 130: 345–346. *Review.*

Summerfield JA, Sumiya M, Levin M et al. Association of mutations in mannose binding protein gene with childhood infection in consecutive hospital series. BMJ 1997; 314: 1229–1232. *A risk factor for infections.*

CARDIOVASCULAR

Curtis N. Kawasaki disease. Early recognition is vital to prevent cardiac complications. BMJ 1997; 315: 322–323. *Review. For diagnostic confusion with Mediterranean spotted fever, see 314: 655–656.*

Professor T.J. David, Booth Hall Children's Hospital, Charlestown Road, Blackley, Manchester M9 7AA, UK

O'Kelly SW, Bove EL. Hypoplastic left heart syndrome. BMJ 1997; 314: 87–88. *Terminal care is not the only option.*

Sharland G. Changing impact of fetal diagnosis of congenital heart disease. Arch Dis Child 1997; 77: F1–F3. *Review. See also pp F41–F46.*

Terai M, Shulman ST. Prevalence of coronary artery abnormalities in Kawasaki disease is highly dependent on gamma globulin dose but independent of salicylate dose. J Pediatr 1997; 131: 888–893. *2 g/kg IVIG combined with at least 30–50 mg/kg per day aspirin provides maximum protection.*

Walsh KP. Interventional cardiology. Arch Dis Child 1997; 76: 6–8. *Review.*

COMMUNITY

American Academy of Pediatrics. Committee on Sports Medicine and Fitness. Adolescents and anabolic steroids: a subject review. Pediatrics 1997; 99: 904–908. *Review.*

Conseur A, Rivara FP, Barnoski R et al. Maternal and perinatal risk factors for later delinquency. Pediatrics 1997; 99: 785–790. *Birth to teenage or unmarried mothers are strongly associated with later risk of juvenile delinquency.*

Crowcroft NS, Strachan DP. The social origins of infantile colic. BMJ 1997; 314: 1325–1328. *Dietary factors contribute little to mothers' reporting of infantile colic, and dietary change should not be the primary intervention.*

Dennison BA, Rockwell HL, Baker SL. Excess fruit juice consumption by preschool-aged children is associated with short stature and obesity. Pediatrics 1997; 99: 15–22. *May contribute to failure to thrive.*

Forsyth R. Support of the head injured child in the community. Baillière Clin Paediatr 1997; 5: 479–487. *Review.*

Gibb DM, Masters J, Shingadia D et al. A family clinic – optimising care for HIV infected children and their families. Arch Dis Child 1997; 77: 478–482. *Describes operation of a clinic in London. See also pp 483–487.*

Holloway JS. Outcome in placements for adoption or long term fostering. Arch Dis Child 1997; 76: 227–230. *Poor outcome in older children. For needs for support see pp 231–235.*

Impicciatore P, Pandolfini C, Casella N et al. Reliability of health information for the public on the world wide web: systematic survey of advice on managing fever in children at home. BMJ 1997; 314: 1875–1881. *Few web sites provided complete and accurate information.*

Jones CM, Taylor GO, Whittle JG et al. Water fluoridation, tooth decay in 5 year olds, and social deprivation measured by the Jarman score. BMJ 1997; 315: 514–517. *The more socially deprived areas benefit more from fluoridation.*

Kessler DA, Natanblut SL, Wilkenfeld JP et al. Nicotine addiction: a paediatric disease. J Pediatr 1997; 130: 518–524. *Review.*

Meates M. Ambulatory paediatrics – making the difference. Arch Dis Child 1997; 76: 468–476. *Review.*

Mellanby AR, Pearson VAH, Tripp JH. Preventing teenage pregnancy. Arch Dis Child 1997; 77: 459–462. *Review.*

Reading R. Poverty and the health of children and adolescents. Arch Dis Child 1997; 76: 463–467. *Review.*

Roberts H. Children, inequalities, and health. BMJ 1997; 314: 1122–1125. *Review.*

Robinson TN, Killen JD. Do cigarette warning labels reduce smoking? Arch Pediatr Adolesc Med 1997; 151: 267–272. *Paradoxical effects among adolescents. See also N Engl J Med 1997; 337: 1044–1051.*

Srivastava OP, Polnay L. Field trial of graded care profile scale: a new measure of care. Arch Dis Child 1997; 76: 337–340. *This provides a measure of care in four areas: physical, safety, love, and esteem.*

Accidents

Anonymous. Ingestion of cigarettes and cigarette butts by children – Rhode Island, January 1994–July 1996. MMWR Morb Mortal Wkly Rep 1997; 46: 125–128. *About one-third of cases had symptoms attributable to nicotine toxicity, but no serious harm in this series.*

Beattie TF. Minor head injury. Arch Dis Child 1997; 77: 82–85. *Review.*

Bratton SL, Dowd MD, Brogan TV et al. Serious and fatal air gun injuries: more than meets the eye. Pediatrics 1997; 100: 609–612. *Air guns are associated with serious and fatal injuries.*

DiGuiseppi C, Roberts I, Li L. Influence of changing travel patterns on child death rates from injury: trend analysis. BMJ 1997; 314: 710–713. *A substantial proportion of the decline in pedestrian traffic and pedal cycling deaths seems to have been achieved at the expense of children's walking and cycling.*

Dixon JJ, Roberts DGV. Head injuries in infants caused by falls from surfaces while restrained in car seats. J R Soc Med 1997; 90: 335–336. *Infants sustained head injuries when falling from a surface where they had been restrained in a car seat.*

Drago DA, Winston FK, Baker SP. Clothing drawstring entrapment in playground slides and school buses. Arch Pediatr Adolesc Med 1997; 151: 72–77. *The only feasible intervention is removal of drawstrings. For rope tree swing injuries see Pediatrics 1997; 99: 548–550.*

Moore F. 'I've just been bitten by a dog'. BMJ 1997; 314: 88–89. *Surgical toilet, appropriate antibiotics, and advice to come back if infection develops. For life-threatening sepsis after dog bite see pp 129–130.*

Mott A, Rolfe K, James R et al. Safety of surfaces and equipment for children in playgrounds. Lancet 1997; 349: 1874–1876. *Bark alone is insufficient to prevent all injuries.*

Toren A, Goshen E, Katz M et al. Bilateral femoral stress fractures in a child due to in-line (roller) skating. Acta Paediatr 1997; 86: 332–333. *The fractures were only visible with an isotope bone scan.*

van Weeghel I, Kendrick D, Marsh P. Accidental injury: risk and preventative interventions. Arch Dis Child 1997; 77: 28–31. *First aid training may not reach those most at risk.*

Wheeler DS, Shope TR. Depressed skull fracture in a 7 month old who fell from bed. Pediatrics 1997; 100: 1033–1034. *The result of a 24 inch fall.*

Wyatt JP, McLeod L, Beard D et al. Timing of paediatric deaths after trauma. BMJ 1997; 314: 868. *Most were either dead when found or died at the scene of the accident.*

Cerebral palsy

Grether JK, Nelson KB. Maternal infection and cerebral palsy in infants of normal birth weight. JAMA 1997; 278: 207–211. *Intrauterine exposure to maternal infection was associated with a marked increase in risk of CP in infants of normal birth weight.*

Hoon AH, Reinhardt EM, Kelley RI et al. Brain magnetic resonance imaging in suspected extrapyramidal cerebral palsy: observations in distinguishing genetic-metabolic from acquired causes. J Pediatr 1997; 131: 240–245. *A useful diagnostic tool.*

Perlman JM. Intrapartum hypoxic-ischemic cerebral injury and subsequent cerebral palsy: medicolegal issues. Pediatrics 1997; 99: 851–859. *Review. For neonatal risk factors in preterm infants see BMJ 1997; 314: 404–408.*

Pharoah POD, Cooke RWI. A hypothesis for the aetiology of spastic cerebral palsy – the vanishing twin. Dev Med Child Neurol 1997; 39: 292–296. *Death of monochorionic cotwin hypothesis.*

Scrutton D, Baird G. Surveillance measures of the hips of children with bilateral cerebral palsy. Arch Dis Child 1997; 76: 381–384. *Review.*

Steinbok P, Reiner AM, Beauchamp R et al. A randomized clinical trial to compare selective posterior rhizotomy plus physiotherapy with physio-therapy alone in children with spastic diplegic cerebral palsy. Dev Med Child Neurol 1997; 39: 178–184. *Improvement in motor function after rhizotomy is more than can be explained by the associated intensive physiotherapy.*

Child abuse

Haviland J, Russell RIR. Outcome after severe non-accidental head injury. Arch Dis Child 1997; 77: 504–507. *Poor outcome in 11 of 13 survivors.*

Hymel KP, Abshire TC, Luckey DW et al. Coagulopathy in pediatric abusive head trauma. Pediatrics 1997; 99: 371–375. *Prothrombin time prolongation and activated coagulation are common complications of paediatric abusive head trauma.*

Lawrenson F. Runaway children: whose problem? A history of running away should be taken seriously: it may indicate abuse. BMJ 1997; 314: 1064. *Review.*

Ng CS, Hall CM, Shaw DG. The range of visceral manifestations of non-accidental injury. Arch Dis Child 1997; 77: 167–174. *Review.*

Olds DL, Eckenrode J, Henderson CR et al. Long-term effects of home visitation on maternal life course and child abuse and neglect. Fifteen-year follow-up of a randomized trial. JAMA 1997; 278: 637–652. *Prenatal and early childhood home visitation reduces abuse, subsequent pregnancies and use of welfare.*

Sinal SH, Lawless MR, Rainey DY et al. Clinician agreement on physical findings in child sexual abuse cases. Arch Pediatr Adolesc Med 1997; 151: 497–608. *Documents incomplete agreement between experienced clinicians.*

Southall DP, Plunkett MCB, Banks MW et al. Covert video recordings of life-threatening child abuse: lessons for child protection. Pediatrics 1997; 100: 735–760. *Report of 33 cases.*

Swanston HY, Tebbutt JS, O'Toole BI et al. Sexually abused children 5 years after presentation: a case-control study. Pediatrics 1997; 100: 600–608. *Many children had ongoing problems.*

Tyagi AK, Willshaw HE, Ainsworth JR. Unilateral retinal haemorrhages in non-accidental injury. Lancet 1997; 349: 1224. *Report of 3 cases.*

Wall N. Judicial attitudes to expert evidence in children's cases. Arch Dis Child 1997; 76: 485–489. *Review.*

Wyatt DT, Simms MD, Horwitz SM. Widespread growth retardation and variable growth recovery in foster children in the first year after initial placement. Arch Pediatr Adolesc Med 1997; 151: 813–816. *Almost half of the children showed significant catch-up growth in the first year after foster care.*

Enuresis

Rona RJ, Li L, Chinn S. Determinants of nocturnal enuresis in England and Scotland in the '90s. Dev Med Child Neurol 1997; 39: 677–681. *Despite the availability of treatment only half of parents consult a doctor.*

Super M, Postlethwaite RJ. Genes, familial enuresis, and clinical management. Lancet 1997; 350: 159-160. *Review.*

Handicap

Goodman R. Psychological aspects of hemiplegia. Arch Dis Child 1997; 76: 177–181. *Review.*

Henderson RC. Bone density and other possible predictors of fracture risk in children and adolescents with spastic quadriplegia. Dev Med Child Neurol 1997; 39: 224–227. *Bone density in the lumbar spine was not predictive of subsequent fracture risk.*

Palisano R, Rosenbaum P, Walter S et al. Development and reliability of a system to classify gross motor function in children with cerebral palsy. Dev Med Child Neurol 1997; 39: 214–223. *A standardised system with many potential applications.*

Immunisation

American Academy of Pediatrics. Immunization of adolescents: recommendations of the advisory committee on immunization practices. Pediatrics 1997; 99: 479–499. *Review.*

Braun MM, Patriarca PA, Ellenberg SS. Syncope after immunization. Arch Pediatr Adolesc Med 1997; 151: 255–259. *Report of 697 cases.*

Chang MH, Chen CJ, Lai MS et al. Universal hepatitis B vaccination in Taiwan and the incidence of hepatocellular carcinoma in children. N Engl J Med 1997; 336: 1855–1859. *With vaccination, the incidence of carcinoma has fallen. See also pp 1906–1907.*

Feder HM, LaRussa P, Steinberg S et al. Clinical varicella following varicella vaccination: don't be fooled. Pediatrics 1997; 99: 897–899. *Vaccination is dangerous during or soon after therapy with oral steroids.*

Feeney M, Clegg A, Winwood P et al. A case-control study of measles vaccination and inflammatory bowel disease. Lancet 1997; 350: 764–766. *Vaccination does not cause bowel disease.*

Joensuu J, Koskenniemi E, Pang XL et al. Randomised placebo-controlled trial of rhesus-human reassortment rotavirus vaccine for prevention of severe rotavirus gastroenteritis. Lancet 1997; 350: 1205–1209. *Highly effective.*

Jones EM, Reeves DS. Controlling chickenpox in hospitals. Vaccination may be the way forward. BMJ 1997; 314: 4–5. *Review. For vaccination in healthy children see Pediatrics 1997; 100: 761–766 and Health Trends 1997; 29: 80–82.*

Lee WM. Hepatitis B virus infection. N Engl J Med 1997; 337: 1733–1745. *Review.*

Moxon ER. Applications of molecular microbiology to vaccinology. Lancet 1997; 350: 1240–1244. *Review.*

Poland GA. Still more questions on pertussis vaccines. Lancet 1997; 350: 1564–1565. *Review. See also pp 1569–1577.*

Ramsay M, Joce R, Whalley J. Adverse events after school leavers received combined tetanus and low dose diphtheria vaccine. Commun Dis Rep CDR Wkly 1997; 7: R65–R67. *Mild local reactions were common.*

Sanchez PJ, Laptook AR, Fisher L et al. Apnea after immunisation of preterm infants. J Pediatr 1997; 130: 746–751. *12 (12%) infants experienced a recurrence of apnoea, and 11 (11%) had at least a 50% increase in the number of apnoeic and bradycardic episodes in the 72 hours after immunisation.*

Taddio A, Katz J, Ilersich AL et al. Effect of neonatal circumcision on pain response during subsequent routine vaccination. Lancet 1997; 349: 599–603. *Circumcised infants showed a stronger pain response to subsequent vaccination.*

Van Damme P, Kane M, Meheus A. Integration of hepatitis B vaccination into national immunisation programmes. BMJ 1997; 314: 1033–1037. *Is cost effective even in countries with low endemicity.*

Wawryk A, Mavronmatis C, Gold M. Electronic monitoring of vaccine cold chain in a metropolitan area. BMJ 1997; 315: 518. *Unacceptable cold was found in 21 of 40 sites.*

Infant feeding

Dungy CI, Losch ME, Russell D et al. Hospital infant formula discharge packages. Do they affect the duration of breast-feeding? Arch Pediatr Adolesc Med 1997; 151: 724–729. *Apparently not, but unclear if findings apply to those of lower socio-economic status.*

Setchell KDR, Zimmer-Nechemias L, Cai J et al. Exposure of infants to phyto-oestrogens from soy-based infant formula. Lancet 1997; 350: 23–27. *Degree of hazard, if any, is unknown.*

Victora CG, Behague DP, Barros FC et al. Pacifier use and short breastfeeding duration: cause, consequence, or coincidence? Pediatrics 1997; 99: 445–453. *Pacifiers seem to contribute to earlier weaning among a group of women uncomfortable with breastfeeding but do not seem to affect breastfeeding duration among self-confident mothers.*

von Schenck U, Bender-Gotze C, Koletzko B. Persistence of neurological damage induced by dietary vitamin B-12 deficiency in infancy. Arch Dis Child 1997; 77:137-139. *Infantile vitamin B-12 deficiency was induced by maternal vegan diet.*

Sudden infant death syndrome (SIDS)

Bacon CJ. Cot death after CESDI. Arch Dis Child 1997; 76: 171–173. *Review.*

Brooke H, Gibson A, Tappin D et al. Case-control study of sudden infant death syndrome in Scotland, 1992–5. BMJ 1997; 314: 1516–1520. *Sleeping prone and parental smoking were risk factors.*

Ford RPK, Mitchell EA, Stewart AW et al. SIDS, illness, and acute medical care. Arch Dis Child 1997; 77: 54–55. *Only 1.3% of all SIDS cases had symptoms suggesting severe illness and had not seen a general practitioner.*

McKenna JJ, Mosko SS, Richard CA. Bedsharing promotes breastfeeding. Pediatrics 1997; 100: 214–219. *And thereby may help to prevent SIDS?*

Mitchell EA, Tuohy PG, Brunt JM et al. Risk factors for sudden infant death syndrome following the prevention campaign in New Zealand: a prospective study. Pediatrics 1997; 100: 835–840. *Prone and side sleeping positions, maternal smoking, and the joint exposure to bed sharing and maternal smoking were associated with increased risk of SIDS.*

Mosko S, Richard C, McKenna J. Infant arousals during mother-infant bed sharing: implications for infant sleep and sudden infant death syndrome research. Pediatrics 1997; 100: 841–849. *Arousals associated with bed sharing might be protective.*

Williams SM, Mitchell EA, Scragg R. Why is sudden infant death syndrome more common at weekends? Arch Dis Child 1997; 77: 415–419. *May be explained in part by the lesser protective effect of sharing a bedroom with an adult.*

Surveillance/screening

Simmers AJ, Gray LS, Spowart K. Screening for amblyopia: a comparison of paediatric letter tests. Br J Ophthalmol 1997; 81: 465–469. *There are problems with the test format and testing procedure in the present school screening system.*

Turner G, Robins H, Wake S et al. Case finding for the fragile X syndrome and its consequences. BMJ 1997; 315: 1223–1226. *Active case finding can reduce the prevalence of this condition. See also pp 1174–1175.*

DERMATOLOGY

Bass JW, Chan DS, Creamer KM et al. Comparison of oral cephalexin, topical mupirocin and topical bacitracin for treatment of impetigo. Pediatr Infect Dis J 1997; 16: 708–710. *Topical bacitracin is unsuitable.*

Liebke C, Wahn U, Niggemann B. Sweat electrolyte concentrations in children with atopic dermatitis. Lancet 1997; 350: 1678–1679. *Significantly higher than in normal children.*

ENDOCRINOLOGY

Elders MJ, Scott CR, Frindik JP et al. Clinical workup for precocious puberty. Lancet 1997; 350: 457–458. *Review.*

Franks S. Polycystic ovary syndrome. Arch Dis Child 1997; 77: 89–90. *Review.*

Le Roith D. Insulin-like growth factors. N Engl J Med 1997; 336: 633–640. *Review.*

Lee MM, Donahoe PK, Silverman BL et al. Measurement of serum mullerian inhibiting substance in the evaluation of children with nonpalpable gonads. N Engl J Med 1997; 336: 1480–1486. *Can be used to determine testicular status in prepubertal children with nonpalpable gonads.*

Styne DM. New aspects in the diagnosis and treatment of pubertal disorders. Pediatr Clin North Am 1997; 44: 505–529. *Review.*

Diabetes

Acerini CL, Patton CM, Savage MO et al. Randomised placebo-controlled trial of human recombinant insulin-like growth factor I plus intensive insulin therapy in adolescents with insulin-dependent diabetes mellitus. Lancet 1997; 350: 1199–1204. *Possibly useful adjunct to therapy. See also pp 1188–1189.*

Baumer JH, Hunt LP, Shield JPH. Audit of diabetes care by caseload. Arch Dis Child 1997; 77: 102–108. *Children under non-specialists had higher admission rates. See also pp 109–114.*

Gardner SG, Bingley PJ, Sawtell PA et al. Rising incidence of insulin dependent diabetes in children aged under 5 years in the Oxford region: time trend analysis. BMJ 1997; 315: 713–717. *The incidence has risen markedly. For low incidence in Pakistan see Arch Dis Child 1997; 76: 121–123.*

Holleman F, Hoekstra JBL. Insulin lispro. N Engl J Med 1997; 337: 176–183. *Review.*

Nyamugundura G, Roper H. Childhood onset insulin dependent diabetes presenting with severe hyperlipidaemia. BMJ 1997; 314: 62–65. *Discussion of management.*

Santiago JV. Nocturnal hypoglycemia in children with diabetes. An important problem revisited. J Pediatr 1997; 131: 2–4. *Review. See also 130: 366–372.*

Simmons D. NIDDM and breastfeeding. Lancet 1997; 350: 157–158. *Review. See pp 166–168.*

Sperling MA. The scylla and charybdis of blood glucose control in children with diabetes mellitus. J Pediatr 1997; 130: 339–341. *Review.*

Growth

Binder G, Grauer ML, Wehner AV et al. Outcome in tall stature. Final height and psychological aspects in 220 patients with and without treatment. Eur J Pediatr 1997; 156: 905–910. *Treatment most effective if started early.*

Brook CGD. Growth hormone: panacea or punishment for short stature? Learning to live with being short is more important for short normal children. BMJ 1997; 315: 692–693. *Review. See also pp 708–713.*

Cole TJ. 3-in-1 weight-monitoring chart. Lancet 1997; 349: 102–103. *Conventional weight centiles augmented with extra lines called thrive lines, where the slope defines a cut-off for failure to thrive.*

Downie AB, Mulligan J, Stratford RJ et al. Are short normal children at a disadvantage? The Wessex growth study. BMJ 1997; 314: 97–100. *Social class has more influence than height.*

Hughes JM, Li L, Chinn S et al. Trends in growth in England and Scotland, 1972 to 1994. Arch Dis Child 1997; 76: 182–189. *Children are becoming taller and fatter.*

Kelly AM, Shaw NJ, Thomas AMC et al. Growth of Pakistani children in relation to the 1990 growth standards. Arch Dis Child 1997; 77: 401–405. *It is not safe to assume that short stature or low body weight in a Pakistani child is due to ethnic background.*

Montgomery SM, Bartley MJ, Wilkinson RG. Family conflict and slow growth. Arch Dis Child 1997; 77: 326–333. *Conflict during childhood was associated with slow growth to age 7 years.*

Oestreich AE. Tanner-Whitehouse versus Greulich-Pyle in bone age determinations. J Pediatr 1997; 131: 5–6. *Review.*

EAR, NOSE AND THROAT

Bangert BA. Imaging of paranasal sinus disease. Pediatr Clin North Am 1997; 44: 681–699. *Review.*

Froom J, Culpepper L, Jacobs M et al. *Antimicrobials for acute otitis media? BMJ 1997; 315: 98–102. Review. See also pp 321–322 and 314: 1526–1529. For duration and recurrence of otitis with effusion, see 314: 350–355*

GASTROENTEROLOGY

Alvarez F. Long-term treatment of bleeding caused by portal hypertension in children. J Pediatr 1997; 131: 798–800. *Review. See also Arch Dis Child 1997; 77: 476–477.*

Duggan C, Nurko S. 'Feeding the gut': the scientific basis for continued enteral nutrition during acute diarrhea. J Pediatr 1997; 131: 801–808. *Review.*

Jones NL, Bourke B, Sherman PM. Breath testing for *Helicobacter pylori* infection in children: a breath of fresh air? J Pediatr 1997; 131: 791–793. *Review. See also pp 815–820.*

Mäki M, Collin P. Coeliac disease. Lancet 1997; 349: 1755–1759. *Review.*

Rautanen T, Kurki S, Vesikari T. Randomised double blind study of hypotonic oral rehydration solution in diarrhoea. Arch Dis Child 1997; 76: 272–274. *Hypotonic ORS was more effective in patients with rotavirus positive than with rotavirus negative diarrhoea.*

Rennels MB. Rotavirus vaccine comes of age. J Pediatr 1997; 131: 512–513. *Review.*

Riordan SM, Williams R. Treatment of hepatic encephalopathy. N Engl J Med 1997; 337: 473–479. *Review.*

Sigurdsson L, Flores A, Putnam PE et al. Postviral gastroparesis: presentation, treatment, and outcome. J Pediatr 1997; 130: 751–754. *Impaired gastric emptying after rotavirus infection.*

Vandenplas Y, Belli D, Benhamou P et al. A critical appraisal of current management practices for infant regurgitation – recommendations of a working party. Eur J Pediatr 1997; 156: 343–357. *Review.*

Ziegler MM. Short bowel syndrome: remedial features that influence outcome and the duration of parenteral nutrition. J Pediatr 1997; 131: 335–336. *Review.*

GENETICS AND MALFORMATIONS

Malformations

Albers N, Ulrichs C, Gluer S et al. Etiologic classification of severe hypospadias: implications for prognosis and management. J Pediatr 1997; 131: 386–392. *Review.*

Slater A. Multiple causes of human kidney malformations. Arch Dis Child 1997; 77: 471–477. *Review.*

Wyllie JP, Madar RJ, Wright M et al. Strategies for antenatal detection of Down's syndrome. Arch Dis Child 1997; 76: F26–F30. *Even if maternal serum screening and fetal echocardiography achieve their predicted potential, around half of all pregnancies affected by Down's syndrome will result in live born babies.*

HAEMATOLOGY

Bolton-Maggs PHB, Moon I. Assessment of UK practice for management of acute childhood idiopathic thrombocytopenic purpura against pulished guidelines. Lancet 1997; 350: 620–623. *Problems were overuse of intravenous immunoglobulin as first-line therapy; children received steroids without marrow examination; inappropriate use of platelet transfusions. See also pp 602-603, 1252–1253.*

Booth IW, Aukett MA. Iron deficiency anaemia in infancy and early childhood. Arch Dis Child 1997; 76: 549–554. *Review. For dietary intervention see pp 144–147.*

Enjolras O, Wassef M, Mazoyer E et al. Infants with Kasabach-Merritt syndrome do not have 'true' hemangiomas. J Pediatr 1997; 130: 631–640. *These are not strawberry (capillary) haemangiomas.*

Sickle cell disease

Bunn HF. Pathogenesis and treatment of sickle cell disease. N Engl J Med 1997; 337: 762–769. *Review. See also Lancet 1997; 350: 725–730.*

Davies SC, Oni L. Management of patients with sickle cell disease. BMJ 1997; 315: 656–660. *Review.*

Fertleman CR, Gallagher A, Rossiter MA. Evaluation of fast track admission policy for children with sickle cell crises. BMJ 1997; 315: 650. *Delivers much faster analgesia.*

Jacobson SJ, Kopecky EA, Joshi P et al. Randomised trial of oral morphine for painful episodes of sickle-cell disease in children. Lancet 1997; 350: 1358–1361. *A reliable alternative to intravenous morphine.*

Solovey A, Lin Y, Browne P et al. Circulating activated endothelial cells in sickle cell anaemia. N Engl J Med 1997; 337: 1584–1590. *The vascular endothelium is activated in sickle cell anaemia. See also pp 1623–1624.*

Wright J, Thomas P, Serjeant GR. Septicemia caused by salmonella infection: an overlooked complication of sickle cell disease. J Pediatr 1997; 130: 394–399. *Of 55 with salmonella, 27 had septicaemia.*

INFECTIOUS DISEASE

Amir J, Harel L, Smetana Z et al. Treatment of herpes simplex gingivostomatitis with aciclovir in children: a randomised double blind placebo controlled study. BMJ 1997; 314: 1800–1803. *Shortens the duration of clinical manifestations.*

Drago F, Ranieri E, Malaguti F et al. Human herpesvirus 7 in pityriasis rosea. Lancet 1997; 349: 1367–1368. *Strongly supports its causative role.*

Duncan A. New therapies for severe meningococcal disease but better outcomes? Lancet 1997; 350: 1565–1566. *Review. See also pp 1590-1593, 1439–1443.*

Dunn MW, Berkowitz FE, Miller JJ et al. Hepatosplenic cat-scratch disease and abdominal pain. Pediatr Infect Dis J 1997; 16: 269–272. *Abdominal pain as a feature of cat-scratch disease.*

Hewlett EL. Pertussis: current concepts of pathogenesis and prevention. Pediatr Infect Dis J 1997; 16: S78–S84. *Review.*

Hoofnagle JH, Di Bisceglie AM. The treatment of chronic viral hepatitis. N Engl J Med 1997; 336: 347–356. *Review.*

Kaplan SL. Prevention of hearing loss from meningitis. Lancet 1997; 350: 158–159. *Review.*

Levy JA. Three new human herpesviruses (HHV6, 7, and 8). Lancet 1997; 349: 558–562. *Review.*

Mandl KD, Stack AM, Fleisher GR. Incidence of bacteremia in infants and children with fever and petechiae. J Pediatr 1997; 131: 398–404. *Petechiae were common in febrile children, seldom associated with bacteraemia.*

Mayon-White RT, Heath PT. Preventive strategies on meningococcal disease. Arch Dis Child 1997; 76: 178–181. *Review. For tobacco smoke as a risk factor see Pediatr Infect Dis J 1997; 16: 979–983.*

Prober CG, Wang EEL. Reducing the morbidity of lower respiratory tract infections caused by respiratory syncytial virus: still no answer. Pediatrics 1997; 99: 472–475. *Review.*

Shann F. Meta-analysis of trials of prophylactic antibiotics for children with measles: inadequate evidence. BMJ 1997; 314: 334–336. *Antibiotics should be given only if a child has clinical signs of pneumonia or other evidence of sepsis. See also pp 316–317.*

Swerdlow DL, Griffin PM. Duration of faecal shedding of *Escherichia coli* 0157:H7 among children in day-care centres. Lancet 1997; 349: 745–746. *Review.*

Vesikari T. Rotavirus vaccines against diarrhoeal disease. Lancet 1997; 350: 1538–1541. *Review.*

Wylie PAL, Stevens D, Drake III W et al. Epidemiology and clinical management of meningococcal disease in west Gloucestershire: retrospective, population based study. BMJ 1997; 315: 774–779. *Early treatment with penicillin is important. See also pp 757–758.*

AIDS

Cohn JA. HIV infection-I. BMJ 1997; 314: 487–491. *Review.*

Evans JA, Gibb DM, Holland FJ et al. Malignancies in UK children with HIV infection acquired from mother to child transmission. Arch Dis Child 1997; 76: 330–333. *HIV infection is a predisposing cause of childhood cancer.*

Shearer WT, Quinn TC, LaRussa P et al. Viral load and disease progression in infants infected with human immunodeficiency virus type 1. N Engl J Med 1997; 336: 1337–1342. *High viral load is associated with increased risk of rapid progression.*

Walsh D, Drumm B. Pediatric HIV infection. Arch Dis Child 1997; 76:293-297. *Review. For zidovudine and didanosine therapy see N Engl J Med 1997; 336: 1704–1712.*

METABOLIC

Boles RG, Chun N, Senadheera D et al. Cyclic vomiting syndrome and mitochondrial DNA mutations. Lancet 1997; 350: 1299–1300. *The authors suggest that all cases with idiopathic cyclic vomiting be evaluated for possible mitochondrial dysfunction.*

Bouchard C. Obesity in adulthood – the importance of childhood and parental obesity. N Engl J Med 1997; 337: 926–927. *Review. See also pp 869–873.*

Cadogan J, Eastell R, Jones N et al. Milk intake and bone mineral acquisition in adolescent girls: randomised, controlled intervention trial. BMJ 1997; 315: 1255–1260. *Increased milk consumption significantly enhances bone mineral acquisition in adolescent girls.*

Morris AAM, Leonard JV. Early recognition of metabolic decompensation. Arch Dis Child 1997; 76: 555–556. *Review.*

MISCELLANEOUS

Chitre VV, Premchandra DJ. Recurrent parotitis. Arch Dis Child 1997; 77: 359–363. *Review.*

Daoud AS, Batieha A, Al-Sheyyab M et al. Effectiveness of iron therapy on breath-holding spells. J Pediatr 1997; 130: 547-550. *Children treated showed significant reduction in the frequency of breath holding spells (88%) compared with the frequency (6%) in the placebo group. For familial nature of breath holding, see J Pediatr 1997; 130: 647–651.*

Gemke RJBJ. Centralisation of paediatric intensive care to improve outcome. Lancet 1997; 349: 1187–1188. *Review. See also pp 1213–1217.*

Goodman TR, McHugh K. Advances in radiology. Arch Dis Child 1997; 77: 265–271. *Review.*

Greenhalgh T. How to read a paper. The medline database. BMJ 1997; 315: 180–183. *Review. For medical databases on the internet, see J R Soc Med 1997; 90: 610–611. For paediatrics and the internet see Arch Dis Child 1997; 77: 179–182.*

Jan MM, S., Camfield PR, Gordon K et al. Vomiting after mild head injury is related to migraine. J Pediatr 1997; 130: 134–137. *History of motion sickness, migraine headaches, and family history of migraine are highly predictive of vomiting after a mild head injury.*

Jenney MEM, Campbell S. Measuring quality of life. Arch Dis Child 1997; 77: 347–350. *Review. See also pp 350–354.*

Jones BM, Hayward R, Evans R et al. Occipital plagiocephaly: an epidemic of craniosynostosis? BMJ 1997; 315: 693–694. *Review.*

Mower WR, Sachs C, Nicklin EL et al. Pulse oximetry as a fifth paediatric vital sign. Pediatrics 1997; 99: 681–686. *Resulted in important changes in the treatment of a small proportion of paediatric patients.*

Platt MJ. Child health statistical review, 1997. Arch Dis Child 1997; 77: 542–548. *Review.*

Schott GD. Influence of age on Henoch Schonlein purpura. Lancet 1997; 350: 1116–1117. *Review. For pulmonary haemorrhage as a complication, see Pediatr Dermatol 1997; 14: 299–302.*

Teach SJ, Yates EW, Feld LG. Laboratory predictors of fluid deficit in acutely dehydrated children. Clin Pediatr 1997; 36: 395–400. *Conventional laboratory studies used to assess dehydration in children are poorly predictive of fluid deficits. See also pp 401–402.*

NEONATOLOGY

American Academy of Pediatrics. Revised guidelines for prevention of early-onset group B streptococcal infection. Pediatrics 1997; 99: 489–496. *Review.*

American Academy of Pediatrics. Noise: a hazard for the fetus and newborn. Pediatrics 1997; 100: 724–727. *Review.*

Barnett CP, Perlman M, Ekert PG. Clinicopathological correlations in postasphyxial organ damage. Pediatrics 1997; 99: 797–799. *The organs of newborns dying of hypoxic encephalopathy may be suitable for use as donor organs.*

Barrington KJ, Finer NN. Care of near term infants with respiratory failure. BMJ 1997; 315: 1215–1218. *Review.*

Bishop NJ, Morley R, Day JP et al. Aluminum neurotoxicity in preterm infants receiving intravenous-feeding solutions. N Engl J Med 1997; 336: 1557–1561. *Prolonged intravenous feeding with solutions containing aluminium is associated with impaired neurologic development.*

Boppana SB, Fowler KB, Vaid Y et al. Neuroradiographic findings in the newborn period and long-term outcome in children with symptomatic congenital cytomegalovirus infection. Pediatrics 1997; 99: 409–414. *CT scan is a good predictor of outcome.*

Carr R, Modi N. Haemopoietic colony stimulating factors for preterm neonates. Arch Dis Child 1997; 76: F128–F133. *Review.*

Carrasco M, Martell M, Estol PC. Oronasopharyngeal suction at birth: effects on arterial oxygen saturation. J Pediatr 1997; 130: 832–834. *Suction was associated with delay in reaching 86% and 92% saturation.*

Chang GY, Lueder FL, DiMichele DM et al. Heparin and the risk of intraventricular haemorrhage in premature infants. J Pediatr 1997; 131: 362–366. *No effect. See also pp 337–338.*

Clark RH, Dykes FD, Bachman TE et al. Intraventricular hemorrhage and high-frequency ventilation: a meta-analysis of prospective clinical trials. Pediatrics 1997; 98: 1058–1061. *HFV is not associated with increased occurrence of IVH or PVL.*

Darnall RA, Kattwinkel J, Nattie C et al. Margin of safety for discharge after apnea in preterm infants. Pediatrics 1997; 100: 795–801. *Supports a 5–10 day apnoea-free period before discharge.*

Deshpande SA, Ward Platt MP. Association between blood lactate and acid-base status and mortality in ventilated babies. Arch Dis Child 1997; 76: F15–F20. *pH or base excess cannot be used as proxy measures for blood lactate.*

Doyle LW. Kangaroo mother care. Lancet 1997; 350: 1721–1722. *Review.*

Doyle LW. Improved outcome into the 1990s for infants weighing 500–999 g at birth. Arch Dis Child 1997; 77: F91–F94. *Survival and disability have increased; 73% had impaired development. See also BMJ 1997; 314: 107–111.*

Ekert P, Perlman M, Steinlin M et al. Predicting the outcome of postasphyxial hypoxic-ischemic encephalopathy within 4 hours of birth. J Pediatr 1997; 131: 613–617. *Age of onset of breathing, administration of chest compressions, and age of onset of seizures were the most important variables.*

Estan J, Hope P. Unilateral neonatal cerebral infarction in full term infants. Arch Dis Child 1997; 76: F88–F93. *Aetiology remains unclear.*

Fadavi S, Punwani IC, Jain L et al. Mechanics and energetics of nutritive sucking: a functional comparison of commercially available nipples. J Pediatr 1997; 130: 740–745. *The Playtex nipple permitted a more rapid rate of milk flow and may be unsuitable for infants unable to safely swallow larger volumes of milk with each suck.*

Field D, Milligan D, Skeoch C et al. Neonatal transport: time to change? Arch Dis Child 1997; 76: F1–F2. *Review.*

Finer N. Inhaled nitric oxide in neonates. Arch Dis Child 1997; 77: F81–F84. *Review.*

Fox H. Ageing of the placenta. Arch Dis Child 1997; 77: F171–F175. *Review.*

Gilbert C, Rahi J, Eckstein M et al. Retinopathy of prematurity in middle-income countries. Lancet 1997; 350: 12–14. *A major cause of potentially preventable blindness in middle-income countries.*

Gotoff SP, Boyer KM. Prevention of early-onset neonatal group B streptococcal disease. Pediatrics 1997; 99: 866–869. *Review.*

Jenni OG, von Siebenthal K, Wolf M et al. Effect of nursing in the head elevated tilt position (15°) on the incidence of bradycardic and hypoxemic episodes in preterm infants. Pediatrics 1997; 100: 622–625. *Nursing in a moderately tilted position (15°) reduces hypoxaemic events in preterm infants.*

Lander A, Redkar R, Nicholls G et al. Cisapride reduces neonatal postoperative ileus: randomised placebo controlled trial. Arch Dis Child 1997; 77: F119–F122. *Cisapride is effective.*

Manson WG, Weaver LT. Fat digestion in the neonate. Arch Dis Child 1997; 76: F206–F211. *Review.*

McCormick MC. The outcomes of very low birth weight infants: are we asking the right questions? Pediatrics 1997; 99: 869-876. *Review.*

Morley CJ. Systematic review of prophylactic vs rescue surfactant. Arch Dis Child 1997; 77: F70–F74. *Review.*

Nelle M, Hoecker C, Linderkamp O. Effects of bolus tube feeding on cerebral blood flow velocity in neonates. Arch Dis Child 1997; 76: F54–F56. *Tube feeding may decrease cerebral perfusion.*

Powls A, Botting N, Cooke RWI et al. Visual impairment in very low birthweight children. Arch Dis Child 1997; 76: F82–F87. *Stereopsis and contrast sensitivity identified impaired vision that was not detected by normal screening and were related to impaired neurodevelopmental outcome.*

Prechtl HFR, Einspieler C, Cioni G et al. An early marker for neurological deficits after perinatal brain lesions. Lancet 1997; 349: 1361–1363. *Spontaneous motor activity can identify infants who require early intervention.*

Raju TNK, Langenberg P, Bhutani V et al. Vitamin E prophylaxis to reduce retinopathy of prematurity: a reappraisal of published trials. J Pediatr 1997; 131: 844–850. *52% reduction in incidence of stage 3 retinopathy.*

Roberts JD, Fineman JR, Morin FC et al. Inhaled nitric oxide and persistent pulmonary hypertension of the newborn. N Engl J Med 1997; 336: 605–610. *Improved systemic oxygenation. See also pp 597–604.*

Roth SC, Baudin J, Cady E et al. Relation of deranged neonatal cerebral oxidative metabolism with neurodevelopmental outcome and head circumference at 4 years. Dev Med Child Neurol 1997; 39: 718–725. *Severities of adverse outcomes at 1 and 4 years of age were closely related to the extent of cerebral energy derangement in the first week of life.*

Schwartz DS, Gettner PA, Konstantino MM et al. Umbilical venous catheterization and the risk of portal vein thrombosis. J Pediatr 1997; 131: 760–762. *Appropriate placement is associated with a low risk.*

Schwartz RP. Neonatal hypoglycaemia: how low is too low? J Pediatr 1997; 131: 171–173. *Review.*

Shah VS, Taddio A, Bennett S et al. Neonatal pain response to heel stick vs venepuncture of routine blood sampling. Arch Dis Child 1997; 77: F143–F144. *Venepuncture is less painful.*

Shukla HK, Hendricks-Munoz KD, Atakent Y, et al. Rapid estimation of insertional length of endotracheal intubation in newborn infants. J Pediatr 1997; 131: 561–564. *Nasal-tragus length and sternal length are good parameters.*

Skinner J. The effects of surfactant on haemodynamics in hyaline membrane disease. Arch Dis Child 1997; 76: F67–F69. *Review.*

Subhedar NV, Ryan SW, Shaw NJ. Open randomised controlled trial of inhaled nitric oxide and early dexamethasone in high risk preterm infants. Arch Dis Child 1997; 77: F185–F190. *Neither treatment prevented lung disease or death.*

Subhedar NV, Shaw NJ. Changes in oxygenation and pulmonary haemodynamics in preterm infants treated with inhaled nitric oxide. Arch Dis Child 1997; 77: F191–F197. *Produces transient improved oxygenation.*

van der Heide A, van der Maas PJ, van der Wal G et al. Medical end-of-life decisions made for neonates and infants in The Netherlands. Lancet 1997; 350: 251–255. *57% of all deaths had been preceded by a decision to forgo life-sustaining treatment.*

Van Overmeire B, Follens I, Hartmann S et al. Treatment of patent ductus arteriosus with ibuprofen. Arch Dis Child 1997; 76: F179–F184. *As effective as indomethacin and may have fewer renal side effects.*

Vannucci RC, Perlman JM. Interventions for perinatal hypoxic-ischemic encephalopathy. Pediatrics 1997; 100: 1004–1014. *Review.*

Vyas J, Kotecha S. Effects of antenatal and postnatal corticosteroids on the preterm lung. Arch Dis Child 1997; 77: F147–F150. *Review.*

Wariyar U, Tin W, Hey E. Gestational assessment assessed. Arch Dis Child 1997; 77: F216–F220. *Antenatal ultrasound is better than postnatal dating.*

Whitfield MF, Eckstein Granau RV, Holsti L. Extremely premature (≤ 800 g) schoolchildren: multiple areas of hidden disability. Arch Dis Child 1997; 77: F85–F90. *Learning disability was present in 60% and major disability in 14%.*

NEPHROLOGY

Anonymous. The management of urinary tract infection in children. Drug Ther Bull 1997; 35: 65–72. *Review.*

Benador D, Benador N, Slosman D et al. Are younger children at highest risk of renal sequelae after pyelonephritis? Lancet 1997; 349: 17–19. *No evidence that infants are at higher risk.*

Brown MR, Cartwright PC, Snow BW. Common office problems in pediatric urology and gynecology. Pediatr Clin North Am 1997; 44: 1091–1115. *Review.*

Craig JC, Knight JF, Sureshkumar P et al. Vesicouretic reflux and timing of micturating cystourethrography after urinary tract infection. Arch Dis Child 1997; 76: 275–277. *No need to wait more than 1 week.*

Dudley JA, Haworth JM, McGraw ME et al. Clinical relevance and implications of antenatal hydronephrosis. Arch Dis Child 1997; 76: F31–F34. *Vesico-ureteric reflux is a common finding.*

Feld LG, Waz WR, Perez LM et al. Hematuria. Pediatr Clin North Am 1997; 44: 1191–1210. *Review.*

Loening-Baucke V. Urinary incontinence and urinary tract infection and their resolution with treatment of chronic constipation of childhood. Pediatrics 1997; 100: 228–232. *Relief of constipation resulted in disappearance of daytime urinary incontinence in 89% and nighttime urinary incontinence in 63%.*

Malone PSJ. The management of urinary incontinence. Arch Dis Child 1997; 77: 175–178. *Review.*

Neuhaus TJ, Calonder S, Leumann EP. Heterogeneity of atypical haemolytic uraemic syndromes. Arch Dis Child 1997; 76: 518–521. *Children with a recurrent, familial, or neonatal course have worse outcomes.*

Postlethwaite RJ, Wilson B. Ultrasonography vs cystourethography to exclude vesicoureteric reflux in babies. Lancet 1997; 350: 1567–1568. *Review.*

Proesmans W. Barter syndrome and its neonatal variant tract infection. Eur J Pediatr 1997; 156: 669–679. *Review.*

Rushton HG. Urinary tract infections in children. Pediatr Clin North Am 1997; 44: 1133–1169. *Review.*

Scott JES, Swallow V, Coulthard MG et al. Screening of newborn babies for familial ureteric reflux. Lancet 1997; 350: 396–400. *Screening identifies at risk babies. See also p 380.*

Shalaby-Rana E, Lowe LH, Blask AN et al. Imaging in paediatric urology. Pediatr Clin North Am 1997; 44: 1065–1089. *Review.*

Strife CF, Gelfand MJ. Renal cortical scintigraphy: effect on medical decision making in childhood urinary tract infection. J Pediatr 1997; 129: 785–787. *Review.*

Vernon SJ, Coulthard MG, Lambert HJ et al. New renal scarring in children who at age 3 and 4 years had normal scans with dimercaptosuccinic acid: follow up study. BMJ 1997; 315: 905–908. *The need for surveillance is much reduced after fourth birthday. See also pp 918–919.*

Wan J, Greenfield S. Enuresis and common voiding abnormalities. Pediatr Clin North Am 1997; 44: 1117–1131. *Review.*

Wingen AM, Fabian-Bach C, Schaefer F et al. Randomised multicentre study of a low-protein diet on the progression of chronic renal failure in children. Lancet 1997; 349: 1117–1123. *Diet did not affect decrease in renal function.*

NEUROLOGY

Dubowitz V. The muscular dystrophies – clarity or chaos? N Engl J Med 1997; 336: 650–651. *Review. See also pp 618–624.*

Ganesan V, Kirkham FJ. Mechanisms of ischaemic stroke after chickenpox. Arch Dis Child 1997; 76: 522–525. *Report of 7 cases. For stroke due to carotid dissection see BMJ 1997; 314: 291–292.*

Strupp M, Brandt T. Should one reinsert the stylet during lumbar puncture? N Engl J Med 1997; 336: 1190. *Reinsertion reduces the incidence of the post-lumbar puncture syndrome. For depth of insertion of needle, see Arch Dis Child 1997; 77: 450.*

Tatman A, Warren A, Williams A et al. Development of a modified paediatric coma scale in intensive care clinical practice. Arch Dis Child 1997; 77: 519–521. *A grimace score is useful in intubated patients.*

Vogel L, Mulcahy MJ, Betz RR. The child with a spinal cord injury. Dev Med Child Neurol 1997; 39: 202–207. *Review.*

Epilepsy

Eriksson KJ, Koivikko MJ. Status epilepticus in children: aetiology, treatment, and outcome. Dev Med Child Neurol 1997; 39: 652–658. *Prompt use of barbiturate anaesthesia is encouraged.*

Koul RL, Aithala GR, Chacko A et al. Continuous midazolam infusion as treatment of status epilepticus. Arch Dis Child 1997; 76: 445–448. *Effective and safe.*

Motte J, Trevathan E, Arvidsson JFV et al. Lamotrigine for generalized seizures associated with the Lennox-Gastaut syndrome. N Engl J Med 1997; 337: 1807–1812. *Effective and well tolerated.*

Neville BGR. Epilepsy in childhood. BMJ 1997; 315: 924–930. *Review.*

van Donselaar CA, Brouwer OF, Geerts AT et al. Clinical course of untreated tonic-clonic seizures in childhood. BMJ 1997; 314: 401–404. *A large proportion of children with newly diagnosed, unprovoked tonic-clonic seizures have a decelerating disease process. See also pp 391–392.*

Vining EPG, Freeman JM, Pillas DJ et al. Why would you remove half a brain? The outcome of 58 children after hemispherectomy. Pediatrics 1997; 100: 163–171. *A valuable procedure.*

Wallace SJ. First tonic-clonic seizures in childhood. Lancet 1997; 349: 1009–1012. *Review.*

Wallace SJ. Nasal benzodiazepines for management of acute childhood seizures? Lancet 1997; 349: 222. *Review.*

OPHTHALMOLOGY

Blaikie AJ, Ellis J, Sanders R et al. Eye disease associated with handling pet tarantulas: three case reports. BMJ 1997; 314: 1524–1525. *The transfer from spider to hand to eye of urticarious hairs from the tarantula may result in devastating occular inflammation.*

Chylack LT. Cataracts and inhaled corticosteroids. N Engl J Med 1997; 337: 46–48. *Review. See also pp 8–14.*

Young JDH, MacEwen CJ. Managing congenital lacrimal obstruction in general practice. BMJ 1997; 315: 293–296. *Review.*

PSYCHIATRY

Berg I. School refusal and truancy. Arch Dis Child 1997; 76: 90–91. *Review.*

Ernst M, Zamethkin AJ, Matochik JA et al. Low medial prefrontal dopaminergic activity in autistic children. Lancet 1997; 350: 638. *Dopaminergic deficit may contribute to the cognitive impairment seen in autism.*

Goodman R. Child mental health: who is responsible? BMJ 1997; 314: 813–817. *Review.*

Heyman I. Children with obsessive compulsive disorder. BMJ 1997; 315: 444. *Review.*

Lainhart JE. Developmental abnormalities in autism. Lancet 1997; 349: 373–374. *Review. See also pp 392–395.*

Levy F. Attention deficit hyperactivity disorder. BMJ 1997; 315: 894–895. *Review.*

Marcovitch H. Managing chronic fatigue syndrome in children. BMJ 1997; 314: 1635–1636. *Review. See also Pediatrics 1997; 100: 270–271.*

Murray L, Cooper PJ. Prediction, detection, and treatment of postnatal depression. Arch Dis Child 1997; 77: 97–101. *Review. See also pp 99–101.*

Rapin I. Autism. N Engl J Med 1997; 337: 97–104. *Review. See also Lancet 1997; 350:1761-1766.*

Robson P. Cannabis. Arch Dis Child 1997; 77: 164–166. *Review.*

Silber TJ. Resumption of menses in anorexia nervosa. Arch Pediatr Adolesc Med 1997; 151: 14–15. *Review. See also pp 16–21.*

Taylor DC. A psychiatric perspective of epilepsy. Arch Dis Child 1997; 77: 86–88. *Review.*

Zimet GD, Owens R, Dahms W et al. Psychosocial outcome of children evaluated for short stature. Arch Pediatr Adolesc Med 1997; 151: 1017–1023. *No significant psychosocial distress or impairment.*

Brownlee KG, Crabbe DCG. Paediatric bronchoscopy. Arch Dis Child 1997; 77: 272–275. *Review.*

Finder JD. Primary bronchomalacia in infants and children. J Pediatr 1997; 130: 59–66. *Should be considered in the differential diagnosis of the persistently wheezing infant.*

Godden CW, Campbell MJ, Hussey M et al. Double blind placebo controlled trial of nebulised budesonide for croup. Arch Dis Child 1997; 76: 155–158. *Clear evidence of benefit.*

Hull J, Chow CW, Robertson CF. Chronic idiopathic bronchiolitis of infancy. Arch Dis Child 1997; 77: 512–515. *Report of 8 infants.*

Klassen TP, Sutcliffe T, Watters LK et al. Dexamethasone in salbutamol-treated in-patients with acute bronchiolitis: a randomized, controlled trial. J Pediatr 1997; 130: 191–196. *No benefit.*

Noble V, Murray M, Webb MSC et al. Respiratory status and allergy nine to 10 years after acute bronchiolitis. Arch Dis Child 1997; 76: 315-319. *The excess respiratory symptoms after acute bronchiolitis are not due to familial or personal susceptibility to atopy.*

Orlow SJ, Isakoff MS, Blei F. Increased risk of symptomatic hemangiomas of the airway in association with cutaneous hemangiomas in a 'beard' distribution. J Pediatr 1997; 131: 643–646. *May be associated with airway haemangioma. See also pp 514–515.*

Rodriguez WJ, Gruber WC, Welliver RC et al. Respiratory syncytial virus (RSV) immune globulin intravenous therapy for RSV lower respiratory tract infection in infants and young children at high risk for severe RSV infections. Pediatrics 1997; 99: 454–461. *Safe but not efficacious. See also Lancet 1997; 349: 743–744.*

Sward-Comunelli SL, Mabry SM, Truog WE et al. Airway muscle in preterm infants: changes during development. J Pediatr 1997; 130: 570–576. *Airway muscle is present at 23 weeks' gestation at all levels of the conducting airways.*

Thomson A. The role of negative pressure ventilation. Arch Dis Child 1997; 77: 454–458. *Review.*

Asthma

Browne GJ, Penna AS, Phung X et al. Randomised trial of intravenous salbutamol in early management of acute severe asthma in children. Lancet 1997; 349: 301–305. *Can curtail progression of attack.*

Cohen HA, Neuman I, Nahum H. Blocking effect of vitamin C in exercise-induced asthma. Arch Pediatr Adolesc Med 1997; 151: 367–370. *Seen in some patients.*

Coren ME, Rosenthal M, Bush A. The use of cyclosporin in corticosteroid dependent asthma. Arch Dis Child 1997; 77: 522–523. *Benefit seen in 2 out of 5 cases.*

Nursoy MA, Bakir M, Barlan IB et al. The course of chickenpox in asthmatic children receiving inhaled budesonide. Pediatr Infect Dis J 1997; 16: 74–75. *Uneventful.*

O'Callaghan C, Barry P. Spacer devices in the treatment of asthma. BMJ 1997; 314: 1061–1062. *Review.*

Sears MR. Epidemiology of childhood asthma. Lancet 1997; 350: 1015–1020. *Review.*

Silverman M, Wilson N. Asthma – time for a change of name? Arch Dis Child 1997; 77: 62–65. *Review. See also Thorax 1997; 52: 953–957.*

Simons FER. A comparison of beclomethasone, salmeterol, and placebo in children with asthma. N Engl J Med 1997; 337: 1659–1665. *Beclomethasone was associated with decreased growth. Salmeterol was less effective. See also pp 1690–1692. For steroids in viral-induced wheezing see BMJ 1997; 315: 858–862.*

Tasche MJA, van der Wouden JC, Uijen JHJM et al. Randomised placebo-controlled trial of inhaled sodium cromoglycate in 1–4 year old children with moderate asthma. Lancet 1997; 350: 1060–1064. *Not more effective than placebo.*

Cystic fibrosis

Balfour-Lynn IM, Klein NJ, Dinwiddie R. Randomised controlled trial of inhaled corticosteroids (fluticasone propionate) in cystic fibrosis. Arch Dis Child 1997; 77: 124–130. *Lack of benefit.*

Balfour-Lynn IM, Martin I, Whitehead BF et al. Heart-lung transplantation for patients under 10 with cystic fibrosis. Arch Dis Child 1997; 76: 38–40. *Outcome similar to older children.*

Button BM, Heine RG, Catto-Smith AG et al. Postural drainage and gastro-oesophageal reflux in infants with cystic fibrosis. Arch Dis Child 1997; 76: 148–150. *Standard physiotherapy was associated with a significant increase in reflux. See also Lancet 1997; 349: 1567–1568.*

Conway SP. Recombinant human DNase (rhDNase) in cystic fibrosis: is it cost effective? Arch Dis Child 1997; 77: 1–3. *Review.*

Davis PB. The decline and fall of pulmonary function in cystic fibrosis: new models, new lessons. J Pediatr 1997; 131: 789–790. *Review. See also pp 809–814.*

Dodge JA, Morison S, Lewis PA et al. Incidence, population, and survival of cystic fibrosis in the UK, 1968–95. Arch Dis Child 1997; 77: 493–496. *The survival of successive cohorts continues to be better than earlier cohorts.*

Fauroux B, Delaisi B, Clement A et al. Mycobacterial lung disease in cystic fibrosis: a prospective study. Pediatr Infect Dis J 1997; 16: 354–358. *Non-tuberculous mycobacteria were found in 7/106 patients over 1 year.*

Fitzsimmons SC, Burkhart GA, Borowitz D et al. High-dose pancreatic-enzyme supplements and fibrosing colonopathy in children with cystic fibrosis. N Engl J Med 1997; 336: 1283–1289. *A strong relation between high daily doses of pancreatic-enzyme supplements and the development of fibrosing colonopathy. See also Arch Dis Child 1997; 77: 66–70.*

Gavin J, Ellis J, Dewar AL et al. Dietary fibre and the occurrence of gut symptoms in cystic fibrosis. Arch Dis Child 1997; 76: 35–37. *A low residue diet might be an important factor in the pathogenesis of gastrointestinal symptoms.*

Gregg RG, Simantel A, Farrell PM et al. Newborn screening for cystic fibrosis in Wisconsin: comparison of biochemical and molecular methods. Pediatrics 1997; 99: 819–824. *IRT/DNA was better than IRT alone.*

Hardin DS, LeBlanc A, Lukenbaugh S et al. Insulin resistance is associated with decreased clinical status in cystic fibrosis. J Pediatr 1997; 130: 948–956. *The combination of insulin resistance and decreased insulin secretion is responsible for CF-related diabetes.*

McIlwaine PM, Wong LT, Peacock D et al. Long-term comparative trial of conventional postural drainage and percussion versus positive expiratory pressure physiotherapy in the treatment of cystic fibrosis. J Pediatr 1997; 131: 570–574. *Documents benefit from PEP mask. See also pp 506–508.*

Robinson WM, Ravilly S, Berde C et al. End-of-life care in cystic fibrosis. Pediatrics 1997; 100: 205–209. *Small doses of opiates seem to be effective.*

Southern KW. ΔF508 in cystic fibrosis: willing but not able. Arch Dis Child 1997; 76: 282. *Review.*

Stern RC. The diagnosis of cystic fibrosis. N Engl J Med 1997; 336: 487–491. *Review. See also Arch Dis Child 1997; 76: 85–91.*

Warren WS, Hamosh A, Egan M et al. False-positive results of genetic testing in cystic fibrosis. J Pediatr 1997; 130: 658–660. *Compound heterozygosity for ΔF508 and F508C, a polymorphism not associated with clinical disease.*

Wine JJ. A sensitive defense: salt and cystic fibrosis. Nat Med 1997; 3: 494–495. *Review.*

RHEUMATOLOGY

Adachi JD, Bensen WG, Brown J et al. Intermittent etidronate therapy to prevent corticosteroid-induced osteoporosis. N Engl J Med 1997; 337: 383–387. *Etidronate prevents the loss of vertebral and trochanteric bone. See also pp 420–421.*

Allgrove J. Biphosphonates. Arch Dis Child 1997; 76: 73–75. *Review.*

Hashkes PJ, Lovell DJ. Recognition of infantile-onset multisystem inflammatory disease as a unique entity. J Pediatr 1997; 130: 513–515. *Review.*

Helms PJ. Sports injuries in children: should we be concerned? Arch Dis Child 1997; 77: 161–163. *Review.*

Kuis W, Heijnen CJ, Hogeweg JA et al. How painful is juvenile chronic arthritis? Arch Dis Child 1997; 77: 451–453. *Review.*

Malleson PN. Management of childhood arthritis. Part 1: acute arthritis. Arch Dis Child 1997; 76: 460–462. *Review. For part 2, see pp 541–544.*

Malleson PN, Sailer M, Mackinnon MJ. Usefulness of antinuclear antibody testing to screen for rheumatic diseases. Arch Dis Child 1997; 77: 299–304. *A positive test is found so frequently in children without a rheumatic disease that it has little or no diagnostic value.*

Murray K, Thompson SD, Glass DN. Pathogenesis of juvenile chronic arthritis: genetic and environmental factors. Arch Dis Child 1997; 77: 530–534. *Review.*

Sathananthan R, David J. The adolescent with rheumatic disease. Arch Dis Child 1997; 77: 355–358. *Review.*

Sills JA. Non-inflammatory musculoskeletal disorders in childhood. Arch Dis Child 1997; 77: 71–75. *Review.*

Stollerman GH. Rheumatic fever. Lancet 1997; 349: 935–942. *Review.*

SURGERY

Davies BW, Stringer MD. The survivors of gastroschisis. Arch Dis Child 1997; 77: 158–160. *Adhesive bowel obstruction is a late complication.*

Jack DB. Diagnosis of appendicitis: getting it right every time? Lancet 1997; 349: 1076. *Review.*

Kass EJ, Lundak B. The acute scrotum. Pediatr Clin North Am 1997; 44: 1251–1266. *Review.*

Kenny SE, Shankar KR, Rintala R et al. Evidence-based surgery: interventions in a regional paediatric surgical unit. Arch Dis Child 1997; 76: 50–53. *Only 11% of interventions were based on randomised controlled trials data.*

Kimber C, Spitz L, Cuschieri A. Current state of antenatal *in utero* surgical interventions. Arch Dis Child 1997; 76: F134–F139. *Review.*

Lee PA, O'Leary LA, Songer NJ et al. Paternity after bilateral cryptorchidism. Arch Pediatr Adolesc Med 1997; 151: 260–263. *Among the married men who had bilateral cryptorchidism, 50% had fathered children, compared with 76% in the control group and 74% in the unilateral group.*

Lloyd DA, Carty H, Patterson M et al. Predictive value of skull radiography for intracranial injury in children with blunt head injury. Lancet 1997; 349: 821–824. *Clinical neurological abnormalities are a reliable predictor of intracranial injury. If imaging is required, it should be with CT and not skull radiography.*

Morrison SC. Controversies in abdominal imaging. Pediatr Clin North Am 1997; 44: 555–574. *Review.*

Rowe DE, Bernstein SM, Riddick M et al. A meta-analysis of the efficacy of nonoperative treatments for idiopathic scoliosis. J Bone Joint Surg 1997; 79: 664–674. *Demonstrates the effectiveness of bracing.*

Russell SCS, Doyle E. Paediatric anaesthesia. BMJ 1997; 314: 201–204. *Review.*

Schoen EJ. Benefits of newborn circumcision: is Europe ignoring medical evidence? Arch Dis Child 1997; 77: 258–260. *Review. See also pp 194–195.*

Sivit CJ. Imaging children with acute right lower quadrant pain. Pediatr Clin North Am 1997; 44: 575–589. *Review.*

Swerdlow AJ, Higgins CD, Pike MC. Risk of testicular cancer in cohort of boys with cryptorchidism. BMJ 1997; 314: 1507–1511. *Biopsy seems to be a stronger risk factor for testicular cancer than any factor previously identified.*

Taddio A, Stevens B, Craig K et al. Efficacy and safety of lidocaine-prilocaine cream for pain during circumcision. N Engl J Med 1997; 336: 1197–1201. *Efficacious and safe. See also pp 1244–1245.*

Thomas DFM. Surgical treatment of urinary incontinence. Arch Dis Child 1997; 76: 377–380. *Review.*

Zaeontz MR, Packer MG. Abnormalities of the external genitalia. Pediatr Clin North Am 1997; 44: 1267–1297. *Review.*

THERAPEUTICS

Anderson JM, Sugerman KS, Lockhart JR et al. Effective prophylactic therapy for cyclic vomiting syndrome in children using amitriptyline or cyproheptadine. Pediatrics 1997; 100: 977–981. *Both work in the majority of patients.*

Anonymous. Aminoglycosides once daily? Drug Ther Bull 1997; 35: 36–37. *Review. See also Lancet 1997; 350: 1412.*

Bembi B, Parma A, Bottega M et al. Intravenous pamidronate treatment in osteogenesis imperfecta. J Pediatr 1997; 131: 622–625. *May be useful. See also Eur J Pediatr 1997; 156: 792–794.*

Markestad T. Use of sucrose as a treatment for infant colic. Arch Dis Child 1997; 76: 356–358. *Beneficial.*

Murphy MS. Sedation for invasive procedures in paediatrics. Arch Dis Child 1997; 77: 281–284. *Review.*

Simon HK, Weinkle DA. Over-the-counter medications. Do parents give what they intend to give? Arch Pediatr Adolesc Med 1997; 151: 654–656. *Poor ability to calculate correct dose of paracetamol.*

Wood AJJ. Outpatient parenteral antimicrobial-drug therapy. N Engl J Med 1997; 337: 829–838. *Review.*

MEDICINE IN THE TROPICS

Addiss DG, Beach MJ, Streit TG et al. Randomised placebo-controlled comparison of ivermectin and albendazole alone and in combination for *Wuchereria bancrofti microfilaraemia* in Haitian children. Lancet 1997; 350: 480–484. *Combined treatment was more effective.*

Brewster DR, Manary MJ. Comparison of milk and maize based diets in kwashiorkor. Arch Dis Child 1997; 76: 242–248. *Milk is superior to a local maize based diet. See also pp 236–241.*

Ceesay SM, Prentice AM, Cole TJ et al. Effects on birth weight and perinatal mortality of maternal dietary supplements in rural Gambia: 5 year randomised controlled trial. BMJ 1997; 315: 786–790. *Supplementation reduced retardation in intrauterine growth.*

Cherian T, Steinhoff MC, Simoes EAF et al. Clinical signs of acute lower respiratory tract infections in malnourished infants and children. Pediatr Infect Dis J 1997; 16: 490–494. *The current WHO algorithm is suitable for diagnosis in undernourished children.*

English RM, Badcock JC, Giay T et al. Effect of nutrition improvement project on morbidity from infectious diseases in preschool children in Vietnam: comparison with control commune. BMJ 1997; 315: 1122–1125. *Significant reduction in respiratory and diarrhoeal infection.*

Hotez PJ, Ghosh K, Hawdon J et al. Vaccines for hookworm infection. Pediatr Infect Dis J 1997; 16: 935–940. *Review.*

Ingenbleek Y, Jung L, Ferard G et al. Iodised rapeseed oil for eradication of severe endemic goitre. Lancet 1997; 350: 1542–1545. *Review.*

Kautner I, Robinson MJ, Kubnle U. Dengue virus infection: epidemiology, pathogenesis, clinical presentation, diagnosis, and prevention. J Pediatr 1997; 131: 516–524. *Review.*

Lang J, Hoa DQ, Gioi NV et al. Randomised feasibility trial of pre-exposure rabies vaccination with DTP-IPV in infants. Lancet 1997; 349: 1663–1665. *Safe and probably effective.*

Levine MM. Oral vaccines against cholera: lessons from Vietnam and elsewhere. Lancet 1997; 349: 220–221. *Review. See also pp 231–235.*

Muhe L, Lulseged S, Mason KE et al. Case-control study of the role of nutritional rickets in the risk of developing pneumonia in Ethiopian children. Lancet 1997; 349: 1801–1804. *Vitamin D or calcium deficiency may be predisposing factors.*

Mulholland K, Hilton S, Adegbola R et al. Randomised trial of *Haemophilus influenzae* type-B tetanus protein conjugate for prevention of pneumonia and meningitis in Gambian infants. Lancet 1997; 349: 1191–1197. *The introduction of HiB vaccines into developing countries should substantially reduce childhood mortality due to pneumonia and meningitis.*

Nacul LC, Kirkwood BR, Arthur P et al. Randomised, double blind, placebo controlled clinical trial of efficacy of vitamin A treatment in non-measles childhood pneumonia. BMJ 1997; 315: 505–510. *No effect on immediate outcome of the pneumonia episode.*

Perez-Schael I, Guntinas MJ, Perez M et al. Efficacy of the rhesus rotavirus-based quadrivalent vaccine in infants and young children in Venezuela. N Engl J Med 1997; 337: 1181–1187. *High level of protection. See also pp 1228–1229.*

Potter AR. Reducing vitamin A deficiency. BMJ 1997; 314: 317–318. *Review. See also Arch Dis Child 1997; 77: 191–194.*

Ross DA, Cutts FT. Vindication of policy of vitamin A with measles vaccination. Lancet 1997; 350: 81–82. *Review. See also pp 101–105.*

Roy SK, Tomkins AM, Akramuzzaman SM et al. Randomised controlled trial of zinc supplementation in malnourished Bangladeshi children with acute diarrhoea. Arch Dis Child 1997; 77: 196–200. *Simple, acceptable, useful and affordable strategy.*

Ruel MT, Rivera JA, Santizo MC et al. Impact of zinc supplementation on morbidity from diarrhoea and respiratory infections among rural Guatemalan children. Pediatrics 1997; 99: 808–813. *The large impact of zinc supplementation on diarrhoea incidence suggests undetected zinc deficiency.*

Sanchez JL, Taylor DN. Cholera. Lancet 1997; 349: 1825–1830. *Review.*

Senanayake MP, Gunawardena MKS, Peiris DSP. Maternal comprehension of two growth monitoring charts in Sri Lanka. Arch Dis Child 1997; 76: 359–361. *Agencies may need to redesign parent held growth charts to achieve better comprehension by mothers.*

Sive AA, Dempster WS, Malan H et al. Plasma free iron: a possible cause of oedema in kwashiorkor. Arch Dis Child 1997; 76: 54–56. *Free circulating iron may contribute to the oedema.*

Steinhoff MC, El Khalek MKA, Khalif N et al. Effectiveness of clinical guidelines for the presumptive treatment of streptococcal pharyngitis in Egyptian children. Lancet 1997; 350: 918–921. *The WHO guideline has a high specificity but a low sensitivity. See also pp 899–900.*

Weber MW, Usen S, Palmer A et al. Predictors of hypoxaemia in hospital admissions with acute lower respiratory tract infection in a developing country. Arch Dis Child 1997; 76: 310–314. *Over half of the children with hypoxaemia could be identified with a combination of extreme respiratory distress, cyanosis, and severely compromised general status.*

Yemaneberhan H, Bekele Z, Venn A et al. Prevalence of wheeze and asthma and relation to atopy in urban and rural Ethiopia. Lancet 1997; 350: 85–90. *Much less common in rural than urban areas.*

Malaria

Brabin BJ, Ganley Y. Imported malaria in children in the UK. Arch Dis Child 1997; 77: 76–81. Review.

Bradley DJ, Warhurst DC. Guidelines for the prevention of malaria in travellers from the United Kingdom. Commun Dis Rep CDR Wkly 1997; 7: R138–R152. *Review.*

Brandts CH, Ndjave M, Graninger W et al. Effect of paracetamol on parasite clearance time in *Plasmodium falciparum* malaria. Lancet 1997; 350: 704–709. *Paracetamol prolongs parasite clearance time. See also pp 678–679.*

Kwiatkowski D, Marsh K. Development of a malaria vaccine. Lancet 1997; 350: 1696–1701. *Review.*

Menendez'C, Kahigwa E, Hirt R et al. Randomised placebo-controlled trial of iron supplementation and malaria chemoprophylaxis for prevention of severe anaemia and malaria in Tanzanian infants. Lancet 1997; 350: 844–850. *Iron supplementation was effective in preventing severe anaemia without increasing susceptibility to malaria.*

Newton CRJC, Crawley J, Sowumni A et al. Intracranial hypertension in Africans with cerebral malaria. Arch Dis Child 1997; 76: 219–226. *Severe intracranial hypertension is associated with a poor outcome.*

Nussenzweig RS, Zavala F. A malaria vaccine based on a sporozoite antigen. N Engl J Med 1997; 336: 128–130. *Review. See also pp 86–91.*

Snow RW, Omumbo JA, Lowe B et al. Relation between severe malaria morbidity in children and level of *Plasmodium falciparum* transmission in Africa. Lancet 1997; 349: 1650–1654. *A critical determinant of life-time disease risk is the ability to develop clinical immunity early in life. See also pp 1636–1637 and 350: 362–364, 813.*

Index

** after page-numbers refers to papers in the
literature review section (Chapter 14)*

A

Abdominal imaging controversies, 252*
Abnormal illness behaviour, 62, 63
Accident prevention groups, 82
Accidental death, coroners' inquest, 74
Accidental falls
    backward, 53
    window barriers, 77
Accidental home injury, 73–82
    information sources, 73–4
    mechanism, 79
    nature and extent of problem, 73–4
    pattern, 74–5
    protection from, 75–8
    types, 79–82
Accidental injury prevention, 232*
ACTH for asthma, 1
Adenovirus and respiratory illness, 28
Adoption outcome, 230*
Adrenal reserve, steroid effects, 5–6
Adrenal suppression, clinical effects, 6
Adrenocorticotrophic hormone see ACTH
Advanced Paediatric Life Support
    courses, 89
    protocols, 102, 105
Aerosol, metered dose, 3
AIDS, programmes after disaster, 225
Air gun injuries, 231*
Air medical physiology, 93–4
Aircraft, partial pressure of oxygen, 93
Airflow, obstruction in small airways, 20–21
Airway
    acute lower, obstruction, 103–4
    acute upper, obstruction, 102–3
    muscle in preterm infants, 249*
    preterm damage, 19
    and ventilatory management, in
      transport, 94–6

Albuterol, 24–5
Alcohol and lower oesophageal sphincter
    pressure, 162–3
Allergy, aminopenicillin, 229*
Aluminum toxicity in preterm infants, 243*
Amblyopia screening, 236*
Ambulances, 92
Ambulatory paediatrics, 231*
Aminoglycosides, 253*
Aminopenicillin allergy, 229*
Aminophylline, 25
Anabolic steroids and adolescents, 230*
Anaemia, 219
    iron deficiency, 239*
Anaesthesia, 252*
Anorexia nervosa
    and dental erosion, 148
    menses resumption, 248*
Antimicrobial-drug therapy, outpatient
    parenteral, 253*
Apnoea
    and gastrooesophageal reflux
      disease, 164
    methylxanthine therapy, 25
    and preterm infant discharge, 243*
Appendicitis
    in CF 187
    diagnosis, 252*
Arterial access, critically ill children, 92
Arthritis
    acute, management, 251*
    chronic juvenile
      genetic/environmental factors, 252*
      pain in, 251*
Asphyxiation, 82
Aspiration and gastrooesophageal reflux
    disease, 163
Aspiration pneumonia, 174
Asthma
    beclomethasone, salmeterol,
      placebo, 250*

and BPD, 20
corticosteroid dependent,
    cyclosporin use, 249*
corticosteroid therapy, 1
effects on growth, 7
epidemiology, 250*
exercise-induced, 31
and gastrooesophageal reflux
    disease, 164
height before therapy, 7
intravenous salbutamol trial, 249*
management in transport, 104
name change, 250*
sodium cromoglycate/placebo trial,
    250*
spacer devices, 250*
vitamin C for, 249*
Attachment disorders, 63–4
Attention deficit hyperactivity disorder,
    248*
Autism, 248*
    developmental abnormalities, 248*
    and dopaminergic activity, 248*
AVPU score, 99

B

Baby walker avoidance, 77
Baclofen, intrathecal, in CP, 133–4
Bacteremia, incidence, 240*
Bag-mask ventilation, 95
Barotrauma, 18
Barrett's oesophagus, 169, 176
Barter syndrome, 246*
Bath mat, non slip, 78
Battered baby syndrome, 40
Beclomethasone
    clinical efficacy, 11
    growth suppression, 8, 9
    inhaled, growth retardation, 8
Beclomethasone dipropionate, 1, 2, 3
    growth studies, 10
Becotide, 1
Beri-beri, 219
Bernstein test, in gastrooesophageal reflux
    syndrome, 167–8, 176
Bile duct strictures, 178
Biliary cirrhosis
    focal, 178
    multilobular, 178, 179–80
Biliary tract disorders in CF, 183–4
Biopsy, oesophageal, 176
Biphosphonates, 251*
Birth, premature, and abnormal lung
    function, 30
Birth trauma and subdural haematoma, 42
Birth weight
    extremely low, 17, 20
        dexamethasone therapy, 30
        outcome, 243*
    very low, 17, 20
        and abnormal lung function, 30
        outcomes, 244*
        visual impairment, 244*
Blood lactate and ventilation, 243*

Blood pressure, direct monitoring 92
Bone
    biochemical markers of metabolism,
        6–7
    density in spastic quadriplegia, 233*
    mineral density measurement, 152
    steroid effects on metabolism, 6–7
Books in third world, 206–7
Botox, 132
Botulinum toxin A in CP, 132–3
Brain
    inertial movements, 40, 51
    perinatal lesions and neurological
    deficits, 244*
Brain injury, 36, 39
    investigations, 45–6
    shaking, or impact, 51–3
Breast feeding
    in disaster, 219
    and pacifiers, 235*
    and SIDS prevention, 235*
    in third world, 196, 197–8
Breath-holding spells, iron therapy, 242*
Breathing
    rapid, demonstration, 200
    work increase in shock, 107
British Paediatric Association Surveillance
    Unit, 58, 66
Bronchial asthma see Asthma
Bronchiolitis, 249*
    dexamethasone for, 249*
    management in transport, 103–4
    sequelae, 249*
Bronchodilators, inhaled, for BPD, 23, 24–5
Bronchomalacia, 21–2, 249*
    bronchodilator therapy, 25
Bronchopulmonary dysplasia, 17–34
    aetiology, 18–20
    and asthma, 31
    clinical findings, 20, 21–2
    complications, 21–2
        monitoring, 26–7
    definition, 18
    diuretic therapy, 23
    genetic aspect, 20
    incidence, 18
    inhaled bronchodilator therapy, 23–5
    nutritional management, 26
    outpatient management, 22–6
    oxygen therapy, 22–3
    pathogenesis equations, 20
    pathophysiology, 20–2
    pharmacologic treatment, 24
    pulmonary abnormalities, 21
    pulmonary outcome, 30–1
    respiratory health, 30–1
    risk factors, 18
    sudden death, 29–30
    viral respiratory illness, 28–9
Bronchoscopy, 249*
    in gastrooesophageal reflux
        syndrome, 167
Bronchospasm, 163, 174
Budapest, National Motor Therapy
    Institute, 130

Budesonide, 1, 3
  clinical efficacy, 11
  growth suppression, 8
Burns, 80
  management in transport, 108–9
  and shock, 105

C

Caffeine, 24, 25
  in cola drinks, 142, 151
Caffeine citrate, 24
Calcium intake
  and bone mass, 153–5
  during childhood, 153
  supplementation trial, 153, 155
Cannabis, 248*
Carbon dioxide, risk in fizzy drinks, 151
Cardiac complications, early recognition, 229*
Cardiology, interventional, 230*
Cardiovascular complications
  of BPD, monitoring, 26–7
  of CLD, monitoring, 26–7
Cat-scratch disease and abdominal pain, 240*
Cataracts, after inhaled corticosteroids, 5, 248*
Catheterisation, in transport, 97
Central venous access
  critically ill children, 92
  in transport, 96–7
Cerebral palsy
  botulinum toxin A, 132–3
  brain MRI, 232*
  feeding disorders in, 129–30
  gait analysis, 136–8
  hip surveillance, 232*
  and hypoxic-ischemic cerebral
    injury, 232*
  intrathecal baclofen, 133–4
  and maternal infection, 232*
  motor function classification system,
    233*
  orthopaedic surgical management,
    135–6
  physical therapy, 130–2
  rhizotomy/physiotherapy trial, 232*
  spastic, aetiology, 232*
  surgery in, 134–8
Chemical incidents, 213
Chickenpox
  in asthmatic children, 250*
  vaccination, 234*
Child abuse, 35–6
  factitious illness by proxy, 57–71
  home visitation long-term effects, 233*
  judicial attitudes, 233*
  life-threatening, video recordings, 233*
  management in transport, 101–2
  retinal haemorrhages, 233*
  scope and scale, 40
  sexual
    clinican agreement, 233*
    effects, 233*
  visceral manifestations, 233*
Child Accident Prevention Trust, 77, 82

Child care
  in disaster and refugee settings, 211–27
  in third world, low technology
    approaches, 193–209
Child in disaster situation, 213–15
Child health
  inequalities, 83
  statistical review, 1997, 242*
Child injury prevention, 75–8, 82–3
Child psychiatry team, 68
Child resistant closures for bottles, 77
Child resistant containers, 78
Child Safety Week, 82
Child-to-Child, 202, 203, 224
Children for Health, 202
Choking, 82
Cholelithiasis, 178
Cholera, 220–1, 255*
  oral vaccines, 254*
Chronic fatigue syndrome management, 248*
Chronic lung disease, 17–34
  aetiology, 18–20
  clinical findings, 20–2
  complications, 22
    monitoring, 26–7
  differentiation from GERD, 174
  gestational age specific incidence, 19
  incidence, 18
  outpatient management, 22–6
  pharmacologic treatment, 24
  risk factors, 18
  in transport, 104
  viral respiratory illness, 28–9
Cigarette ingestion, 231*
Cigarette warning labels efficacy, 231*
Ciprofloxacin, 221
Circulatory failure, 105, 107
Circumcision
  benefits, 253*
  lidocaine-prilocaine cream for, 253*
Cisapride, 168, 175, 186
  neonatal postoperative ileus
    reduction, 244*
Co-trimoxazole, 220–2
Coeliac disease, 238*
Cola drinks
  and caffeine, 151
  childhood consumption and
    osteoporosis risk, 156
  consumption, 141, 144
    increasing, 151–6
  and dietary load of phosphorus, 156
  gastritis risk, 151
  kidney stone risk, 151
  milk and fizzy beverages
    ethnic consumption, 145
    weekly consumption, 145
  nutritional contribution, 142
Cold water on burns, 76
Colloid therapy, critically ill children, 92
Coma, management in transport, 100–1
Coma scale development, 247*
Communicable disease in disaster, 219–22
Community development, health worker's
    place, 201–5

Congenital heart disease, fetal diagnosis, 230*
Congenital lacrimal obstruction, management, 248*
Constipation and urinary incontinence/infection, 246*
Convention on the Rights of the Child 1994, 215
Conversion disorder, 61
Cor pulmonale, 22
Corticosteroids
　for BPD, 30
　inhaled
　　bioavailability, 2–3
　　dose availability, 3
　　effects on growth, 7–11
　　　long-term, 11
　　　medium-term, 8–11
　　　short-term, 8
　　effects on inflammation, 2
　　ethical difficulties in controlled trial, 9
　　growth studies, 10
　　ideal pro-drug, 3–4
　　inhaler device, 3
　　pharmacokinetics, 2
　　pharmacological differences, 3
　　pharmacology, 2–4
　　side-effects, 2–3, 4–11
　　　biochemical measurements, 5–6
　　toxicity, 1, 4–11
　　molecular differences, 11–12
Cortisol, steroid suppression of production, 5
Cough, persistent, in GERD, 174
Coughs and colds, in third world, 200
Craniosynostosis, 242*
Cretinism, 219
Critically ill children
　diagnostic groups, 85–86
　stabilisation and transport, 85–113
　transport practice principles, 86
Cromolyn sodium, 24–5
Crouch gait diplegia, 137–8
Croup
　budesonide for, 249*
　severe, 103
Cryptorchidism, paternity after, 252*
Cushingism
　after corticosteroids, 1
　after inhaled corticosteroids, 4
Cushing's triad, 99
Cyclic vomiting syndrome
　and DNA mutations, 241*
　prophylactic therapy, 253*
Cycling injuries, boys, 74
Cystic fibrosis
　ascites in CF, 181
　ΔF508, 251*
　diagnosis, 251*
　dietary fibre and gut symptoms, 251*
　end-of-life care, 251*
　fluticasone propionate trial, 250*
　gastrointestinal and hepatobiliary problems, 173–92
　genetic testing results, 251*
　and GERD 173–8

heart-lung transplantation, 250*
incidence and survival, 250*
insulin resistance, 251*
mycobacterial lung disease, 250*
newborn screening, 251*
pancreatic-enzyme supplements and fibrosing colonopathy, 250*
postural drainage
　and gastrooesophageal reflux, 250*
　and GERD, 175–6
　vs physiotherapy trial, 251*
pulmonary function in, 250*
recombinant human DNase cost effectiveness, 250*
salt and, 251*
Cystic fibrosis transmembrane regulator, 173, 178, 184
Cytomegalovirus infection, 243*

D

Davis/Bamford report, 125
Death
　accidental, coroners' inquest, 74
　from trauma, distribution, 98
　rates from travel injuries, 231*
　sudden, in BPD, 29–30
　timing after trauma, 232*
Declaration of the Rights of the Child, 224
Decompression sickness, 94
Deglutition in CP, 129
Dehydration assessment, 242*
Delinquency, maternal and perinatal risk factors, 230*
Dengue virus infection, 254*
Dental decay, from soft drinks, 146–7
Dental erosion, 147–50
　and acidic soft drinks, 148–9
　dietary factors, 149–50
　survey, 148
Department of Health: Sub-committee on Nutritional Surveillance 1989, 144
Depression, postnatal, 248*
Dermatitis, sweat electrolyte concentrations, 236*
Developmental pattern, in accidental home injury, 75
Dexamethasone, for BPD, 30
Diabetes
　audit by caseload, 237*
　blood glucose control, 237*
　and breastfeeding, 237*
　hyperlipidaemia, 237*
　insulin dependent increase, 237*
　insulin lispro, 237*
　insulin-like growth factor 1 and insulin therapy, 236*
　nocturnal hypoglycemia, 237*
Diagnostic and Statistical Manual: American Psychiatry Association, 57
Diarrhoea
　in disaster, 220–2
　enteral nutrition basis, 238*
　in third world, 199

vomiting, and shock, 105
zinc supplementation, 255*
Dietary factors in dental erosion, 149–50
Diffuse axonal injury, 35, 39, 46
DIOS *see* Distal intestinal obstruction
syndrome
Direct Recording Scale, 203, 204–5
Disability, hidden, in extremely premature
schoolchildren, 245*
Disaster
child care, 211–15
health care priorities, 217–24
postemergency phase, 224–5
principles in health care delivery, 217
programming 216–17
rapid assessment, 215–17
strategy and activity scheme, 216
Distal intestinal obstruction syndrome, 184–6
treatment questions, 186
Distraction Test Screen, 117
Diuretics, for BPD, 23–24
Dog bite treatment, 231*
Double fractures, 37
Down syndrome, antenatal detection, 239*
Drawstring entrapment in slides and
buses, 231*
Drinks (*see also* Cola drinks; Milk; Soft
drinks; Water)
adolescent weekly range, 144
Drought, 211
Drowning
near
management in transport, 107–8
prognostic factors, 108
prevention, 81
DSM-IV research criteria for factitious
disorder by proxy, 59–60
Dual-energy x-ray absorptiometry (DXA),
152, 154, 155
Dysbarism, 93
Dysentery, 220–1
Dysphonia, 4
Dysplasia, bronchopulmonary *see*
Bronchopulmonary dysplasia
Dysport 132

E
Earthquakes, 211–13
Eczema, and asthma, 8
Education
for accidental home injury
prevention, 76
conductive, 130
for hearing-impaired, costs, 124
ELBW *see* Birth weight, extremely low
Electrocution, 79
Emergency Public Health, 213
End-of-life, medical decisions, 245*
Endoscopic retrograde
cholangiopancreatography (ERCP), 183
Endoscopy, in GERD, 176
Endotracheal intubation
critically ill children, 92
insertional length estimation, 245*

in transport, 95
route, 96
Endotracheal tube, blockage, 96
Enforcement, for accidental home injury
prevention, 76
Engineering, for accidental home injury
prevention, 76
Entrapment, 82
Enuresis
determinants, 233*
genes and clinical management, 233*
and voiding difficulties, 246*
Environment, stimulating, in third world,
201
Epiglottitis, 102
suspected, management in
transport, 103
Epilepsy, 247*
psychiatric perspective, 248*
ERCP (Endoscopic retrograde
cholangiopancreatography), 183
Escherichia coli faecal shedding, 240*
Ethics in disaster, 225
European Standard EN 71 Safety of Toys, 79
European Toy Safety Directive, 79
Exercise testing, in BPD, 31
Exposure and accidental home injury, 75
Extubation, accidental, 96
Eye disease and tarantulas, 248*

F
Factitious illness by proxy, 57–71
case management approach, 68
as child abuse, 61
co-morbidity, 60
development of hypotheses, 62–3
diminishing coping strategies, 64
effects on child's health and
development, 60
elements, 58
emotional harm, 60
fabrication of illness in child, 59
family patterns, 62
framework for assessment, 58–60
initial assessment approach, 59
origins and preterred terminology, 57
predisposing risk factors, 61–4
prognosis overview, 66–8
prognostic factors, 67
psychiatric disorders classification, 59
psychiatric risk factors, 61–2
psychodynamic hypotheses, 63
reports of series of cases, 58
treatment, 64–6
Falls
accidental, 79, 80–1
and skull fracture, 36
Feeding
in convalescence, in third world,
200–1
supplementary, 218–19
Feeding disorders in CP, 129–30
Feeding formula discharge packages and
breast-feeding, 235*

Femoral stress fractures in skating, 232*
Fibrosing colonopathy in CF, 187–9
    abdominal pain, 188–9
    aetiology and pathogenesis, 188–9
Fire blanket, 80
Fire deaths, 80
Fire and heater guards, 78
Fires
    Home Office information, 74
    house, 80
    smoke detector, 76, 77, 78
Flixotide, 1
Floods, 211
Fluid and drug therapy, in transport, 96–7
Fluoride, 149
Fluticasone, clinical efficacy, 11–12
Fluticasone propionate, 1, 3
Fluticasone/cromoglycate trial, 9, 10
Food distribution in disaster, 218
Fostering, long term, outcome, 230*
Fragile X syndrome, 236*
Fruit juice
    and dental erosion, 149
    excess consumption and short
        stature, 230*
    pH, 143
Fundoplication, 130, 169
Furosemide, 24

G

Gait analysis
    components, 137
    in CP, 135–8
Gallstones, 183
Gastritis, after cola fizzy drinks, 151
Gastrooesophageal reflux, 161–72
    algorithms for evaluation, 166
    clinical presentations, 163–5
    conservative therapy, 168–9
    in CP, 129–30
    in cystic fibrosis, 173–8
    defense mechanisms, 175–6
    dental erosion, 147
    diagnosis, 165, 167–8
    endoscopy and biopsy, 165, 167
    epidemiology, 161–2
    factors preventing, 175
    investigations, 176–7
    management, 177–8
    pathophysiology, 162–3
    pharmacotherapy, 168–9
    radiography, 165
    respiratory sequelae, 163
    respiratory symptoms, 174
    surgery, 169
Gastrografin, 185, 186
Gastroparesis, postviral, 238*
Gastroschisis survivors, 252*
Gastrostomy, 130
Geneva Convention, 224
Genitalia, external, abnormalities, 253*
GERD see Gastrooesophageal reflux disease
Gestational assessment, 245*
Glasgow Coma Scale, 95, 100

Glass injuries, 81
Global malnutrition rate, 218
Glucose and inhaled corticosteroids, 5
Goitre, 219
    rapeseed oil for, 254*
Gonads, nonpalpable, evaluation, 236*
Graded care profile scale, 231*
Growth
    adequate measurement in third
        world, 202
    bone age determinations, 238*
    effects
        of asthma, 7
        of inhaled corticosteroids, 7–8
            short-term, 8
    failure
        in BPD, 27–8
        in CLD, 27–8
    and family conflict, 237*
    monitoring charts, 255*
    monitoring in third world, 203
    Pakistani children, 237*
    retardation in foster children, 233*
    short stature outcome, 237*
    short stature psychosocial outcome,
        248*
    stunting by long-term
        corticosteroids, 1
    tall stature outcome, 237*
    trends 1972–94, 237*
Growth hormone, 237*
Gynecology problems, 246*

H

H2-receptor antagonists for GERD, 168
Haemolytic uraemic syndrome
    heterogeneity, 246*
Haemophilus influenzae, 220
Haemophilus influenzae type-B vaccines for
    pneumonia and meningitis, 254*
Haemopneumothorax, and shock, 105
Haemopoietic colony stimulating factors, 243*
Haemorrhage
    oesophageal or gastric variceal, 182
    and shock, 105
Hall Report on hearing, 125
Hand skill measures in CP, 131
Harness/walking reins, 78
Head, shaking, and brain movement, 40
Head injury
    abusive, coagulopathy, 232*
    blunt, skull radiography, 252*
    infantile and car seats, 231*
    minor, 231*
    non-accidental, outcome, 232*
    support in community, 230*
    vomiting and migraine, 242*
Health of the Nation, 82, 83
Health Promotion in our Schools, 202
Health services, for hearing, 115–6
Health Technology Assessment
    programme, 116
    report, 126

Health Visitor Distraction Test, 116, 117–18,
  120–1, 123, 126
    costs, 123–4
    targeted, 125–6
Health worker in community
  development, 201–5
Hearing
  impairment
    early detection, 116
    effects, 115
    language abilities, 121–2
  permanent impairment
    age distribution, 120
    age of identification, 123
    craniofacial abnormality, 119, 123
    epidemiology, 118–21
    family history, 119, 123
    loss assessment, 120
    outcomes, 121–2
    prevalence, 119
    register, 126
    screening programmes, 117
  screening, 115–28
    current practice, 116–18
    options, 124, 125–6
    performance, 122–3
    programmes cost, 124
    sensitivity, 122–3
  sensorineural loss, 115
Hearing aid fitting, 120–1, 122
Heartburn, 174
  and soft drinks acidity, 151
Heimlich valves, 94
Helicobacter pylori breath testing, 238*
Helicopters, 93
Hemangioma of airway, 249*
Hematuria, 246*
Hemiplegia, psychological aspects, 233*
Hemispherectomy, 247*
Hemophagocytic lymphohistiocytosis,
  229*
Henoch Schonlein purpura, age influence,
  242*
Heparin and intraventricular haemorrhage,
  243*
Hepatic disorders, in cystic fibrosis, 178–83
Hepatic encephalopathy, treatment, 238*
Hepatic steatosis 178–9
Hepatitis, chronic viral, treatment, 240*
Hepatitis B
  infection, 234*
  vaccination
    hepatocellular carcinoma, 234*
    in national programmes, 234*
Hepatobiliary disorders in cystic fibrosis, 178
Hepatocellular failure, 182–3
Herpes simplex gingivostomatitis, aciclovir
  treatment, 240*
Herpesvirus 7, in pityriasis rosea, 240*
Herpesviruses, three new human, 240*
HIV
  in disaster, 223
  family clinic, 230*
  malignancies in child, 241*
  pediatric infection, 241*

HIV-1
  infection, 241*
  viral load and disease in infants, 241*
HIV/AIDS, teaching material in third
  world, 205
HLA-A2 haplotype and BPD, 20
Hoarseness, 174
  in gastrooesophageal reflux disease,
    164–5
Home Accident Surveillance System:
  Department of Trade and Industry, 73
Home safety, 73–84
Hookworm infection vaccines, 254*
Hot water, temperature reduction, 77
Hyaline membrane disease, surfactant
  effects, 245*
Hydrochlorthiazide, 24
Hydronephrosis, antenatal, 246*
Hypaque, 185
Hypertension, in BPD, 26–7
Hypocalcaemia and phosphoric acid
  containing soft drinks, 150–1
Hypochondriasis, 61
Hypoplastic left heart syndrome, 230*
Hypospadias, classification, 239*
Hypothermia
  management in transport, 108
  prevention in transport, 91
Hypoxia
  in BPD, 29–30
  ground versus air transport, 93
Hypoxic-ischemic encephalopathy
  outcome, 243*
  perinatal interventions, 245*

I

ICD-10 Classification of Mental and
  Behavioural Disorders: WHO, 59
Imidazoles, 168
Immunisation
  adolescents, 234*
  after disaster, 225
  apnoea in preterm, 234*
  circumcision effects, 234*
  in disaster, 220
  infantile, in third world, 198
  influenza, 28
  measles, and inflammatory bowel
    disease, 234*
  pertussis, 29
  syncope after, 234*
Immunodeficiency, severe combined, 229*
Impetigo, drug treatment, 236*
Incubators, for mobile intensive care, 91
Inequalities and health, 231*
Infant, head shaking, 40
Infant and pre-school child, in third world,
  198–201
Infantile colic
  social origins, 230*
  sucrose for, 253*
Infectious diseases, Vietnam, nutrition
  improvement morbidity effect, 254*

Inflammatory cascade, preterm lung damage, 19–20
Inflammatory disease, infantile-onset multisystem, 251*
Influenza and respiratory illness, 28
Inhaler device, 3
Injury prevention, recent advances 82
Inotrope therapy, critically ill children, 92
Insulin-like growth factor 1 and milk supplementation, 154
Insulin-like growth factors, 236*
Intensive care
    centralisation, 242*
    mobile
        equipment and monitoring, 90–2
        ethos, 86–90
International aid, 211–13
International Society of Child and Adolescent Injury Prevention, 82
Intestinal disorders, 184–9
Intracranial pressure, raised, 99–100
Intrahospital transfers, 97
Intussusception in CF, 186
Invasive procedures, sedation, 253*
Ipratropium bromide, 24–5
Iron, and oedema, 255*
Isoproterenol, 25

J

Joint muscles in CP, 135–6

K

Kangaroo mother care, 195, 243*
Kasabach-Merritt syndrome, 239*
Kawasaki disease, coronary artery abnormalities, 230*
Kettle, coiled flex, 78, 80
Kitchen fires, 80
Knemometry, 8
    fluticasone assessment, 11–12
    short-term studies, 9
Kwashiorkor, diet in, 254*

L

Landing surfaces and fracture, 38–9
Lansoprazole, 169
Laryngoscopy, in gastrooesophageal reflux syndrome, 167
Latrines, in disaster, 221
Lennox-Gastaut syndrome, lamotrigine for, 247*
Leptomeningeal fractures, 36
Lipophilicity, 2
Lumbar puncture method, 247*
Lung
    infection and feeding problems in CP, 129
    injury aetiology, 18–20
    preterm, corticosteroid effects, 245*
    surfactant deficiency, 19

M

Malaria
    cerebral, intracranial hypertension, 256*
    chemoprophylaxis in Tanzania, 256*
    in disaster, 222–3
    imported in UK, 255*
    morbidity and *Plasmodium falciparum* transmission, 256*
    paracetamol effect, 255*
    prevention in UK visitors, 255*
    vaccine
        based on sporozoite antigen, 256*
        development, 256*
Malnutrition
    and immune system, 229*
    measurement, 218
Mannose binding protein gene mutation and infection, 229*
Maternal dietary supplements, effects on birth weight and perinatal mortality, 254*
Maternal-infant bed sharing and SIDS, 235*
Measles
    in disaster, 222
    infecting dose, 198
    prophylactic antibiotic trials, 240*
    vaccination
        in disaster, 218
        and vitamin A, 255*
    vaccine in third world, 198
Medécins sans Frontières, 213
Medications over-the-counter, 253*
Medline database, 242*
Meningitis
    in disaster, 223
    hearing loss prevention, 240*
    pneumococcal, and chronic subdural effusion, 43
Meningococcal disease
    management, 241*
    new therapies, 240*
    preventive strategies, 240*
    recognition, 106
Meningococcal shock, 107
Meningoencephalitis, suspected, 101
Mental health
    in disaster, 224
    responsibility, 248*
MERLIN, 213
Metabolic decompensation, 241*
Metaproterenol, 25
Methacholine challenge, 30, 31
Methylxanthines, 24, 25
Microgallbladder, 178, 184
Micronutrient deficiency, 219
Micturating cystourography timing, 246*
Milk
    cola and fizzy beverages
        ethnic consumption, 145
        weekly consumption, 145
    consumption surveys, 142–5
    declining intake, 151–6
    higher consumption by boys, 144
    intake and bone minerals, 241*
    nutritional contribution, 142
    supplementation trials, 153–5
Molecular microbiology, application to vaccinology, 234*

Monitoring system, portable, 91
Motor function measure scores, 132, 134–5
Munchausen's syndrome by proxy *see* Factitious illness by proxy
Muscular dystrophies, 247*
Musculoskeletal disorders, non-inflammatory, 252*

N

National Child Dental Survey, 148
National Diet and Nutrition Survey 1995, 143
Neonatal care in third world, 194–8
Neonatal cerebral infarction, 243*
Neonatal cerebral oxidative metabolism, deranged, relation to neurodevelopment, 244–5*
Neonatal cholestasis, 178–9
Neonatal fat digestion, 244*
Neonatal hypoglycaemia, 245*
Neonatal infection in third world, 195
Neonatal Intensive Care, and hearing impairment, 119
Neonatal pain response to blood sampling, 245*
Neonatal tests for hearing, 116, 117–18
        costs, 124
        specificity, 122
Neonatal transport, 244*
Neonatal transport medicine, 85
Neonatal weight gain, 196, 197–8
Neurological failure
        assessment, 99
        non-traumatic causes, 99–109
Neutrophils, 19
Nicotine addiction, 230*
Nipples, commercially available, 243*
Nitric oxide
        and dexamethasone, preterm infant trial, 245*
        inhaled, 244*
        and persistent pulmonary hypertension, 244*
Noise
        ground versus air transport, 93
        as hazard, 242*
Nursing in tilted position, neonatal benefits, 244*
Nutrition
        in BPD, 20, 26
        in disaster, 218–19
        supplements in growth failure, 27–8
Nutritional status
        evaluation in CF, 180–1
        measurement in disaster, 218

O

Obesity, 241*
Obsessive compulsive disorder, 248*
Octreotide, 182
Oesophageal pH monitoring, 167
Oesophagitis, 161, 163, 174, 176
Oesophagogastroscopy, 130
Oesophagoscopy, 174

Omeprazole, 168
Oral rehydration
        in disaster, 221
        in third world, 199
        trial, 238*
Organ damage, postasphyxial, 242*
Oronasopharyngeal suction at birth, 243*
Oropharyngeal thrush, 4
Osteogenesis imperfecta, pamidronate therapy, 253*
Osteoporosis, 6–7
        childhood origins, 152–3
        childhood risk factors, 151–2
        etidronate therapy, 251*
        risk and childhood cola drinks, 156
Otitis media
        antimicrobials for, 238*
        effects, 115
Otoacoustic emissions, 117
Oxygen
        in BPD management, 22–3, 30
        in growth failure, 27
        home therapy, 30
        increase at altitude, 93–4
        lung injury, 18–19
        for mobile intensive care, 91
        respiratory syncytial virus, 28

P

Paediatric Advanced Life Support courses, 89
Paediatric Intensive Care Society, 86
Paediatric intensive care unit (PICU), 85
Paediatric risk of mortality (PRISM) score, 85, 87, 88
        decrease, 110
Paediatric transfer team, 85, 86
Paediatric Transport Medicine, 98
Pain, right lower quadrant, imaging, 253*
Paranasal sinus disease imaging, 238*
Parotitis, recurrent, 241*
Patent ductus arteriosus, ibuprofen treatment, 245*
Pellagra, 219
Peritonitis
        bacterial, 181–2
        and shock, 105
Permanent Hearing Impairment *see* Hearing, permanent impairment
Personality disorder, 61–2, 63, 67–8
Pertussis, 240*
        vaccines, 234*
pH
        monitoring, 130
        oesophageal monitoring, 167
        studies in CF, 174–5, 176
Pharmacological agents affecting lower oesophageal sphincter pressure, 162
Pharyngitis, streptococcal, treatment, 255*
Phosphorus
        dietary load and cola drink consumption, 156
        and hypocalcaemia, 150–1
Physical therapy trials in CP 130–2

Piaget, Jean, 203
Placenta, ageing, 244*
Play pen, 78
Playground safety, 231*
Pneumonia, 220
    vitamin A therapy, 254*
Pneumothorax, tension, and shock, 105
Poisoning prevention, 81
Polio epidemic after aerial bombardment, 212
Polycystic ovary syndrome, 236*
Portable Auditory Response Cradle, 117
Portal hypertension
    bleeding treatment, 238*
    in CF, 180
Poverty and child health, 231*
Preconceptual care in third world, 193–4
Product safety standards, 83
Protease inhibitors, lung deficiency, 19
Protective reflexes, 38
Psychosocial needs in disaster, 224
Puberty
    in asthma with steroid therapy, 11
    disorder management, 236*
    precocious, 236*
Pulmicort, 1
Pulmonary artery hypertension, 22
Pulmonary function tests, 20–2
    in BPD, 30
Pulmonary oedema, 21–2, 27, 102, 103
Pulmonary vascular disease, 22
Pulse oximetry, 242*
Pyelonephritis, renal sequelae risk, 246*

Q

Quality of life measurement, 242*

R

Rabies vaccination, 254*
Radiology, advances in, 242*
Rape, 223
Re-bleeding, and subdural haematoma, 42–3
Reflux oesophagitis, 129
Refugee camp, 214
Regurgitation, current management practices, 238*
Rehabilitation after disaster, 225
Relief agencies, 211–13
Renal failure and low-protein diet, 247*
Renal malformation causes, 239*
Renal scarring, new, 246*
Renal stones and cola drinks, 151
Respigam, 29
Respiratory distress syndrome, 18–20, 103
Respiratory dysfunction, reflux-associated, mechanisms, 164
Respiratory emergencies, management in transport, 102–4
Respiratory failure, near term infants, 243*
Respiratory illness
    acute, in disaster, 220
    in BPD, 28–9

Respiratory syncytial virus, infection morbidiry reduction, 240*
Respiratory syncytial virus disease, 28–9
Respiratory syncytial virus IGIV, 29
Respiratory syncytial virus immune globulin therapy, 249*
Respiratory tract infections
    clinical signs in malnourished, 254*
    hypoxia predictors, 255*
Retinal haemorrhages, 44–5
Retinopathy
    of prematurity, 244*
    vitamin E prophylaxis, 244*
Rheumatic disease
    adolescent, 252*
    antibody screening, 252*
Rheumatic fever, 252*
Rhinitis, and asthma, 8
Rhizotomy, selective posterior, 134–5
Rib fractures, 45
Rickets and pneumonia risk, 254*
Rotavirus gastroenteritis, vaccination for prevention, 234*
Rotavirus vaccine, 238, 241*
    efficacy, 254*
Runaway children and abuse, 232*

S

Safety
    home *see* Home safety
    low cost measures, 78
    practical advice, 78
Safety equipment
    for accidental home injury prevention, 77
    recommended, 78
Safety gates/barriers, 78
Safety glass or film, 78
Safety solutions not recommended, 77–8
Salmeterol, growth studies, 10
Salmeterol/beclomethasone, trials, 9
Salmonella typhi, multiple resistant, 222
Sandifer's syndrome, 165
Scalds, 80
School Entry Screen for hearing, 116, 117–18
    effectiveness, 123
School refusal and truancy, 248*
Scoliosis, non-operative treatment efficacy, 252*
Scrotum, acute, 252*
SCUBA diver, air transport, 94
Scurvy, 219
Sedatives during transport, 95–6
Seizures
    first, 247*
    nasal benzodiazepines for, 247*
    untreated, 247*
Septic shock, 103
Septicaemia, and shock, 105
Sex in accidental home injury, 74
Sexual health, in disaster, 223
Shaken brain injury
    engineering explanations, 50–1
    MR image, 50

outcome, 46–7
timing of symptom onset, 47–50
Shaken impact theory, 52
Shigella spp., 220
Shock, 105, 107
classification of causes, 105
management in transport, 107
phases, 105
Short bowel syndrome, 238*
Sickle cell disease
crisis admission evaluation, 239*
endothelial cells, 239*
management, 239*
morphine trial, 239*
septicemia caused by infection, 240*
treatment, 239*
Skull fractures, 36–9
depressed, 232*
and linear, 37
force needed, 36, 38
incidence, 38
speed and energy of impact, 39
Slide projection in third world, 205
Smoke detectors, 76, 77, 78, 80
Smoke inhalation, 108–9
Social class, in accidental home injury, 74, 83
Social learning models, 63
Sodium cromoglycate, 24–5
Soft drinks
acidic, and dental erosion, 148–9
acidity and heartburn, 151
as calorie source, 150
composition, 141–2
dental decay 146–7
effects of excessive consumption,
141–60
pH, 143
surveys, 142–5
Somatizing disorders, 61
Soy-based infant formula, 235*
Spastic diplegia, intrathecal baclofen, 134
Spastic hemiplegia, classification, 136
Spinal cord injury, 247*
Spironolactone, 24
Spoon, two-ended, 199
Sports injuries, 251*
Squash drinking syndrome, 150
Stabilisation time, 88
Stadiometry, fluticasone assessment, 11–12
Stairgate, 75, 76, 77, 80
Status epilepticus, 247*
Strangulation, 82
Streptococcal infection group B
prevention, 242*
neonatal, 244*
Streptococcus pneumoniae, 220
Stress factors in accidental home injury, 75
Stroke after chickenpox, 247*
Subdural haematoma, 39–53, 49
causes, 42
epidemiology, 40–2
investigations, 4–6
presenting signs and symptoms, 45
Suckling, 196–8
Sudden infant death syndrome

after CESDI, 235*
at weekends, 236*
GP care, 235*
risk factors, 235*
study in Scotland, 235*
Supervision, for accidental home injury
prevention, 76
Surfactant
prophylactic vs rescue, 244*
replacement therapy, 30
therapy, 17, 18
Surgery
antenatal, 252*
evidence-based, 252*
Syndrome
Barter, 246*
battered baby *see* Child abuse 40
chronic fatigue, 248*
cyclic vomiting, 241, 253*
Down, 239*
distal intestinal obstruction, 184–6
fragile X, 236*
gastrooesophageal reflux, 167–8, 176
haemolytic uraemic, 246*
hypoplastic left heart, 230*
Kasabach-Merritt, 239*
Lennox-Gastaut, 247*
Munchausen's *see* factitious illness
by proxy
polycystic ovary, 236*
respiratory distress, 18–20, 103
Sandifer's, 165
short bowel, 238*
squash drinking, 150
sudden infant death, 235*, 236*
toxic shock, 103

T

Teaching Aids at Low Cost, 205–6
Teenage pregnancy, prevention, 231*
Testicular cancer in cryptorchidism, 253*
Tetanus/diphtheria vaccine reactions, 234*
Tetracosactrin test, 5
Theophylline, 24, 25
Theophylline/beclomethasone, growth
retardation trial, 9, 10
Third world, child care low-technology
approaches, 193–209
Thrombocytopenic purpura, UK practice
assessment, 239*
TIPS *see* Transjugular intrahepatic
portosystemic shunting, 182
Toxic shock syndrome, 103
Toy injuries, 79, 80
Toy Safety Standard, 82
Tracheal aspiration of food, 129
Tracheal intubation, rapid sequence, in
transport, 95
Tracheitis, bacterial, 103
Tracheobroncheal tree, abnormalities, 20,
21–2
Tracheomalacia, 21–2
bronchodilator therapy, 25
Tramline fractures, 36

Transaminases, serum elevation in CF, 179
Transfer, theoretical and practical aspects,
    86–109
Transfer log, 88, 90
Transjugular intrahepatic portosystemic
    shunting (TIPS), 182
Transport
    of critically ill children, 85–113
    ground versus air, 92–3
        stresses, 93
Transport team
    communication, 88
    composition, 88
    operational time intervals, 89
    specialised and non-specialised, 109–10
    utilising response time, 89–90
Trauma, and subdural haematoma, 42
Trauma injuries, after disaster, 213
Trauma patients, transfer, 98–9
Troleandomycin, 168
Tube feeding and cerebral bloodflow, 244*
Turbohaler, 3
Typhoid fever, 222
Typhus, in disaster, 223

Varicella after varicella vaccination, 234*
Vector control in refugee camps, 223
Ventilation
    high-frequency, and intraventricular
        hemorrhage, 243*
    lung injury, 18–19
    negative pressure, 249*
Ventilators, portable mechanical, 91
Ventilatory intervention, 96
Vesicoureteric reflux, ultrasonography vs
    cystourethography, 246*
Vibration, ground versus air transport, 93
Vibrio cholerae, 220
Videofluoroscopy in tracheal aspiration,
    129–30
Viral disease and respiratory failure, 21
Viral respiratory illness, 28–9
Vitamin A deficiency, 219
    reduction, 255*
Vitamin B–12 deficiency, 235*
Vitamin C deficiency, 219
VLBW see Birth weight, very low
Volutrauma, 18
Vomiting in third world 199–200

U

UK National Diet and Nutrition Survey,
    147, 148
UK National Screening Committee, 126
Umbilical catheterisation and portal vein
    thrombosis risk, 245*
Umbilical stump, care in third world, 195
UN Children Fund, 211
UNICEF, and third world child care, 193–209
UNICEF/WHO/UNESCO: Facts for Life, 202
Universal Declaration of Human Rights, 224
Ureaplasma urealyticum, and BPD, 20
Ureteric reflux screening, 246*
Urinary incontinence
    management, 246*
    surgery, 253*
Urinary tract infections, 246*
    management, 245*
    renal cortical scintigraphy, 246*
Urology
    imaging, 246*
    problems, 246*
Ursodeoxycholic acid, 180, 183
US Food and Drug Administration, 29
US National Health and Nutritional survey
    1971–74, 146

W

Warmth, neonatal, in third world, 194–5
Wars, 211–13
Water
    consumption by infants and
        preschool children, 144
    in disaster, 221
    pH, 143
Water fluoridation in social deprivation,
    230*
Weight, neonatal gain, 196, 197–8
Weight-for-age charts, 203
Weight-monitoring chart, 237*
Wheeze
    asthma prevalence in Ethiopia, 255*
    beclomethasone trial, 9
    exercise-induced, 31
Whiplash shaking, 51
WHO and third world child care, 194–5,
    198
Window falls, prevention, 80–1
Window locks, 78
World wide web, health information
    reliability, 230*
Wuchereria bancrofti microfilaraemia,
    ivermectin and albendazole for, 253*

V

Vaccine cold chain monitoring, 235*
Vaccines see Immunisation

Z

Zinc supplementation and Guatemalan
    morbidity, 255*

Recent Advances in Paediatrrics
Edited by T J David

If you wish to place an order for an earlier vlolume, please contact your local medical bookseller or the Sales Promotion Department, Harcourt Brace and Company Ltd, 24–28 Oval Road, London NW1 7DX, UK

Contents of Volume 15

1. **Bronchiolitis**
    L I Landau

2. **Identification and management of large airway disease in the first year of life**
    M P Rothera, T J Woolford

3. **Superantigen disease**
    N Curtis, M Levin

4. **Thalassaemia**
    Nancy F Olivieri

5. **Congenital hypothyroidism**
    M D C Donaldson, D B Grant

6. **Coeliac disease**
    J A Walker-Smith

7. **Cholera**
    Nicola S Crowcroft

8. **Nitric oxide: physiology, pathophysiology and potential clinical applications**
    R H Mupanemunda, A D Edwards

9. **Strategies to assist breastfeeding in preterm infants**
    Paula Meier, Linda Brown

10. **Persistent pulmonary hypertension of the newborn**
    Marlene Rabinovitch

11. **Evaluating headaches**
    M B O'Neill

12. **Sleep problems and disorders**
    P Hill

13. **Paediatric literature review – 1995**
    T. J. David

ISBN 0443 05849-0

Recent Advances in Paediatrrics
Edited by T J David

Contents of Volume14

1. The continuing enigma of cot death
   C Morley

2. Childhood diabetes in the community
   P G F Swift

3. Home oxygen therapy
   M P Samuels, D P Southall

4. Child physical abuse: risk indicators and prevention
   H L MacMillan, A C Niec, D R Offord

5. Unintentional injury prevention
   E M L Towner, S N Jarvis

6. Television and its effects on children's behaviour
   M M Davies

7. Extended role nurses in neonatal intensive care
   J Pinelli, B Paes

8. Pathophysiology of the respiratory distress syndrome
   H M Berger, R M W Moison, D van Zoeren-Grobben

9. Advances in epilepsy: seizures and syndromes
   P S Baxter, C D Rittey

10. Growth and endocrine sequelae following treatment of childhood cancer
    S M Shalet

11. Vitamin A deficiency: a paediatric priority in the tropics
    K P West

12. Trachoma
    S West, L Bobo

13. Paediatric literature review – 1994
    T. J. David

ISSN 0-309-0140

Recent Advances in Paediatrrics

Edited by T J David

Contents of Volume13

1. **Lessons of experience**
   D. Hull

2. **Birth asphyxia**
   M. I. Levene

3. **Pathogenesis of respiratory disease in cystic fibrosis**
   C. Koch, N. Høiby

4. **House dust mite avoidance regimens for the treatment of asthma**
   T. A. E. Platts-Mills, M. L. Hayden, J. A. Woodfolk, R. S. Call, R. Sporik.

5. **The mechanism of fever**
   M. J. Kluger

6. **A population approach to weight monitoring and failure to thrive**
   C. Wright

7. **Strategies to improve immunisation uptake**
   B. W. Taylor

8. **Bullying: another form of abuse?**
   J. L. Dawkins, P. D. Hill

9. **Identification and early intervention in pervasive developmental disorders**
   P. Szatmari

10. **Cytokines and adhesion molecules in acute inflammation**
    A. H. Finn

11. **Recent advances in paediatric rheumatology**
    J. E. Davidson, R. M. Laxer

12. **Retinopathy of prematurity**
    E. Ziavras, J. J. Javitt

13. **Paediatric literature review – 1993**
    T. J. David

ISBN 0443 051003

Recent Advances in Paediatrrics
Edited by T J David

Contents of Volume12

1. Mortality, morbidity and health-related behaviour in childhood.
    Dunnell

2. Medico-legal reports about children.
    Bamford

3. Gastrostomy feeding.
    Grunow, Chait, Savoie, Mullan, Pencharz

4. Accidental hypothermia.
    Corneli

5. HIV infection.
    Newell, Gibb

6. Malaria.
    Greenwood

7. Molecular pathophysiology of meningitis
    Saez-Llorens, McCracken

8. Passive smoking.
    Couriel

9   Fragile X
    Hirst & Davies

10. Sickle cell disease
    Serjant

11. Fatty acids in human and formula milk
    Innis

12. Language disorders
    Rosenbloom

13. Management of atopic eczema
    David

14. Literature review
    David

ISBN 0443 048711